- Almost 50 percent of all adults in the United States will have at least one diagnosable psychiatric episode in their lifetime.

- Depression is not a sign of weakness. Winston Churchill and Abraham Lincoln both suffered from clinical depression.

- Only 35 percent of Americans with emotional problems currently get help.

BUT MEDICAL HELP **IS** AVAILABLE.

NOW YOU CAN CONSULT THE

CONSUMER'S GUIDE TO PSYCHIATRIC DRUGS

FOR COMPREHENSIVE, ACCURATE AND

UP-TO-DATE INFORMATION

BEFORE, AFTER, AND WHILE SEEKING

MEDICAL HELP.

CONSUMER'S GUIDE TO PSYCHIATRIC DRUGS

Straight Talk for Patients and Their Families

John D. Preston, Psy.D.
John H. O'Neal, M.D.
Mary C. Talaga, R.Ph., Ph.D.

POCKET BOOKS

New York   London   Toronto   Sydney

Pocket Books
A Division of Simon & Schuster, Inc.
1230 Avenue of the Americas
New York, NY 10020

First Pocket Books paperback edition January 2009

POCKET and colohon are registered trademarks of
Simon & Schuster, Inc.

For information about special discounts for bulk purchases,
please contact Simon & Schuster Special Sales at 1-800-456-6798
or business@simonandschuster.com.

Cover design by Richard Yoo
Cover photo by Microzoa © Getty Images

Manufactured in the United States of America

10 9 8 7 6 5 4 3

ISBN-13: 978-1-4165-7912-0
ISBN-10:   1-4165-7912-5

*To the readers of this book, for whom
our words are written with compassion and hope.*
Mary C. Talaga, R.Ph., Ph.D.

*To my patients, who have been my best teachers.
May this book assist others, who, like them,
seek help for emotional suffering.*
John H. O'Neal, M.D.

*To my brother Tom
and to our new light in the world: Aurora.*
John D. Preston, Psy.D.

Acknowledgments

We would like to thank both our literary agent, Marilyn Allen, and our editor, Kathy Sagan, for all of their efforts, excellent suggestions, and encouragement. And a heartfelt thanks to our patients. It is from you that we have learned our most valuable lessons about suffering, healing, and hope.

Contents

Introduction   1

PART ONE:
PSYCHIATRIC DIAGNOSES AND TREATMENT   7

1. Psychiatric Medication: A Historical Perspective   9
2. Seeking Treatment   21
3. Emotions and the Brain   28
4. Managing Your Medications   44
5. Depression   65
6. Bipolar Disorders   111
7. Anxiety Disorders   144
8. Schizophrenia and Other Psychotic Disorders   165
9. Sleep Disorders   180
10. ADHD, Eating Disorders, Dementia,
    and Other Disorders   190
11. Medication During Childhood, Adolescence,
    Pregnancy, and Old Age   212
12. Natural Remedies   226

PART TWO:
A GUIDE TO PSYCHIATRIC DRUGS   235

Appendix 1. Directory of Brand Names   519
Appendix 2. Caffeine Consumption Questionnaire   523
Appendix 3. General References   525
Appendix 4. Resources   529
Appendix 5. Recommended Reading   531
Index   533

Introduction

Chances are good that because you are reading this book, either you or a family member has begun or is considering medical treatment for an emotional or psychiatric disorder. Our intention is to present a lot of practical, useful information in the hope of answering many of the questions you may have about psychiatric treatment. We believe strongly that everyone has a right to acquire important information about treatment and treatment options.

In the past, it was common practice for you to be examined by a doctor, given a prescription for a certain medication, told how to take it, and sent on your way. The arrangement was one of "powerful doctor" and "passive patient." As a result, many, if not most, patients felt inhibited about asking questions regarding their treatment.

Fortunately, times have changed, and in our view, it is not only legitimate for you to inquire about your treatment, it actually makes the most sense to informed consumers. Accurate information not only is your right but can enhance your treatment outcome and increase the likelihood of treatment success.

It is important for anyone receiving psychiatric medication treatment to know at the very least the following treatment-related information:

- What is the diagnosis?
- What are the recommended treatments for this disorder?
- If psychiatric medications are recommended:
  1. Are the recommended medications standard and well-established treatments?
  2. Are the particular medications addictive?
  3. What can you expect from the medical treatment? This should include the following: (a) What are the common side effects? (b) Are any of the side effects dangerous? (c) How long must you wait to notice the positive benefits of the medication? (d) Are there any potential drug–drug interaction problems? (That is, is it dangerous to take this medication along with other prescription or over-the-counter drugs?) (e) Can you drink alcohol while taking this medication?
  4. Assuming that the medication is effective for you, how long will you have to take it?
  5. Are there any dangers in taking this medication for an extended period of time?
- Is psychotherapy recommended in addition to medication?

Of course, additional questions may come up that will be important to address, and we encourage you to assert your right to inquire about any aspect of your treatment.

Possibly as many as 85 percent of all prescriptions for psychiatric medications are written by primary care and family practice doctors. And, as you well know, a typical office visit with a doctor is brief. It may be difficult, if not impossible, to ask all of your questions during such a short visit. Also, if you are like most of us, other questions may come to mind after your visit to the doctor or in the days that follow. It is our hope that this book will address many of those concerns.

THE SPECTRUM: FROM HAVING A BAD DAY
TO HAVING A NERVOUS BREAKDOWN

In the chapters that follow we will be writing about several common emotional and psychiatric problems. Some of these disorders are serious but fairly rare (e.g., schizophrenia). Many, however, are common, especially depression and anxiety disorders. It is important to understand that among these disorders, a great deal of variability exists with regard to severity. Most of us experience occasions of mild depression or anxiety. These times may last only a day or two, or they may be present for longer periods, causing discomfort but not debilitation. Sometimes however, anxiety and depression can become extremely severe.

At this severe end of the spectrum, these disorders may become all consuming and have the potential to ruin a person's life. Not only is there great personal and emotional suffering, but there also can be a collapse into a sort of paralysis and a total inability to function. Dysfunction may take the form of fearfulness that is so intense the person cannot leave home or be left alone: or depression so engulfing that the person is literally bedridden. Depression can also cause such an extreme disorganization of thinking that the individual is convinced he or she is going crazy.

While a number of people can and do experience serious, chronic psychotic illness, the percentage of such disorders in the general population is only about 1 percent. A much higher percentage of people go through very serious bouts of anxiety and depression that result in significant dysfunction. At the extreme end of this spectrum, these emotional disorders are what some of us grew up calling a "nervous breakdown" or "mental breakdown." Furthermore, these disorders can and do happen to many people who have gone through much of their lives functioning quite well. In fact, such grave versions of these kinds of psychiatric reactions can, under certain circumstances, strike otherwise mentally healthy individuals (as is often the case with bipolar disorder or post-traumatic stress disorder).

The good news is that current treatments for psychiatric disorders have a well-established record of effectiveness. The bad news is that many people suffer and never seek treatment. It is critical to understand that emotional and psychiatric problems are very common, that most problems can be treated successfully, and that someone suffering from such a problem can take action by seeking treatment.

HOW TO USE THIS BOOK

This book is divided into two parts. Part One consists of Chapters 1 through 12, which discuss psychiatric diagnoses and the specifics of medication treatment. Part Two is a compendium of psychiatric medications and provides detailed information on specific medications.

The first four chapters of this book address some general issues to help you learn more about the use of psychiatric medications. Our clients routinely ask about specific issues that relate to psychiatric diagnosis, the biology of emotional illnesses, and how medications work. Thus, we have attempted to speak to many of these concerns.

What follows are chapters devoted specifically to groups of psychiatric disorders such as depression, anxiety disorders, and others. In each of these chapters we provide a great deal of specific information about treatment, including the following:

- Signs and symptoms
- How the diagnosis is made

- The role of a medical evaluation in diagnosis
- Theories about the biology of the disorder (to help explain how medications appear to work)
- Specifics of medical treatment, for example: (1) standard medical treatments, (2) details regarding treatment (e.g., recommended doses, what to expect, common side effects), (3) precautions, (4) treatment options when first-line treatments are ineffective
- Frequently recommended nonmedical treatments (e.g., types of psychotherapy)

Self-help references (books and support groups) can be found at the back of the book.

As is the case in all areas of medicine, there are several generally accepted, standard treatments for any particular disorder or disease. Rarely is only one approach or one medication the treatment of choice. This is certainly the case in the treatment of psychiatric disorders. Thus, this book presents the major points regarding standard psychiatric treatment for each particular disorder.

Treatment decisions will be influenced by several unique factors (particular symptoms, one's age, medical status, and so forth) and may vary from person to person. We provide general information about all the available treatments because we strongly believe that people have the right to know as much as possible about their disorder and its treatment. However, be advised that particular treatment decisions will be unique for each individual.

Although we recommend that you read Chapter 1 for some background, it is also fine to skip ahead and turn to the particular chapter that is relevant to your current concerns.

LIFE IS HARD

We, the authors, do not know of anyone—friends, family, our patients, and ourselves—who has not been through difficult times, often very difficult times. Life brings joys and blessings, as well as hardships. All of us are entitled to find ways to reduce suffering for ourselves and for our loved ones. Sometimes, professional help can be a godsend, whether in the form of counseling or as treatment with psychiatric medications. Too many people suffer needlessly, either putting off seeking treatment or rejecting such options outright. We encourage our readers to take action to reduce emotional suffering. We also encourage you to become knowledgeable about currently available treatment choices. This is your right.

PART ONE

PSYCHIATRIC DIAGNOSES AND TREATMENT

CHAPTER 1

Psychiatric Medication: A Historical Perspective

Since the beginning of recorded history, it has been obvious that human beings are subject to a host of emotional pains. Some of these are mild, temporary, and simply annoying, while others are prolonged and a source of agony and disability. A recent and extremely thorough study carried out by the National Institute of Mental Health has shown that 48 percent of all adults in the United States will have a diagnosable psychiatric disorder at least once in their lifetimes. This may seem like a surprisingly large percentage; yet, it appears to be quite accurate (see table below).

PREVALENCE OF PSYCHIATRIC DISORDERS IN THE UNITED STATES		
DISORDER	PER YEAR	LIFETIME
Mood disorder	11%	19%
Anxiety	17%	25%
Substance abuse	11%	26%
Psychotic disorders	1%	1%

Many individuals will have two or more disorders at the same time (e.g., depression and alcohol abuse). This is referred to as co-morbidity or co-occurrence. Only 35 percent of those affected receive any form of treatment.

Yet, despite a growing awareness of psychological disorders, a good deal of negative stigma still exists surrounding psychiatric problems. In our society, emotional and psychological problems continue to be a source of shame. As a result, many of those living through difficult times are likely to keep their psychological pain private, sharing their personal feelings with no one except their closest relatives. What has become abundantly clear, however, is that the vast majority of human beings are affected by stressful and painful life events, and that many of us experience a sufficient amount of distress for this to be correctly seen as a type of psychiatric disorder.

Part of the negative stigma associated with psychological disorders comes from misconceptions and inaccuracies regarding mental and emotional illnesses, such as the common notion that if you are mentally ill, you have a weakness of character or intellect. Two cases in particular underscore how far this idea is from the truth. Both Winston Churchill and Abraham Lincoln suffered from bouts of severe clinical depression. Yet, no one would question that these men were intellectually gifted, had strength of character, and were able to exert enormous influence over the histories of their nations and the lives of countless people.

Psychiatric disorders, however, can and certainly do have a marked impact on our quality of life. In the midst of emotional illnesses, not only do people experience overwhelming anguish but their basic functioning can be affected. Severe emotional disorders can, at least temporarily, adversely transform otherwise normally capable people.

Many people suffering from such disorders find it difficult

to function in their day-to-day lives as productive employees, nurturing parents, and loving husbands, wives, or partners.

NEW APPROACHES TO AGE-OLD PROBLEMS

In the early part of the twentieth century, two important events changed attitudes about psychiatric treatment and the entire landscape of mental illness and emotional suffering.

The first was a shift toward more humane treatment for people with mental illnesses. Prior to this time, those afflicted with serious psychiatric disorders were often subject to horrific "treatments," such as prolonged confinement in asylums. Some patients were continuously restrained in straitjackets and treated more like criminals than sick people. The twentieth century brought an increased understanding of emotional disorders as either an extension of normal human emotional responses to difficult life circumstances or as a type of illness deserving treatment—not punishment, blame, or shame.

The second event that helped change attitudes about emotional illnesses was the development of the first truly effective psychological treatment: psychotherapy or, as it is sometimes called, talk therapy.

PSYCHOLOGICAL TREATMENT

This psychological approach was ushered in by the work of Sigmund Freud, and it has been expanded and modified in many ways during the past one hundred years. Since the 1970s, hundreds of published research studies have demonstrated that, in general, psychotherapy is an effective treatment for a number of emotional and psychiatric disorders.

Also, the past three decades have seen the development of specific psychological therapies designed to treat certain types of disorders (e.g., cognitive therapy for the treatment of depression). Psychotherapy is often the treatment of choice for many psychological problems, although it has demonstrated only limited success with more severe mental illnesses.

THE DISCOVERY OF PSYCHIATRIC MEDICATIONS

In the mid-1950s, the first effective medications for treating very severe mental illnesses, such as schizophrenia and manic-depressive illness, were developed. They were hailed as godsends because at that time, no other form of therapy existed other than psychotherapy for the more severe forms of mental illness, and that often didn't work.

But these early psychiatric medications had their problems. Many came with a large variety of unwanted side effects, and, especially in the early years, the drugs often were subject to overuse or misuse. The medications helped many patients, but they were also responsible for some disasters, especially when some patients were treated inappropriately.

During the five decades since their inception, psychiatric medications have undergone significant changes. The development of new medical and scientific technologies has provided researchers with a much clearer understanding of the functioning of the brain and the biology of mental illness. Newer, safer, and more effective medications have been developed. A great deal of information has also been acquired about how to prescribe treatments appropriately and how to avoid or minimize problems with side effects. Recently, new vistas have opened regarding the use of psychiatric medications for what are considered to be the less severe emotional disorders.

COMMON CONCERNS ABOUT
PSYCHIATRIC MEDICATION

When we look at the history of the development and use of psychiatric drugs for treating mental and emotional disorders (which produce all of the real-life consequences just described), the public's opinion and the media's attention have often been anything but positive. Why? Two good reasons have brought medication treatment under scrutiny and negative press.

THE "CHEMICAL STRAITJACKET"

The first has to do with the realities of early psychiatric medication treatment, especially as it was conducted during the 1950s and 1960s. At that time, in a great many well-publicized cases, psychiatric patients received grossly inappropriate treatment with the then-new psychiatric drugs. The most common abuse was the use of excessively high doses of tranquilizing medications, mainly to impose behavioral controls on agitated or troublesome patients. This took place primarily in state mental hospitals.

Typically, the medications were the early versions of antipsychotic drugs. They were helpful in reducing psychotic symptoms, such as hallucinations, but they were notoriously loaded with unpleasant side effects. When used in extremely high doses, they did achieve behavioral control, but often at great cost in human terms. Many patients frequently were over-sedated and seemed like "zombies." At this time the term "chemical straitjacket" came into use.

These decades were also a time of great social change, when free speech, personal freedom, racial equality, and civil rights became paramount values. The whole idea of restraining human beings with drugs (often completely against their will) sounded suspiciously Orwellian and provoked outcries of protest.

Although the use of psychiatric drugs did result in significantly more people being released from state hospitals, the necessity of ongoing chemical restraint caused many to question whether the newly released patients were really better off.

Many opponents of psychiatric medication treatment (most notably Dr. Thomas Szasz) argued that the new drugs were robbing people of their humanity and individuality. The question was raised: Were these new discoveries truly medical breakthroughs, or were they simply a new technology for mind control?

MOTHER'S LITTLE HELPERS

The second reason that medication treatment was not well received began to emerge in the 1960s, when the minor tranquilizers, such as Miltown, Librium, and Valium were widely prescribed by family practice doctors. They were dispensed as treatment for a variety of maladies such as frayed nerves, insomnia, tearfulness, and generalized sadness or disappointment with life. These drugs became known as "mother's little helpers" (popularized as such in the Rolling Stones' song). They were seen as a panacea for many of life's woes—"Just swallow one or two and mellow out." Eventually, the darker side of using drugs in this way became apparent.

Questions were raised: Could it be that the main effect of the tranquilizers, so prescribed, was to induce a state of relative, albeit temporary, oblivion for unhappy housewives? Might this state of drug-induced numbness be a way to keep women in their place and perpetuate the status quo of the male-dominated society? If women were sufficiently anesthe-tized, maybe they would either not notice, or find a way to tolerate, an obnoxious or dissatisfying lifestyle (e.g., spousal abuse or passive subservience). In a broader less politicized scheme, the question could be stated as: Do psychiatric medi-cations inhibit autonomy? Do they somehow conceal or hide one's inner, truer self?

JILL'S STORY

Jill, a thirty-four-year-old librarian, was the mother of two young children. Her early life had been like that of many peo-ple growing up in small-town America. She came from a stable and loving family, had the ordinary experiences of youth, and could not recall any remarkably traumatic or stressful times. After high school she attended a nearby college. Upon gradu-ation, she found a job with a university library. In the years that followed, Jill married and had children. She had a good life and was grateful for it. At the age of twenty-four, she would have thought it impossible that ten years later she would be completely unable to leave her home or be alone for more than a few minutes without experiencing overwhelming surges of panic. She would have been incapable of imagining that in a decade she would be contemplating suicide every day.

But Jill had her first panic attack at the age of thirty. She experienced a sudden eruption of intense, overwhelming fear. Her heart began to race, and she felt short of breath and dizzy. She became convinced that she was going to die at any moment. This episode came on for no apparent reason; she was sitting in a coffee shop with a friend when panic en-gulfed her.

In the following week she had four additional attacks, each identical to the first. She and her husband were sure that she had some kind of serious medical problem. Later that week she was admitted to the emergency room with chest pains and an overwhelming sense of dread and panic. After a careful evaluation, she was told that she had experienced an anxiety attack, given reassurance that nothing was medically wrong with her, and sent home. But she did not feel reassured at all. She was still frightened out of her wits.

During the next three months as the attacks continued, Jill did what many other people in her situation do. She began to develop intense fears about leaving her home. She had attacks at home, too, but it was familiar turf and she felt safer there. She started frequently calling in sick to work. She did not get further medical attention, but she did start to drink a lot of alcohol in an attempt to quell her nerves. In five short months her life was transformed. She quit her job, stopped attending social functions, and became less and less involved in the lives of her two kids. Her life was focused on the ever-present dread, "When will the next attack occur?"

Four years later, Jill was an emotional cripple. She was unable and unwilling to leave her house. To her great shame, her husband had to hire a "baby-sitter" to be with her during the day because she could not bear to be alone. Jill's life had been completely transformed. She was chronically depressed and lived in constant fear about the next anxiety attack.

Jill's story is not uncommon. She was suffering from severe panic disorder, and it ruined her life. This kind of disorder rarely goes away without treatment. Fortunately for Jill, she finally did seek professional help. In utter desperation, she made an appointment with a therapist. After a careful evaluation she was told that she was suffering from a treatable emotional illness. The therapist recommended a treatment that included psychiatric medications and a type of psychotherapy called cognitive-behavior therapy. This combined approach is a standard and very effective treatment for panic disorder. Initially, Jill was reluctant to take medications, so it was important for the therapist to spend a good deal of time answering her questions about the drugs. It was also crucial for her to know that the choice of whether to try medication was entirely hers. On her second visit to the therapist she decided to follow her therapist's recommendation for the medication. After two months of treatment, Jill was radically different. The panic attacks stopped, and for the first time in years she was able to reenter her normal life. She was able to attend school functions with her children, visit her parents, and go out on a "date" with her husband. Eventually, she returned to work and pursued the career she had loved. She was able to reclaim her life.

Although it is true that initially far too many instances occurred in which psychiatric medications were misused to stifle aliveness, free choice, and autonomy, in Jill's case we see just the opposite. The medication helped free her from an engulfing disorder and enabled her to reclaim her true self.

These days, when people are treated with modern psychiatric medications, one of the most common remarks therapists hear once the drugs begin to take effect is this: "I am beginning to feel like myself again." This is a very important point to emphasize. Although some medications do have unpleasant side effects, and some misuse of these drugs certainly continues, the goal of appropriate psychiatric treatment is twofold: to reduce human suffering and to promote the development and expression of autonomy. This is a far cry from the chemical straitjackets of the mental hospitals' back wards in the 1950s.

DRUG ADDICTION

Prior to the mid-1950s, some drugs were used in psychiatry, although most were ineffective—and many were recognized as potentially addictive and dangerous. Such drugs included alcohol, marijuana, bromides, barbiturates, and amphetamines. Cultural awareness of escalating drug abuse in the 1960s sensitized the medical profession as well as the general public to the hazards of drug addiction. As the poet Robert Bly noted at the time, "The drugged state is the fastest-growing state in the union."

Unfortunately, some of the next drugs developed in the mid-1950s and early 1960s were tranquilizers, which were found to be habit-forming. Increasingly, in those years, when psychiatric drugs were portrayed in the media, they were discussed as if they were all the same—that they all had terrible side effects, were habit-forming, and were being used to achieve behavioral control. This journalistic misrepresentation continues, to some degree, to this day and can influence some patients who would readily benefit from drug therapy to stay away from it.

MEDICATIONS AND THE MEDIA

Research studies and clinical experience certainly have a bearing on therapists' prescribing practices. However, in recent years the media have also had a profound effect on public opinion and ultimately on medical practice. In the late 1980s, negative media attention was focused on the drug Ritalin, a widely prescribed stimulant medication used to treat attention deficit hyperactivity disorder (ADHD). Psychiatrist Andrew Brotman, summarizing the work of Safer and Krager (1992), stated, "The media attack was led by major national television talk show hosts and in the opinion of the authors, allowed anecdotal and unsubstantiated allegations concerning Ritalin to be aired. There were also over twenty lawsuits initiated throughout the country, most by a lawyer linked to the Church of Scientology" (Brotman 1992).

In their study of the effects of the negative media and litigation blitz conducted in Baltimore County, Maryland, Safer and Krager found that the use of Ritalin had dropped significantly. In the two-year period during and just following the negative media attention, the number of prescriptions written for Ritalin decreased by 40 percent. (The use of Ritalin had increased five-fold during the prior six-year period).

Furthermore, this decrease occurred at a time when research on ADHD and stimulant treatment continued to strongly support the overall safety and effectiveness of such medication. The authors stated that 36 percent of the children who discontinued Ritalin experienced major academic maladjustments (such as failing grades or being suspended), and an additional 47 percent who discontinued treatment encountered mild to moderate academic problems. While Ritalin use decreased, there was a significant (fourfold) *increase* in the prescription of tricyclic antidepressants (such as Tofranil) among hyperactive children. Apparently, physicians discontinued Ritalin and then prescribed antidepressants. It is important to note that tricyclic antidepressants, although often used to treat ADD in the 1990s, tend to have more troublesome side effects than Ritalin and have been implicated in six reports of cardiac deaths in children. Brotman concluded, "When there are reports in the media that lead to stigmatization of a certain drug . . . there tends to be a move to other medications which have less notoriety, even if they may, in fact, be more problematic" (1992).

More recent concerns have been raised regarding a possible

increase in suicidality in children and teenagers taking antidepressants. Since 1990 the suicide rates in the United States among young people ages 10 to 24 have dropped by 29 percent. However, in the wake of concerns about suicide and antidepressant use in children and adolescents, prescriptions for antidepressants for youngsters have dropped by 30 percent, and ironically, suicide rates in this age group have increased by 8 percent (Lubell et al. 2007). This topic is covered in greater detail in Chapter 5, Depression.

Media coverage can certainly call attention to the serious problems seen with particular medications, which in turn can lead to careful investigations by the FDA and other regulatory agencies. But the media can also present sensationalized reports that fail to provide accurate information, and may have adverse consequences in prescribing practices and patient care.

All medications produce some side effects. But reports of serious side effects, even if seen very infrequently, must be taken seriously and investigated systematically. There certainly is a place for skepticism and scrutiny. However, it is also important to consider the negative effect of unsubstantiated reports in the press.

Several discrete classes of psychiatric medication exist, and each class is quite different with regard to chemical composition, side effects, and potential for addiction. As an informed patient, you need to know about the various classes and have accurate information regarding possible side effects and addiction potential.

CHAPTER 2

Seeking Treatment

WHO CAN PRESCRIBE PSYCHIATRIC MEDICATIONS?

In most states the only people who can prescribe psychiatric medications are physicians and dentists (although for dentists, prescribing is limited to the dentist's scope of practice). In a few states such medications may be prescribed or furnished by appropriately trained nurse practitioners. In Louisiana and New Mexico specially trained psychologists may write prescriptions. The legal right to prescribe, however, does not imply that all such professionals are trained in the treatment of emotional and psychiatric disorders.

As noted in Chapter 1, many prescriptions for psychiatric medications are written by primary care and family practice doctors. Some of these general practitioners are well trained in the diagnosis and treatment of emotional problems and have years of experience carrying out such treatment. In fact, primary care physicians see, on average, between two and three people daily who are suffering from major depression and, two patients each day who have severe anxiety disorders. Lots of patients visit their family doctor when they are experiencing psychological distress, for the following reasons:

- They already have a relationship with their physicians and have learned to trust them.
- Many folks are reluctant to see a mental health professional because of the negative stigma.
- Many psychiatric disorders cause significant physical symptoms, such as fatigue, aches and pains, sexual dysfunction, and insomnia, and thus may not even be recognized as emotional in origin. Rather, they are assumed by the patient to be symptoms of some sort of physical illness.

Although many people do seek treatment from their primary care doctors, the ability to accurately diagnose psychiatric disorders in this setting is not ideal. The fast pace and brief nature of a visit to a general medical doctor (the average office visit with a physician is about 10 minutes!) makes it harder to focus on the psychological component. While some physicians have developed ways to accurately identify their patients' emotional problems, some studies show that as many as 50 to 90 percent of patients who present with psychiatric disorders in a primary care setting go either undiagnosed or misdiagnosed. While the diagnosis and treatment of psychiatric problems in primary care settings are improving, they still have a long way to go.

If you suspect that you (or a relative) are suffering from a psychiatric disorder and you want to consult your primary care doctor, it is strongly recommended that you first contact him or her and ask directly *if* they have experience in treating emotional disorders (e.g., depression or anxiety). If your doctor doesn't, it is wiser to ask for a referral to a mental health specialist. If you are treated by your family practice doctor, we highly recommend that you also ask for the name of a good psychotherapist. Psychiatric medication treatment is almost always more effective if it is taken in conjunction with psycho-therapy.

MENTAL HEALTH SPECIALISTS

Professionals who have special training in the diagnosis and treatment of psychological disorders include the following, along with their degrees and certification:

- Psychiatrists (M.D., D.O.)
- Psychologists (Ph.D., Psy.D., or Ed.D.)
- Clinical social workers (M.S.W. or L.C.S.W.)
- Licensed counselors (most have a master's degree: either M.A. or M.S.)
- Some pastoral counselors

Although these professionals are all licensed to provide mental health treatment, their training and experience can vary tremendously. Thus, when seeking a referral, you should be sure to determine if a particular specialist has experience in the area for which you are seeking treatment.

This book provides a fairly comprehensive overview of psychiatric disorders so that you will have a basic understanding of particular problems you or your family member may be experiencing. In part, this will help you locate appropriate professional help.

We strongly encourage you that in choosing a therapist, you speak to him or her by phone first, before making an appointment. Ask about the therapist's areas of expertise, fees, and more. This call will also give you a quick sense of how the therapist comes across. Many of our clients have remarked that screening a therapist by phone made them feel more at ease and confident that a particular therapist could help them.

If you think that psychiatric medication may be warranted in your treatment, ask therapists whether they use drugs as a part of their approach. Also, you should know that some psychiatrists are trained primarily in psychopharmacology or medication treatment, and may not have much expertise or practice in psychotherapy. So be prepared to ask psychiatrists if they provide psychotherapy in addition to medication treatment. If they do not, most of these doctors will be glad to provide the names of qualified therapists.

Finally, it is also important to note that pharmacists can be very helpful in providing you with information about prescriptions, especially about potential drug–drug interactions. Nowadays, many states mandate a pharmacist consultation whenever a patient receives a new prescription or requires a change in an existing one. It is your right to receive this valuable information—take advantage of this resource!

TAKING POSITIVE ACTION: THE NAME OF THE GAME

Almost all varieties of psychological disorders and emotional stress are accompanied by some feelings of powerlessness. All patients in the throes of significant distress have tried their best to manage those feelings and, to a greater or lesser degree, have felt either frustrated or overwhelmed as the stress continues and the symptoms either persist or become worse. The main antidote for feeling powerless is to take action. For many thousands of people, the first step in regaining control over their lives is to decide to seek out mental health treatment. Often that is a lifesaving decision. It can mean the difference between enduring months of emotional pain or getting back on their feet quickly.

With major psychological disorders, wishing, hoping, and

gritting one's teeth rarely works. And yet, only 35 percent of those afflicted seek help. The decision to get treatment not only may be the smart thing but also is the courageous thing to do. And when a patient is informed about his or her choices, that patient will be the one in charge. Knowledge really is empowering.

COSMETIC PSYCHOPHARMACOLOGY

"Cosmetic psychopharmacology" is a term coined by Dr. Peter Kramer, a psychiatrist and the author of the best-selling book *Listening to Prozac* (1993). Dr. Kramer points out that most psychiatric medications were originally developed to treat the more severe mental and emotional disorders, such as schizophrenia, major depression, and bipolar disorder. In fact, a perusal of most psychiatric textbooks prior to the 1990s reveals that these illnesses were clearly the major focus of psychiatric drug treatment. However, in the past two decades, new discoveries have been made that have broadened the focus of psychiatric medication treatment.

In particular, some psychiatric medications have been successful in treating such minor emotional disorders as mild depression and even in changing what heretofore were thought to be aspects of personality, such as shyness (not disorders or diseases, per se). Three factors have brought this about.

First, many of the new drugs (especially the new generation of antidepressants) have relatively few side effects. Add to that the fact that antidepressants are nonaddictive and generally safe, even for long-term use, and it may come as no surprise that physicians have been willing to try these medications even on people who do not have grave mental disorders.

Second, the advent of managed care has placed an increased emphasis on mandated brief treatment for many psychiatric problems. Since many disorders (even minor adjustment disorders and stress reactions) require at least medium-length psychotherapy (i.e., a few months of therapy), some health insurers and others have advocated the use of psychiatric drugs (with or without psychotherapy) in an attempt to speed up recovery. Although this is often a short-sighted approach, some people have responded well to it.

Finally, when patients are treated with psychiatric medications for more serious disorders, behaviors that had previously been believed to be character traits, or aspects of temperament or personality, also appeared to change, sometimes significantly. For example, some patients treated for depression have reported that in addition to relief from bad feelings, they have also experienced changes in their thinking and behaving that are new to them, such as an increased assertiveness, less social anxiety, a decreased tendency to fret and to worry, a more relaxed and casual approach to work, a less rigid approach to life, an enhanced ability for productivity, and more. Changes in the individuals' personalities were also noticeable. Most interesting of all, many of have reported that "this is my real self" (even though they may have never felt or acted that way in the past).

This certainly raises all sorts of questions regarding how we define the self. Is the self that set of personality characteristics that endures over the decades of life, or is it the more recent experiences that simply "feel" better, such as less shyness in social settings?

Peter Kramer describes several cases in which people were treated not for major mental illnesses but for what may be seen as personality quirks. He invented the clever term "cosmetic psychopharmacology" to describe this particular use of psychiatric medications. Is it possible to use chemicals in the same way we might put on a power tie to wear to an important business meeting? This aspect of psychiatric medication treatment has obviously sparked considerable controversy.

The use of drugs for "cosmetic" purposes most likely accounts for some of the increase in the prescriptions for the newer generation of medications. In this book, however, we have chosen to focus on the most important targets of psychiatric medication treatment: the serious and more often debilitating psychological symptoms that accompany mental or emotional disorders.

Suffice it to say that this is a complex matter of medical ethics and personal choice. For the moment, improving one's personality may be viewed as a possible positive side effect.

CHAPTER 3

Emotions and the Brain

IN THE BEGINNING OF PSYCHIATRY

When modern psychiatry originated in the late 1800s, all psychiatrists were trained primarily in neurology (the study of diseases of the nervous system). The majority of psychiatrists of that time believed that serious mental illnesses, especially psychotic disorders such as schizophrenia and severe depression, were most likely caused by some kind of brain disorder or disease. In those days, because there were no effective treatments for serious mental illnesses, most patients were kept confined in asylums. Physicians of that time must have felt enormously frustrated and impotent, as they could do little to alleviate the intense suffering of those who were afflicted with psychiatric disorders. Thus, much time was spent in neuroanatomy laboratories studying the brains of deceased mental patients. The hunt was on for visible evidence of disease or trauma to the brain.

One important discovery was made back then: many people suffering from very severe psychotic disorders were, in fact, experiencing the effects of syphilitic infection that had spread to the brain. (This was long before the development of antibiotics, so many people were so afflicted.) Beyond this one finding, however, little else was learned about the brain or mental illness. Researchers were stumped, and millions of people worldwide continued to suffer, with no help in sight.

THE REBIRTH OF BIOLOGICAL PSYCHIATRY

During the first half of the twentieth century, psychiatry moved away from the biology lab and into the mental health clinic. Failure to find any promising leads in the realm of neurology led psychiatrists to explore a new, nonmedical approach for treating emotional problems: psychotherapy (or, as previously noted, what many called talk therapy).

Psychotherapy was launched by the famous Austrian neurologist Sigmund Freud under the name of psychoanalysis. Along with several related disciplines, it flourished during the first fifty or sixty years of the twentieth century. Although it had its limitations and certainly did not help everyone, it was rightly heralded as a breakthrough because no other treatments existed. It was, in many ways, a godsend.

Psychotherapy had one limitation that immediately became apparent to most mental health professionals: Severe mental illnesses did not respond well at all to psychotherapeutic techniques. In one of his last papers, Freud wrote in 1940 that he believed it would eventually be discovered that the most severe disorders (e.g., schizophrenia) are caused by some kind of brain malfunction. He speculated further that one day researchers would find medications that would prove helpful in treating these very severe disorders.

That breakthrough arrived in the early 1950s. In 1954, purely by accident, it was found that a drug being used to reduce the adverse effects of general anesthesia also had antipsychotic properties. When this medication, now known by the trade name Thorazine, was given for several weeks to people with chronic schizophrenia, there were dramatic changes in their behavior. The drug tranquilized very agitated patients, but more importantly, it was often effective in reducing hallucinations and greatly improving the patients' ability to think logically and coherently.

When viewed in a historical context, this discovery was truly miraculous. In the years before the development of Thorazine, most seriously disturbed patients were relegated to lifetime confinement in state mental hospitals. These hospitals, often referred to as snake pits, were grim, bleak repositories for thousands of lost souls. By 1955, for the first time, the populations of mental hospitals began to decline as many patients improved enough to be able to return to their families and communities.

Human beings who had been completely out of touch with reality, who were badly regressed and beyond hope, were coming back to life. And somehow this remarkable change was due to specific chemical molecules producing some types of change in brain functioning. These early drugs also had numerous side effects, sometimes serious, and clearly did not "cure" schizophrenia. But it was undeniable that the drugs did make a significant difference. For the first time there was hope that treatments could be developed to help those who had suffered so much.

The knowledge that chemicals could so alter psychiatric symptoms ignited a growing interest in brain functioning and mental illness. Remember—the first psychiatric drug (like several others thereafter) was discovered only by accident. Early researchers had no true understanding about how these medications worked, but they quickly began to speculate. And the search was on, once again, to find out more about the biology of emotional and mental illness.

NEW WINDOWS INTO THE BRAIN

Multitudes of theories were proposed, and as is the case in all areas of science, many of them were ultimately rejected. Nevertheless, investigations continued at a frantic pace. A good deal of the research was supported by pharmaceutical companies. By the mid-1970s, psychiatric drugs were among the top money-makers in the pharmaceutical industry. Besides the introduction of antipsychotics, drugs were also developed to treat anxiety, depression, and bipolar (manic-depressive) disorder. Gradually, the newer medications proved more effective and less likely to have debilitating side effects than the earlier drugs. Research in the neurosciences was re-invigorated by the development of exciting new technologies, including these new high-tech tools:

- CT (computerized tomography) and MRI (magnetic resonance imaging) scans, which are sophisticated devices for photographing the human brain
- PET (positron emission tomography), SPECT (single photon emission computerized tomography), and fMRI (functional magnetic resonance imaging) scans, which allow the researcher to watch actual metabolic functioning as it occurs in the living brain
- Gene mapping

President George H. W. Bush designated the 1990s as the "decade of the brain," and rightly so; in that decade, knowledge about brain functioning took a quantum leap.

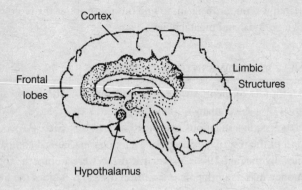

THE BASIC BRAIN

The following discussion presents some very basic concepts about the brain that will help you understand more about the biology of emotional and mental disorders. Of course, a comprehensive discussion of these topics is beyond the scope of this book; however, at the end of the book are some excellent references for readers interested in a more extensive discussion.

It may be helpful to think of the brain as organized in layers or levels. Neuroscientist Robert Ornstein used the metaphor of a ramshackle house to describe the organization in 1984. Imagine that a small and very basic house has just been built. Some years later, a few rooms are added to the basic structure. A few years after that, more additions are constructed. The original house is not torn down; it is still there and still intact, but more and more modern rooms have been added. So it is with the human brain.

THE REPTILIAN BRAIN

In human beings, the oldest and most basic parts of the brain are called the brain stem, the hind-brain, and the mid-brain. (These parts are analogous to the first story of the ramshackle house.) The structure and functioning of these parts of the brain are identical to those found in many lower species. In particular, they are similar to the brain of reptiles. Thus, these parts are sometimes referred to as the reptilian brain, and they monitor several vital functions necessary for life, including heart rate, breathing, and blood pressure.

THE CENTRAL CORE OF THE BRAIN

The second story of this biological house is represented by the central core of the brain. It contains two important brain centers: the hypothalamus and the limbic system.

FUNCTIONS OF THE HYPOTHALAMUS

The first important part of the brain's central core is a tiny structure called the hypothalamus. This pea-sized but very complex structure controls or influences many important biological functions, such as control of biological drives like sex, hunger, and thirst; control of the biological rhythms that influence sleep cycles and energy levels; functioning of the immune system; and regulation of emotions.

Some psychiatric disorders are thought to involve a malfunction of the hypothalamus. Such malfunctions can result in symptoms like insomnia, significant fatigue, appetite loss or increase, decreased sex drive, and in some instances an impaired immune system, which can result in poor health and decreased resistance to disease.

FUNCTIONS OF THE LIMBIC SYSTEM

The second group of brain structures in the central core of the brain that surround the hypothalamus are collectively known as the limbic system. These structures play an important role in emotional behavior; together, the system is commonly called the emotional brain—and for good reason.

One of these brain structures, the amygdala, is responsible for threat appraisal. When an individual is confronted with danger, this automatic and lightning-fast system perceives the threat. Other limbic system brain structures are responsible for igniting a fight-or-flight response along with other emotional reactions. So when you feel angry or afraid, this feeling is set in motion by chemical activity taking place in one or more brain structures of your limbic system. In a sense, this system is the launching pad for felt emotions.

The limbic system also contributes to emotional behavior, because certain parts operate as emotional control centers in that they play an important role in inhibiting and controlling emotional reactions. For instance, at one time or other we all have been treated rudely by another person. In such moments, it is perfectly understandable to become irritated or angry. However, for several good reasons, most of us do not punch out the offending person. We find a way to contain and hold our anger in check.

The ability to accomplish this type of emotional self-control depends in part on the appropriate functioning of several structures in the limbic system. Most major psychiatric disorders involve some loss of emotional control (e.g., anger is felt as being "out of control"; intense sadness is experienced as engulfing). Evidence is accumulating that suggests this loss of control can often be traced to subtle but important malfunctions in the limbic centers. It should come as no surprise to learn that the limbic system is the locale in the brain where most psychiatric medications appear to do their work.

THE CORTEX

The cortex is the highest level of the brain. It exists in many animals, but it is relatively undeveloped in most species, with the exception of primates (monkeys, apes, and humans). The cortex is the site of perception, information processing, thinking, reasoning, and all the higher human cognitive abilities. One part of the cortex deserves special attention: the frontal lobes.

THE FRONTAL LOBES

In terms of human evolution, the frontal lobes are thought to be the most recent and advanced addition to the brain. (In our house metaphor, the frontal lobes would be the penthouse, or the last room added to the ramshackle house.)

Several important functions are associated with the frontal lobes—in particular, the prefrontal cortex, or the front half of the frontal lobes. Those functions include inhibiting emotional reactions, maintaining attention and concentration, thinking complex thoughts, and problem solving.

The interconnections between the frontal lobes and certain limbic system structures are rich and complex. These brain areas work together to inhibit and control strong emotional reactions. One very common problem in people who have suffered serious damage to the prefrontal cortex is the tendency to express very intense emotional reactions—especially irritability and anger. Such people may know that it is not appropriate to express anger in many situations, and they may feel embarrassed or remorseful after a display of aggression. They often report, however, that they find it very hard, if not impossible, to keep from lashing out in anger. Similarly, some people who have sustained injuries to the prefrontal cortex notice that even mildly upsetting events can provoke intense sadness and floods of tears.

Other individuals, despite average or above-average intelligence, have difficulty maintaining focused attention and concentration, and they fail to thrive academically or in their occupation. For some of them, the prefrontal cortex has been implicated (e.g., in those with attention deficit hyperactivity disorder).

Although it is likely that many brain areas are involved in schizophrenia, a great deal of research points to the role of the prefrontal cortex, which has been shown to be extremely inactive (hypometabolic) in many people who have been diagnosed with this terrible disorder. Disorganized thinking is its hallmark.

In another part of the frontal cortex, the lateral or outside surface, malfunctioning can produce states of pronounced loss of vitality and decreased motivation, as is the case in some forms of major depression.

Evidence is convincing in many psychiatric disorders that the frontal cortex is dysfunctional. In most cases, the problem is not brain damage in the usual sense of the term, because the data suggest little evidence of actual tissue damage. The research findings do indicate, however, that problems can be traced to chemical abnormalities in these various regions of the brain. This brings us to yet another level of investigation—malfunctions at the level of the cell.

BRAIN CELLS AND ABNORMAL CHEMISTRY

Normal brain functioning is dependent on the appropriate action of nerve cells, often called neurons. Each and every brain structure is made up of thousands, if not millions, of neurons. They are responsible for turning particular brain centers on and off, somewhat akin to the way a television set works with electricity. Some nerve cells carry energy that turns the system on, while others operate like a brake to slow it down or turn it off. In addition, multitudes of neurons carry out the fine-tuning of the system, much like the various controls on a TV set that adjust for brightness, color, volume, and so forth. With more than 100 billion nerve cells and over 100 trillion interconnections, it is amazing how well this incredibly complex system functions—at least most of the time.

The nerve cells that have been implicated as malfunctioning in various psychiatric disorders generally represent only a tiny percent of all brain neurons. Thus, when it is determined that a person has an emotional disorder that can be traced to a biological cause, one can assume that the vast majority of brain cells are functioning normally and that the presumed malfunctions involve only a tiny percentage of the total. Yet, a dysfunction in these very few brain neurons can wreak havoc, resulting in intense suffering, marked disability, and at times life-threatening psychiatric problems.

HOW NERVE CELLS WORK

Every nerve cell functions by producing and releasing a particular chemical substance called a neurotransmitter. Sometimes these chemical substances are called messenger molecules because they influence other nerve cells and aid in the communication processes between these cells. Each nerve cell receives numerous messages from other nerve cells and subsequently sends messages to its neighboring nerve cells. These chemical messages can have an impact on the functioning of an individual nerve cell. They can turn the cell on, causing the cell to fire a nerve impulse. Conversely, they can apply brakes, causing the cell to become inactive. They can also cause an adjacent cell to produce and release hormones, at times or to grow or to die.

Remarkably, these very complex processes continue through all the decades of one's life. Most of the time they work well. But it is no surprise that the system can also break down. Let's look at a specific example.

The drug reserpine was used for many years to treat hypertension (high blood pressure). It was fairly effective, but many people who took it became seriously depressed. In most instances, these people were mature, solid individuals with no history of prior mental illness or emotional problems. Yet, some of them became suicidally depressed. Eventually it was discovered that this intense reaction was caused by the effect of reserpine on a very limited number of nerve cells situated in the limbic system and hypothalamus. When the drug was discontinued, the patients recovered from their depression. Antidepressant medications were also used and were effective in treating these patients' depressive symptoms.

Note: The neurotransmitting chemical that is released by a particular nerve cell is also the name given to that nerve cell. Thus, a dopamine nerve cell is a cell that manufactures and releases the transmitter dopamine.

Any of several chemical and environmental factors can derail the functioning of neurotransmitters. The list of nerve cells that have been implicated in major psychiatric disorders is growing. Currently, it includes the following:

- Serotonin (abbreviated 5-HT)
- Dopamine (DA)
- Norepinephrine (NE)
- Corticotropin-releasing factor (CRF)

- Gamma-aminobutyric acid (GABA)
- Glutamate

Some of the factors that have been found to interfere with appropriate nerve cell functioning include the following:

- Specific prescription medications (used to treat many illnesses)
- Recreational drugs (e.g., alcohol, cocaine)
- Hormonal fluctuations (especially female sexual hormones, as may occur premenstrually, postpartum, and with menopause)
- Diseases that cause changes in body chemistry which interfere with brain functioning (e.g., thyroid disease)
- Stress (especially intense and prolonged stress)
- Genetic factors (disorders believed to be caused by genetic vulnerability tend to run in families, and blood relatives may be at increased risk for developing the disorder)

Since so many different factors can cause psychological symptoms, it is important to have a thorough medical evaluation to rule out possible physical conditions or other causes that might be contributing to any current psychological symptoms.

ANDY'S CASE

Andy, a fifty-four-year-old mechanic, was accompanied by his wife to a mental health clinic. He was so tense and anxious that his wife did most of the talking. "Doctor, I don't know what's wrong with my husband. He's never been this way before, but during the last six months he has become a bundle of nerves." Her description was accurate. Andy was incredibly rigid as he sat trembling in his chair. He too was perplexed by his problem. He reported feeling "very nervous all the time" and was plagued by insomnia and fitful, restless sleep.

As they talked, the therapist noted that Andy repeatedly used a nasal spray. The third time Andy used the spray, the therapist inquired about it. It turned out that Andy had begun to use it six months earlier during the hay fever season, and his use had continued well past that time of the year. To keep his nasal passages open, he found it necessary to use the spray many times each day. The decongestant was immediately suspected to be the cause of his anxiety.

Chronic overuse of nasal or oral (e.g., Sudafed) decongestants are known to cause anxiety symptoms. With the help of his primary care doctor, Andy was able to wean himself from the nasal spray successfully. Two weeks later, he was himself again. "I thought I was going nuts. It's hard to believe that a little nasal spray can change a man so much!"

HOW PSYCHIATRIC MEDICATIONS WORK

As mentioned in Chapter 1, psychiatric medications are not all alike. In some cases, particular drugs are believed, in one sense, to "cure" the problem with certain malfunctioning nerve cells (i.e., to return the neurons to a state of normal functioning). Other medications do not result in lasting changes in cellular functioning but rather operate to improve cell functioning temporarily (e.g., the medications may work when they are taken and will provide symptom relief, but if they are discontinued, the symptoms may return). In most cases, the goal of psychiatric medication treatment is to restore the brain to a state of normal cellular functioning, which will contribute a great deal to reducing emotional suffering.

At the same time, no pills have ever been invented to mend broken hearts or to fill empty lives. No medication can teach people how to love one another, nor can drugs insulate us from some of the inevitable challenges and tragedies of life. One fact is clear, however: When the brain is not functioning appropriately, the task of dealing with difficult life circumstances is amplified enormously.

GETTING "HIGH" ON LIFE: THE BRAIN'S PLEASURE CENTERS

Neuroscientists have identified several places in the brain that are known as pleasure centers. These brain areas are a part of an internal biological reward system. They have evolved to generate emotional states that are experienced by people and other animals as pleasant. Biologic pleasure centers are activated by the release of particular neurochemicals (e.g., dopamine, endorphins) that are "turned on" by certain kinds of life experiences. Under normal circumstances, events such as watching a funny movie, enjoying a tasty meal, or making love can evoke a whole range of feelings, from joy to a heightened sense of aliveness to blissful euphoria.

Pleasure centers can also be activated artificially. A person might have a completely awful and unsatisfying life and yet may temporarily feel on the top of the world by drinking champagne or taking cocaine. (Of course, we are certainly *not* recommending this pathway to euphoria. There are significant risks in using alcohol and drugs.)

Conversely, in major depression, a considerable body of evidence suggests that the pleasure centers have become chemically inactivated. This results in a symptom known as *anhedonia* (an inability to experience either pleasure or a feeling of vitality). Thus, even if a wonderfully satisfying event were to take place in the life of a person with serious depression, it would most likely not cause any positive emotions at all. Typically, the response of the depressed individual would be to feel nothing. This is only one of the symptoms that make the life of a seriously depressed person so intolerably painful. Anhedonia has been likened to watching a sunset but seeing no color. Fortunately, antidepressant medications have a good track record in bringing the pleasure centers back on line as well as in combating a variety of other depressive symptoms (see Chapter 5).

CAN PSYCHOTHERAPY CHANGE BRAIN FUNCTIONING?

This question has been subject to a good deal of speculation. In 1992, a now-classic study performed by Baxter and colleagues addressed the question by looking at the neurobiology of people suffering from obsessive-compulsive disorder (OCD) (see Chapter 7). It had been found that people with severe OCD had a specific metabolic abnormality in a particular part of the brain. This was revealed with the use of a positron emission tomography (PET) scan.

In the study, OCD patients were randomly assigned to two treatment groups. One group received standard drug treatment for OCD (serotonergic antidepressants such as Prozac—a proven treatment). The other group received a specialized form of psychotherapy (behavior therapy, first using exposure and then response prevention). All the participants had evidence of abnormal PET scans prior to treatment. After four months of treatment, both groups showed a significant amount of improvement in their obsessional symptoms. They were then evaluated by a second PET scan. Remarkably, *both* groups (those who received drugs and those who received only psychotherapy) demonstrated that brain functioning had normalized and no longer showed evidence of aberrant metabolism.

Additional studies have shown that psychotherapy changes the brain: improving sleep, demonstrated with sleep-related brain wave activity as measured with electroencephalography (EEG) (Thase et al. 1998), normalizing brain metabolic changes in major depression (Zwillich 1999), and reducing social anxiety (Shear et al. 1991).

In studies of both humans and animals, negative experiences, such as prolonged intense stress, have been demonstrated to cause marked changes in brain functioning. So it should come as no surprise that positive experiences might also affect brain functioning (i.e., improve it). The data right now are limited, but there is reason to believe that psychotherapy can alter brain functioning. One key element that may account for this is the experience of mastery. We eagerly await additional research that may shed more light on this theory.

Exercise is yet another way to significantly change and normalize brain functioning. This has been demonstrated in studies of depression and anxiety. At the heart of change in many emotional disorders is a normalizing of chemistry and metabolic activity in the brain. As we have seen, some nonmedical approaches can also be successful (more details in Chapter 12). Such research also accounts for the findings that combined psychotherapy and medication treatments often yield the best results.

CHAPTER 4

Managing Your Medications

The information presented here by no means describes all the complex interactions that take place within the human body when medications are taken. Our intention is not to provide the detail of a textbook but rather to describe and explain some important principles you can use to make sure you get the most benefit out of your medications. By understanding the factors that can affect how a medicine acts in your body, you will be more able to provide your doctor with accurate information to guide him or her in selecting the right drug for you at the right dose. Be sure to ask your doctor or pharmacist for any specifics that might help you understand your medicines better.

In modern medicine, drugs play a fundamental role in the treatment of most diseases or symptoms. This has not always been the case. Prior to the early 1900s, relatively few useful medicines were available. Breakthrough discoveries and technological advances have provided the tools to better understand human physiology and to produce purer and more reliable chemical compounds. It is important to recognize that even as sophisticated as our knowledge of drugs is at the present time, we still do not know a great deal about them. A quick glance through any standard pharmacology reference will confirm this. In discussions about medicines used to treat psychiatric conditions, it is especially important to keep in mind that existing knowledge is limited. Even though tremendous strides have been made in understanding how the brain works, we still do not have the capability to measure all of its functions.

Conversely, because of our modern sophisticated technology, it is tempting to assume that we know exactly what effects a drug will have on the body. Today, new biological discoveries are made, and new drugs developed, at a remarkable pace. Medications are advertised extensively on television, in magazines, and on the internet. There's a tendency to accept each new development as the final and best answer to long-standing questions regarding human behavior and mental health conditions. It is important, however, to maintain a healthy skepticism until new information has been confirmed over a length of time or until new drugs have produced a well-established record of safety and effectiveness. Even the most rigorous clinical trials do not approximate all the effects of the wide use of a drug in diverse populations after it has been released into the marketplace.

Psychopharmacology deals primarily with drugs intended to help symptoms that are categorized under the three main types of disorders: (1) mood disorders, such as depression; (2) anxiety; and (3) psychotic disorders, such as schizophrenia. The use of these medications is relatively recent, with widespread use not beginning until the 1950s and 1960s. Since then, the commercial growth of psychiatric drugs has been phenomenal, which indicates how commonly these conditions occur and how great the need is to treat them. Much of the basic research aimed at understanding how psychiatric medications work has added to the overall knowledge base of emotional and mental illnesses.

HOW MEDICATIONS WORK:
BASIC PHARMACOLOGY

At a very basic level, pharmacology is the science of how drugs interact with the body to produce certain effects. A drug is broadly defined as "any substance that brings about a change in biologic function through its chemical actions." The actions that drugs take extend from the microscopic, or molecular, level to individual organs, such as the heart and brain, to the body as a whole organism. Included in the study of pharmacology is knowledge about the origins and chemical properties of drugs, as well as a thorough understanding of the biology and chemistry of the body.

DRUGS AND RECEPTORS
At the molecular level, most drugs interact with specific receptors to produce their therapeutic effects. Receptors are structures located primarily on the outside surface of nerve cells. To understand the interaction, an often-used analogy is that of a lock and key, where the receptor acts as the lock and the chemical as the key. Various drug receptor systems are located throughout the body.

SIDE EFFECTS
The effects of drugs can be those that are intended, called the therapeutic effects, or unintended, known as side effects. Although side effects often are bothersome and can sometimes create serious problems, some side effects are actually beneficial. Many of these are the most noticeable when a medication is first started or when the dose is increased. Most of them diminish over time. However, side effects that persist or get worse should never be ignored.

The published information about a given drug's side effects is fairly extensive. Generally, when reading about them, you will note that they are categorized by how often they occur. Usually these groupings of side effects are designated as frequent or common, infrequent, or rare.

In Part Two of this book, we cover most of the common side effects of each drug as well as most of the infrequent and rare ones that could be potentially serious. Since we do not reproduce all of the literature that drug manufacturers are required to report, our lists are not all inclusive. We do provide the most important information you need in order to benefit from the medication. If you have any questions at all about the possible side effects of the medication you are taking, you should consult your doctor.

BASIC PHARMACOKINETICS

To better understand and benefit from medications of any type, it is important to have a working knowledge of some of the processes that take place when medications are ingested. The principles summarized in the following pages apply to medications in general. It is important to remember, however, that every person is biologically unique. Even though medications generally follow somewhat predictable patterns, it is obvious that some people will react differently than others to the same medication.

Once a drug enters the body, a cascade of actions is set in motion. Certain bodily organs or systems process a medication differently. Basically, the body will *absorb, distribute, metabolize,* then *excrete* the drug. Collectively these processes are called pharmacokinetics. What follows is a very brief description of these four functions, intended to help you understand the complexities involved in predicting how medicines act in the body.

ABSORPTION

Most drugs are absorbed in the stomach or small intestine. The presence of food, milk, or other medications in the stomach can affect a given medicine. It is important to find out how your medication should be taken in relation to meals. If the absorption of a medicine is known to be impaired when food is present in the stomach, then it might be advisable to take that medicine on an empty stomach. By contrast, the presence of food sometimes increases the amount of a drug that is absorbed, in which case it may be preferable to take the medicine at mealtimes. Certain medications can irritate the stomach and should be taken with food or milk to lessen this effect and prevent damage to the stomach lining.

As a drug travels throughout the body it encounters various membranes that it must cross. One of the most important of these barriers is called the *blood–brain barrier*. This barrier serves to limit the substances that pass into the brain. It is one way the body protects the brain from damage caused by chemicals or other toxins. Some medications pass freely into the brain, whereas others have more limited accessibility.

The total amount of a medication that is ingested may not equal the amount that ultimately becomes available at the place in one's body for which it is intended. This principle is called *bioavailability*. For example, if a medication is known to break down and be inactivated by the acidic environment of the stomach, only a small percentage of the original dose will reach the bloodstream. In this case, less than 100 percent of the drug will be bioavailable. By contrast, a drug injected directly into the bloodstream is considered to be nearly 100 percent bioavailable because it reaches the bloodstream intact.

Bioavailability is also the benchmark used to compare products made by different manufacturers, or to compare generic and brand name products. With most generic drugs, bioavailability closely matches that of the original brand name product. Such generic products can provide an economical advantage over more costly brand name drugs. Certain medications, however, are not readily formulated into generic products, and the brand name product may be superior. From a practical standpoint, it may be more important not to make frequent switches between products.

DISTRIBUTION

Once a medication reaches the bloodstream, it is distributed to various areas or organs in the body. The distribution pattern varies from drug to drug. For most medicines, the distribution process is very straightforward; for others, the pattern is more complex. For example, more complicated processes apply to medicines that are stored in fatty areas of the body. A drug can remain for long periods of time in fatty areas, somewhat like being stored in a reservoir. When the drug is in these storage areas, is not readily available to produce any action; rather, it has been deposited and is inactive.

The amount of medicine in the reservoir will vary in order to reach a balance with the amount that is in the bloodstream. If the amount in the bloodstream drops, then some of the medicine will be released from the storage area. If the amount in the bloodstream is stable and adequate, none will be released from the storage area, and the amount in the reservoir can continue to accumulate.

For people taking antidepressants and antipsychotics, understanding how drug distribution works can be very important. To a large degree, these types of medicines are stored in fatty areas. This means that even after a medication is discontinued, the portion that has been stored will gradually re-enter the bloodstream until all of it is eliminated from the body. In such instances, there can be continuing effects from the medication for several weeks or longer after it has been discontinued.

This information is important to remember when stopping antidepressants or antipsychotics. In essence, a person can continue to experience the benefits or side effects of the medicine even though it is not being taken as a daily dose. After the medicine is discontinued, symptoms may return several weeks later. It is important to watch out for signs that they might be returning, and not just in the first few days after stopping a medicine but for as long as eight weeks afterward.

METABOLISM

This process, which occurs primarily in the liver, is also known as *biotransformation*. Most medications are metabolized, or chemically altered, to varying degrees by the liver. The actual process takes place through the action of enzymes that break down molecules from their original size to smaller ones that can then be eliminated by the kidney more easily.

The extent and rate of metabolism for a given drug is generally consistent, within a range, from person to person. However, some people may be exceptionally fast metabolizers, while others may be especially slow. In these instances, there is less predictability about determining the dosage or frequency of a given drug, and adjustments are often necessary. Slow metabolizers, for instance, might be extremely sensitive to the side effects of a medication, even at a low or average dosage. Antidepressants and antipsychotics are classes of medications that are especially prone to differences in metabolizing capability. There is some evidence that there may be a genetic influence in people who are slow metabolizers.

People who have damaged livers may have impaired metabolic ability, which can lead to a buildup of medication in the body. To prevent serious side effects from excessively high levels of a medication in the blood, it may be necessary for such people to take smaller amounts of medicine or less frequent doses. Because the liver is called upon to metabolize most medications, there are times when multiple drugs will compete for the same enzymes. This competition is the source of one of the most common types of drug interactions. Usually one drug wins this contest over the other. The result is that one medication will build up in the body because the liver is busy metabolizing the other. Adjusting the dose of one or both of the interacting medications may become necessary.

EXCRETION

Excretion is the final step in the process by which drugs are eliminated from the body. The first step, metabolism, happens via the liver, as described above.

Excretion takes place primarily through the kidneys. If there is kidney damage, medications can accumulate to levels that are higher than desired or even dangerous. If the kidneys are working in a less than ideal manner, adjustments in medication may be necessary to avoid unnecessary or dangerous side effects.

HALF-LIFE

A measure of a medication's action that is related to excretion is called *half-life*. The half-life is the amount of time required for the blood level of a drug to drop by 50 percent. A drug's half-life is used to decide how often it should be taken and also to determine correct dosages. For instance, drugs with short half-lives will require more doses throughout a 24-hour period because they will leave the body faster. Medicines with longer half-lives will not need to be taken as frequently because they will stay in the body longer.

GETTING THE MOST OUT OF YOUR MEDICATIONS

Getting the maximum benefit from your medicines requires that you and your doctor work together. Your doctor will ask many specific questions before prescribing a medication. The following list highlights some of the key steps you can take to work effectively with your doctor in managing your medicines.

WHAT YOUR DOCTOR NEEDS TO KNOW

Your doctor will need the following information: your complete medical history; everything to which you are allergic; the names and dosages of all the medicines you take, including over-the-counter products; your past experiences with medicines, both positive and negative; how much alcohol you drink on a daily or weekly basis; all the recreational drugs you use. If you are pregnant, think you might be pregnant, or are considering becoming pregnant, you should discuss this with your doctor.

WHAT YOU CAN DO TO MANAGE YOUR MEDICINES

Take the medicine exactly as prescribed. Taking more than prescribed can be dangerous. Missing doses can mean that you don't get better. If you do not understand the directions, ask your doctor or pharmacist to clarify them for you. If you have trouble remembering to take your medicine, ask a family member or health care provider to help you set up a system.

Be sure you understand exactly why you are taking a given medication. If your questions are not answered to your satisfaction, be persistent with your doctor or pharmacist to get the information you need. This is your right.

Understand how long it should take to begin to feel better.

Do not hesitate to contact your doctor if you experience unexpected side effects or if you are not getting better within the time frame indicated by your doctor.

Avoid seeing too many different doctors who might prescribe many kinds of medicine. If you have an established need to see several physicians, be sure each doctor is aware of what the other doctors are prescribing for you.

If you are having difficulties taking a medicine because it is hard to swallow, find out whether it is available in a liquid form. Also, some tablets are suitable for crushing, and the contents of some capsules can be mixed in a liquid. Check with your doctor or pharmacist first before doing either.

Read the label on the medicine bottle every time you take a dose to be sure you are taking the correct medication. Some people have many bottles of medicine that can be mixed up easily. Become familiar with what your medicine looks like. If you receive a prescription that doesn't "look right" to you, be sure to double-check it with your pharmacist. Never take your medicine in the dark when you cannot see exactly what you are swallowing.

Do not switch medication bottles. Keep your medicine in the original bottle in which it came. Never put all your medicines together in one bottle. If you need help in keeping your medicines straight, you can purchase pill reminder boxes to help you keep track.

Make sure you put the lids back on tightly. By law, child-resistant lids are required for prescription medicines to prevent children from accidental poisonings. Some adults find these hard to use and will compensate by not putting the lids on securely. Such people can ask for a waiver and receive lids that are not child-resistant. In any case, it is essential to prevent ingestion by children because accidental overdoses can be fatal to them.

Know whether your prescription has refills. Sometimes your doctor will want to check with you before authorizing your refills. Keep track of when you are close to running out of your medicine, and allow ample time to get your refills. Be familiar with how to get your prescriptions refilled. Sometimes people run into problems with this and will go for several days without taking their medicine. In that amount of time it is possible for symptoms to return. Taking medicine consistently, without any lapses in treatment, is the best way to ensure that you (or your loved one) will get better—and stay that way.

Follow the storage instructions. In general, most drugs should be kept in a cool dry place, away from high temperatures, in an area of low humidity, and out of direct light. The bathroom medicine cabinet is one of the worst places to store your medications because of the humidity and temperature of the bathroom. If you do not store your medicine appropriately, it may deteriorate or undergo a physical change to become a harmful chemical.

Do not take medications past the expiration date on the bottle. The expiration date is accurate, assuming that proper storage instructions are followed.

Keep taking your medicines as prescribed. Sometimes people decrease their dosage or discontinue their medication altogether because the cost is prohibitive. However, taking less than an adequate dose will not provide the relief that is sought. If you are unable to afford an expensive medicine, your doctor and pharmacist will often work with you to find a more affordable drug. If you do not have insurance that pays for your prescriptions, find out how much your medicines will cost you each month.

USEFUL TIPS ABOUT PSYCHIATRIC MEDICATIONS

If the treatment of your mental health condition requires medication, you can do a lot to make sure you get better. Do not view the prescribing of your medicine as a passive process. Your doctor's decision is based not only on his or her observations and examination of you but also on your ability to provide complete and honest information. No matter how insignificant a concern or question might seem to you, it is important that your doctor hear what is on your mind.

Be open with your doctor if you have not been taking your medicine as prescribed. The doctor will try to work with you to figure out why you are having problems with it. Sometimes, when people are depressed, they may have trouble remembering whether they took their medication. Some people may feel so bad about themselves that they don't believe they deserve to get better. Others might feel so hopeless about their chances of recovery that they have little faith in the medicine's effectiveness. All of these possibilities are typical in a depression. Your doctor will understand the difficulties you face and help you work through them.

Some people are fearful of taking medicines to treat depression, anxiety, or psychotic disorders. If you are afraid in this regard, share your concerns with your doctor. In some cases these concerns are based on faulty information or misconceptions. Your doctor or pharmacist can provide you with factual information that can clear up any misunderstandings and often will allay your fears.

Occasionally, some people become suspicious of everyone and everything involved in their treatment, especially if their problem is a psychotic disorder such as schizophrenia. At those times, people may think that their medicine is intended to harm them or that someone can change their medicine in such a way as to "poison" them. In these situations it can be quite difficult to provide reassurance. If you have ever thought this way, or if you have a loved one who thinks this way, it is important to know that prescription medications are manufactured under very tight quality control conditions. It would be nearly impossible for an individual doctor, nurse, or pharmacist to change the ingredients in a prepared tablet or capsule. In addition, most medications are required by law to have clear identifying markings on them. If you are familiar with what your medicine normally looks like, you'll be able to notice immediately if you receive something else.

Medications have an established role in the treatment of most mental health conditions. They can produce remarkable results and provide relief from the most painful and debilitating of symptoms. These drugs are among the most widely prescribed in the world, and millions of people take them safely every day. There are abundant reasons to expect that your experience with these medications will be positive and that you will find relief from your symptoms.

A multitude of drugs are used to treat psychiatric symptoms. These will be described in detail in the chapters that follow. The following charts briefly summarize the various medications and medication classes, typical doses (adolescent and adult doses), and common side effects. This is a "quick reference" that represents currently available medications. Since new medications periodically come on the market, \you can access updated copies of these charts by going to *www.psychceu.com/quickreference.doc.html* for free downloads.

QUICK REFERENCE TO
PSYCHIATRIC MEDICATION®

To the best of our knowledge recommended doses and side effects listed below are accurate. However, this is meant as a general reference only, and should not serve as a guideline for prescribing of medications. Please check the manufacturer's product information sheet or the P.D.R. (Physicians' Desk Reference) for any changes in dosage schedule or contraindications. (Brand names are registered trademarks.)

BIPOLAR DISORDER MEDICATIONS			
NAMES			
GENERIC	BRAND	DAILY DOSAGE RANGE	SERUM[1] LEVEL
lithium carbonate	Eskalith, Lithonate	600–2400 mg	0.6–1.5
olanzapine/ fluoxetine	Symbyax	6/25– 12/50 mg[4]	[2]
carbamazepine	Tegretol, Equetro	600–1600 mg	4–10+
oxcarbazepine	Trileptal	1200–2400 mg	[2]
divalproex	Depakote	750–1500 mg	50–100
gabapentin	Neurontin	300–2400 mg	[2]
lamotrigine	Lamictal	50–500 mg	[2]
topiramate	Topamax	50–300 mg	[3]
tiagabine	Gabitril	4–12 mg	[3]

1. Lithium levels are expressed in mEq/l, carbamazepine and valproic acid levels expressed in mcg/ml
2. Serum monitoring may not be necessary
3. Not yet established
4. Available in: 6/25, 6/50, 12/25, and 12/50mg formulations

ANTIDEPRESSANTS

NAMES		USUAL DAILY DOSAGE RANGE	SEDATION	ACH[1]	SELECTIVE ACTION ON NEUROTRANSMITTERS[2]		
GENERIC	BRAND				NE	5-HT	DA
imipramine	Tofranil	150–300 mg	mid	mid	++	+++	0
desipramine	Norpramin	150–300 mg	low	low	+++++	0	0
amitriptyline	Elavil	150–300 mg	high	high	++	++++	0
nortriptyline	Aventyl, Pamelor	75–125 mg	mid	mid	+++	++	0
protriptyline	Vivactil	15–40 mg	mid	mid	++++	+	0
trimipramine	Surmontil[3]	100–300 mg	high	mid	++	++	0
doxepin	Sinequan, Adapin[3]	150–300 mg	high	mid	++	+++	0
clomipramine	Anafranil	150–250 mg	high	high	0	+++++	0
maprotiline	Ludiomil	150–225 mg	high	mid	+++++	0	0
amoxapine	Asendin	150–400 mg	mid	low	+++	++	0
trazodone	Desyrel	150–400 mg	mid	none	0	++++	0
nefazodone	Serzone	100–300 mg	mid	none	0	+++	0
fluoxetine	Prozac[4], Sarafem	20–80 mg	low	none	0	+++++	0

					NE[2]	5-HT[2]	DA[2]
bupropion-X.L.	Wellbutrin-X.L.[4]	150–400 mg	low	none	++	0	++
sertraline	Zoloft	50–200 mg	low	none	0	+++++	+
paroxetine	Paxil	20–50 mg	low	low	+	+++++	0
venlafaxine-X.R.	Effexor-X.R.[4]	75–350 mg	low	none	++	+++	+
desvenlafaxine	Pristiq	50–400 mg	low	none	++	+++	+
fluvoxamine	Luvox	50–300 mg	low	low	0	+++++	0
mirtazapine	Remeron	15–45 mg	mid	mid	+++	+++	0
citalopram	Celexa	10–60 mg	low	none	0	+++++	0
escitalopram	Lexapro	5–20 mg	low	none	0	+++++	0
duloxetine	Cymbalta	20–80 mg	low	none	++++	++++	0
atomoxetine	Strattera	60–120 mg	low	low	+++++	0	0
MAO Inhibitors							
phenelzine	Nardil	30–90 mg	low	none	+++	+++	+++
tranylcypromine	Parnate	20–60 mg	low	none	+++	+++	+++
selegiline	Emsam (patch)	6–12 mg	low	none	+++	+++	+++

1. ACH: Anticholinergic Side Effects: dry mouth, constipation, trouble urinating, blurry vision
2. NE: Norepinephrine, 5-HT: Serotonin, DA: Dopamine (0 = no effect, + = minimal effect, +++ = moderate effect, +++++ = high effect)
3. Uncertain, but likely effects
4. Available in standard formulation and time release (XR, XL, or CR). Prozac available in 90mg time released/weekly formulation

ANTIPSYCHOTICS

NAMES							
GENERIC	BRAND	DOSAGE RANGE[1]	SEDATION	ORTHO[2]	EPS[3]	ACH EFFECTS[4]	EQUIVALENCE[5]
Low Potency							
chlorpromazine	Thorazine	50–800 mg	high	high	++	++++	100 mg
thioridazine	Mellaril	150–800 mg	high	high	+	+++++	100 mg
clozapine	Clozaril	300–900 mg	high	high	0	+++++	50 mg
mesoridazine	Serentil	50–500 mg	high	mid	+	+++++	50 mg
quetiapine	Seroquel	150–600 mg	mid	mid	+/0	+	50 mg
High Potency							
molindone	Moban	20–225 mg	low	mid	+++	+++	10 mg
perphenazine	Trilafon	8–60 mg	mid	mid	++++	++	10 mg
loxapine	Loxitane	50–250 mg	low	mid	+++	++	10 mg
trifluoperazine	Stelazine	2–40 mg	low	mid	++++	++	5 mg
fluphenazine	Prolixin[5]	3–45 mg	low	mid	+++++	++	2 mg

thiothixene	Navane	10–60 mg	low	mid	++++	++	5 mg
haloperidol	Haldol[5]	2–40 mg	low	low	+++++	+	2 mg
pimozide	Orap	1–10 mg	low	low	+++++	+	1–2 mg
risperidone	Risperdal	4–16 mg	low	mid	+	+	1–2 mg
paliperidone	Invega	3–12 mg	low	mid	+	+	1–2 mg
olanzapine	Zyprexa	5–20 mg	mid	low	+/0	+	1–2 mg
ziprasidone	Geodon	60–160 mg	low	mid	+/0	++	10 mg
aripiprazole	Abilify	15–30 mg	low	low	+/0	+	2 mg

1. Usual daily oral dosage
2. Orthostatic Hypotension Dizziness and falls
3. Acute: Parkinson's, dystonias, akathisia. Does not reflect risk for tardive dyskinesia. All antipsychotics may cause tardive dyskinesia, except clozapine
4. Anticholinergic Side Effects: dry mouth, constipation, trouble urinating, blurry vision
5. Dose required to achieve efficacy of 100 mg chlorpromazine

ANTIANXIETY			
NAMES			
GENERIC	BRAND	SINGLE DOSE DOSAGE RANGE	EQUIVA-LENCE[1]
Benzodiazepines			
diazepam	Valium	2–10 mg	5 mg
chlordiazepoxide	Librium	10–50 mg	25 mg
prazepam	Centrax	5–30 mg	10 mg
clorazepate	Tranxene	3.75–15 mg	10 mg
clonazepam	Klonopin	0.5–2.0 mg	0.25 mg
lorazepam	Ativan	0.5–2.0 mg	1 mg
alprazolam	Xanax XR	0.25–2.0 mg	0.5 mg
oxazepam	Serax	10–30 mg	15 mg
Other antianxiety agents			
buspirone	BuSpar	5–20 mg	
gabapentin	Neurontin	200–600 mg	
hydroxyzine	Atarax, Vistaril	10–50 mg	
propranolol	Inderal	10–80 mg	
atenolol	Tenormin	25–100 mg	
guanfacine	Tenex	0.5–3 mg	
clonidine	Catapres	0.1–0.3 mg	
prazosin	Minipress	5–20 mg	

1. Doses required to achieve efficacy of 5 mg of diazepam

ANTI-OBSESSIONAL

NAMES

GENERIC	BRAND	DOSE RANGE[1]
clomipramine	Anafranil	150–300 mg
fluoxetine	Prozac[1]	20–80 mg
sertraline	Zoloft[1]	50–200 mg
paroxetine	Paxil[1]	20–60 mg
fluvoxamine	Luvox[1]	50–300 mg
citalopram	Celexa[1]	10–60 mg
escitalopram	Lexapro[1]	5–30 mg

1. Often higher doses are required to control obsessive-compulsive symptoms than the doses generally used to treat depression.

SLEEPING PILLS

NAMES

GENERIC	BRAND	SINGLE DOSE DOSAGE RANGE
flurazepam	Dalmane	15–30 mg
temazepam	Restoril	15–30 mg
triazolam	Halcion	0.25–0.5 mg
estazolam	ProSom	1.0–2.0 mg
quazepam	Doral	7.5–15 mg
zolpidem	Ambien	5–10 mg
zaleplon	Sonata	5–10 mg
eszopiclone	Lunesta	1–3 mg
ramelteon	Rozerem	4–16 mg
diphenhydramine	Benadryl	25–100 mg

PSYCHO-STIMULANTS

NAMES		
GENERIC	BRAND	DAILY DOSAGE[1]
methylphenidate	Ritalin	5–50 mg
methylphenidate	Concerta[2]	18–54 mg
methylphenidate	Metadate	5–40 mg
methylphenidate	Methylin	10–60 mg
methylphenidate	Daytrana (patch)	15–30 mg
dexmethylphenidate	Focalin	5–40 mg
dextroamphetamine	Dexedrine	5–40 mg
lisdexamfetamine	Vyvanse	30–70 mg
pemoline	Cylert	37.5–112.5 mg
d- and l-amphetamine	Adderall	5–40 mg
modafinil	Provigil, Sparlon	100–400 mg

1. Note: Adult Doses
2. Sustained release

OVER THE COUNTER

NAME	DAILY DOSE
St. John's Wort[1, 2]	600–1800 mg
SAM-e[3]	400–1600 mg
Omega-3[4]	1–9 g

1. Treats depression and anxiety
2. May cause significant drug–drug interactions
3. Treats depression
4. Treats depression and bipolar disorder

CHAPTER 5

Depression

INTRODUCTION

Many people will occasionally say that they feel depressed. This can refer to a host of unpleasant emotions such as feeling "blue," moodiness, sadness, disappointment, discouragement, being unmotivated, or just feeling out of sorts. For most of us, feeling down in the dumps occasionally or being saddened temporarily is a normal part of human life. These are understandable reactions to a myriad of difficult life experiences.

In the United States, however, every year 10 percent of the population experiences a much more debilitating mood disorder: major depression, also referred to as clinical depression. Over the life span of the average American, the prevalence of major depression is even higher, affecting 17 percent. One out of six Americans will at some point in their lives suffer with this form of severe emotional disorder (Kessler et al. 1994). With such a high incidence, it is hard to imagine that anyone has not either experienced depression personally or known close friends or relatives who have had episodes of clinical depression. The bottom line is that depression is extremely common.

Major depression differs from minor bouts of sadness in several ways, but its main characteristics are as follow:

- It is extremely severe.
- If not treated, it generally lasts for months.
- It often results in significant disability. In addition to tremendous personal suffering, during episodes of major depression otherwise capable people often cannot function at work or in school, marriages fall apart, and loving parents find it nearly impossible to nurture and guide their children.
- Rates of alcohol abuse and other types of substance abuse go up.
- For untreated or undertreated people, suicide is a risk (the lifetime mortality risk from suicide is 10 percent).
- Chronic depression contributes to poor physical health, especially heart disease.

Clinical depression is obviously much more than a mere case of the blues. It is a common and often devastating emotional illness. The real tragedy is that only one third of people who experience a major depression ever receive treatment. Most somehow grit their teeth and suffer for months and months as the average length of an episode of depression is from nine to fifteen months unless it is treated. Yet, according to the National Institute of Mental Health, most people experiencing major depression can be successfully treated (NIMH 2007).

High rates of treatment success are due to the development of several effective types of therapy, including some types of psychotherapy (cognitive therapy or interpersonal therapy) and medical treatments,* which are discussed in detail later in this chapter.

A RECURRING ILLNESS

For a third of people experiencing a major depression, the episode will be a once-in-a-lifetime event. However, for the other two thirds, the disorder will recur (APA 2000). In this group, many will experience ongoing chronic depression, while most will be plagued with recurring episodes of the illness. Although this may sound bleak, the good news is that medical treatments for depression also have been shown to be effective in reducing relapse rates. Thus, when considering treatment, it is important to focus not only on resolving the current episode but also on taking steps to prevent new ones.

NOT EVERYONE WILL UNDERSTAND

It is very common for those going through a depression to hear comments from concerned friends or family that reveal a misunderstanding of the nature of clinical depression. For example, many people make statements like these: "You just

---

* Treatment guidelines are drawn largely from the following sources:
  American Psychiatric Association: Practice Guidelines
  www.psychiatryonline.com/pracGuide/pracGuideHome.aspx

  Texas Department of Mental Health: Texas Medication Algorithm Project
  www.dshs.state.tx.us/mhprograms/TMAPover.shtm

  Sequenced Treatment Alternatives to Relieve Depression: STAR-D: National Institute of Mental Health
  www.nimh.nih.gov/health/trials/practical/stard/index.shtml

need to look on the bright side." "Just try to snap out of it." "You need to try harder—you need to pull yourself up by your bootstraps." They may even say, "Don't worry—be happy." Their intentions may be good, but many people simply do not understand.

True clinical depression drags people into a kind of emotional paralysis from which it is difficult to escape, despite considerable effort. It must be emphasized that depression can affect anyone in any walk of life. It knows no social or economic barriers. It can occur to anyone regardless of level of intelligence or strength of character. During the past three decades, discoveries have been made in the medical and neurological sciences that have helped us understand more about the role the brain plays in emotional disorders. This is especially true when it comes to understanding the underlying biological basis of some types of depression. As a result, the medical treatments for depression have improved enormously. Nevertheless, it is important to consider several issues that have been raised regarding psychiatric medications.

MAKING THE DIAGNOSIS

Before looking at diagnosis per se, it is important to understand the distinctions between three human experiences: sadness, grief, and clinical depression. Sadness is an experience common to most human beings. It is considered a normal healthy emotional reaction to minor losses and disappointments. This kind of sadness is very transient, lasting only several minutes, a few hours, or at most a few days. It is unpleasant, but typically it does not interfere with one's functioning. People feel sad, but they can continue to work, raise their kids, and go about the tasks of everyday life. Normal minor bouts of sadness do not knock people off of their feet.

By contrast, grief is a much more intense and sometimes devastating human experience. However, it is a normal and inevitable emotional reaction that people in all cultures experience in the aftermath of a major loss, the death of a loved one, or a divorce. Grief tends to have a major disruptive effect on the lives of sufferers and can result in prolonged periods of sadness, mourning, and loneliness. Mental health professionals however, make a distinction between uncomplicated bereavement and complicated grief reactions. Uncomplicated bereavement is considered a very painful, albeit healthy, normal response to a major loss. It often results in prolonged mourning, which can last anywhere from a few months to several years. We want to emphasize that normal grieving may last a very long time—broken hearts do not mend quickly. By contrast, complicated grief reactions can become especially severe and can disintegrate into clinical depression.

The essential feature of uncomplicated bereavement is that it seems to be a necessary part of emotional healing. Some amount of mourning seems to be necessary for people to come to terms with major losses. Two other important features separate uncomplicated bereavement from the kind of grief that turns into clinical depression. The first is that during normal grieving, despite tremendous personal suffering, the grieving person's self-esteem and sense of self-worth remain relatively intact. This is not the case with complicated grief that becomes major depression. In more severe depressions, grieving people almost always experience a significant erosion in their sense of self-worth.

The second marker is a set of symptoms that are commonly a part of major depression and that are absent in uncomplicated bereavement. They are significant agitation, early morning awakening, serious weight loss, suicidal ideations or attempts, anhedonia (loss of the ability to experience any pleasure), and marked impairment of social, interpersonal, academic, or occupational functioning.

The vast majority of individuals encountering major losses grieve but do not become seriously depressed and do not need psychological or psychiatric treatment. However, about 25 percent will, in fact, go on to develop clinical depression (complicated grief reactions) and certainly may need and benefit from mental health treatment (Zisook 1996). Medication treatment may be indicated when grief turns into depression.

Clinical depressions are characterized by their intensity, duration, impact on functioning, and a host of specific symptoms that are outlined below.

HOW DEPRESSION IS DIAGNOSED

A great deal of media attention has recently been paid to the biological basis of depression, often referred to as a type of chemical imbalance in the brain. Thus, one might assume that laboratory tests are now used to diagnose depression. However, at the time this book goes to press, such tests are used only for research purposes, not in clinical settings. There are times when standard medical lab tests should be done, for example to rule out thyroid disease, which can cause depression. But no specific tests exist for depression per se. Currently, the diagnosis of depression is based on three main sources of data: the particular signs and symptoms, the patient's own history (e.g., the onset of symptoms and any history of prior depressions), and the patient's family history of emotional problems (in some mood disorders, like major depression, vulnerability to the disorder is genetically transmitted).

SIGNS AND SYMPTOMS OF DEPRESSION

It is useful to consider two main sets of depressive symptoms. The first set is referred to as core symptoms, which are seen in nearly all types of depression:

- Mood of sadness, despair, emptiness
- Anhedonia (loss of the ability to experience pleasure)
- Low self-esteem, lack of self confidence
- Apathy, low motivation, social withdrawal
- Excessive emotional sensitivity
- Negative, pessimistic thinking
- Irritability
- Suicidal ideas

Note: Some degree of decreased capacity for pleasure (anhedonia) may be seen in all types of depression. However, in depressions that involve a biochemical disturbance, this loss of ability to experience pleasure can become so pronounced that the patient feels almost no moments of joy or pleasure. Such people are said to have a nonreactive mood, which means that they are unable to get out of their depressed mood even temporarily.

A second group of depressive symptoms is called the biological or physical symptoms, which in psychiatric literature are also referred to as vegetative symptoms. As will be discussed shortly, some types of depression are believed to involve significant changes in physical functioning. The biological symptoms of depression are these:

- Appetite disturbance: decreased or increased, with accompanying weight loss or gain
- Fatigue
- Decreased sex drive

- Restlessness, agitation, or psychomotor retardation (slowing down and inability to feel enough energy, thus likely to stay in bed or on the couch)
- Impaired concentration, forgetfulness
- Pronounced anhedonia: total loss of the ability to experience pleasure
- Sleep disturbance such as early morning awakening (for example, waking up at 4 a.m. and unable to return to sleep), frequent awakenings throughout the night, or hypersomnia (excessive sleeping)

Note that initial insomnia (difficulty in falling asleep) may occur with depression but is not diagnostic of a major depressive disorder. Initial insomnia can occur with anyone experiencing stress in general. Initial insomnia alone is more characteristic of anxiety disorders than of depression.

When a person is being evaluated for possible depression, the mental health professional or primary care physician should ask specifically about the presence or absence of both core symptoms and biological symptoms. Not all depressed people will have all these symptoms, but they usually will have several. In general, for a diagnosis of depression to be made, such symptoms must be present for at least two weeks.

Some types of depression appear to be associated with an underlying biological cause—a neurochemical disorder. In most cases, these disorders tend to recur, and thus a history of prior episodes suggests that the disorder may be due, at least in part, to some form of biological vulnerability. Also, the more biologically based depressions tend to run in families. Consequently, obtaining a family history to see if there are blood relatives who have had mood disorders or alcoholism may provide important clues to the diagnosis. Depressions that include not only the core symptoms but also one or more of the biological symptoms are likely to be caused, at least in part, by an underlying neurochemical disturbance. If there is also a history of prior episodes and/or a family history of depression, then the evidence is even stronger that biology may be involved. This is important because individuals who likely have an underlying biological disorder also tend to respond best to antidepressant medications.

WHY IT'S IMPORTANT TO SCREEN FOR BIPOLAR DISORDER

Serious depressions come in two varieties: unipolar and bipolar. In the latter, depressions occur along with episodes of mania (extreme states of agitation, hyperactivity, racing thoughts, and sometimes psychotic symptoms) or hypomania (milder episodes of increased energy, euphoric mood, decreased need for sleep). More details regarding the diagnosis of bipolar disorder are covered in the next chapter.

For 60 percent of teenagers and adults and 70 percent of children suffering from bipolar disorder, their first mood episode is serious depression. It has been well documented that antidepressant medications are risky to use in treating bipolar depression. Most often, they are generally ineffective in treating bipolar depression, yet they can cause the depressed person to switch from a state of depression to mania, and over time they can worsen the course of bipolar disorder. It must be emphasized that manic episodes can be very problematic and sometimes dangerous (see Chapter 6). The following clinical features may suggest a higher risk of bipolar disorder:

- Depressive symptoms that include hypersomnia (excessive sleeping), severe fatigue, increased appetite, carbohydrate craving, and weight gain; these symptoms are often referred to as atypical symptoms

- Seasonal (late fall and winter) depressions
- Psychotic symptoms (e.g., delusions or hallucinations)
- A family history of bipolar disorder

While the list above is helpful, we also recommend taking the self-administered Mood Disorder Questionnaire found on *www.bipolarhelpcenter.com* and then sharing the results with your therapist or physician.

OTHER DIAGNOSTIC ISSUES

Depression can be caused by many factors. Usually it is a response to stressful life experiences, especially two major types of stressors. The first are losses: the loss of a loved one to death or divorce, the loss of a job, the loss of status, money, health, etc. The second are life events that result in persistent feelings of helplessness or powerlessness. When people encounter unrelieved and mounting stress, they sometimes begin to think, "No matter what I do, I can't seem to solve these problems." Such a perception of powerlessness often provokes depression.

In addition to life stresses, certain biological changes can trigger depression. These include various physical diseases and medical conditions that often change body chemistry and ultimately affect the delicate chemical balance of the emotional brain.

Medical disorders that can cause depression include the following:

- Addison's disease
- Anemia

- AIDS
- Asthma
- Chronic infection (mononucleosis, tuberculosis)
- Chronic fatigue syndromes
- Chronic pain
- Diabetes
- Hyperthyroidism
- Hypothyroidism
- Influenza
- Malnutrition
- Porphyria
- Syphilis
- Ulcerative colitis
- Congestive heart failure
- Cushing's disease
- Infectious hepatitis
- Malignancies (cancer)
- Multiple sclerosis
- Rheumatoid arthritis
- Sleep apnea
- Systemic lupus erythematosus
- Uremia

If it is determined that a particular physical illness may be causing depression, then the approach of choice is generally to focus on treating the particular disease (e.g., thyroid disease). When the disorder is successfully treated, the depressive symptoms will typically subside.

At times, antidepressant medication and psychotherapy may also play an important role as part of the total treatment package. Additionally, various medications and recreational drugs can cause depression.

DRUGS THAT CAN CAUSE DEPRESSION

TYPE	GENERIC NAMES	BRAND NAMES
Alcohol	Wine, beer, spirits	Various brands
Antianxiety drugs	Diazepam, alprazolam, and others	Valium, Xanax
Antihypertensives (for high blood pressure)	Propranolol, Methyldopa, Guanethidine, Clonidine, Hydralazine	Inderal, Aldomet, Ismelin , Catapres, Apresoline
Anti-Parkinsonian drugs	Levodopa/carbidopa, Amantadine, Levadopa	Sinemet, Symmetrel, Dopar, Larodopa
Birth control pills	Progestin-estrogen combinations	Various brands
Corticosteroids and other hormones	Cortisone, Estrogen	Cortone, Premarin, Ogen Estrace, Estraderm
	Progesterone and derivatives	Provera, Depo-Provera, Norlutate, Norplant, Progestasert

The majority of people treated with these medications do not experience depression, although a small percentage might. If there have been no major stressful life events in recent times, and the depressive symptoms emerge in the weeks following the beginning of treatment with these medications, then the drug may be suspected as a cause. If you or a family member is receiving medical treatment, is taking one of the drugs listed, and has become depressed, it is important not to discontinue the medication. Rather, you should contact your physician and share your concerns with him or her.

ALCOHOL

Alcohol is one of the most common drugs to cause depression and thus deserves special attention. It is a seductive drug, and many people certainly notice that minutes after drinking alcohol they feel more relaxed or experience a lifting of tension, sadness, or despair. Thus, the immediate effect is one of emotional relief. It is no surprise that when life becomes stressful, a great many people turn to alcohol for respite. This rapid and temporary relief is misleading, however, because over a period of weeks, ongoing alcohol use almost always worsens depression.

Daily moderate to heavy alcohol use also interferes with the actions of antidepressant medications. Many individuals who either fail to respond to antidepressants or experience only partial relief when treated with them have been found to be using alcohol simultaneously. This is one of the most common reasons why medical treatment for depression fails. Thus, anyone suffering from depression who is also drinking alcohol should discuss this with the therapist or physician. If treatment for depression is to be successful, alcohol use must be controlled.

Caution: If someone had been drinking a moderate to heavy amount of alcohol on a daily basis, stopping abruptly can be dangerous. Discontinuation should be monitored medically.

IS A MEDICAL EXAM NECESSARY?

Because some depressions are triggered by underlying medical illnesses, it makes good sense to see your family physician to rule out possible medical causes. Even people experiencing major life stressors may also have an underlying medical condition that may either intensify depressive symptoms or interfere with adequate treatment response.

DEPRESSION AND THE BRAIN

In the past two decades, numerous advances in medicine and the neurosciences have been made—both in new technologies and new discoveries. It is now widely accepted that in many if not most cases of clinical depression, several well-documented changes take place in brain function. Here are a few highlights of some important findings.

- Brain imaging techniques (PET, fMRI, and SPECT scanning) have revealed that in the majority of people suffering from major depression the brain becomes significantly hypometabolic. This means that the neurochemical activity of the brain falls well below normal levels of activity. This does not occur throughout the brain, rather, it affects primarily those parts that govern the ability to be self-motivated (e.g., the frontal cortex). The reduced activity in these regions is the likely cause of the apathy, low motivation, and loss of vitality that are commonly reported.
- Other findings reveal that the hypothalamus (the part of the brain that regulates many biological drives and rhythms) becomes significantly dysfunctional. This accounts for some of the biologically based symptoms discussed earlier, such as sleep disorders, loss of sex drive, pronounced fatigue, and changes in appetite. These brain abnormalities have been observed not only in brain imaging studies but also in laboratory analyses of spinal fluid and measures of stress hormones.

- Current theory holds that such changes in brain functioning are due to abnormalities in two or three specific groups of nerve cells in the central nervous system. The brain is composed of 100 billion nerve cells, and scores of different types of nerve cells make up its incredibly complex organization. Interestingly, only a tiny fraction of brain nerve cells are believed to be responsible for the biological malfunctions that underlie depression. Probably only about 1 or 2 percent of the total nerve cells in the brain malfunction in depression.

- The three types of nerve cells believed to be implicated in major depression are serotonin neurons (5-HT), norepinephrine neurons (NE), and dopamine neurons (DA). All effective antidepressants are known to affect one or more of these classes of nerve cells and in general restore their normal cellular functioning.

Currently, several additional molecules are being investigated: CRF (corticotrophin-releasing factor), cortisol, and substance P. These naturally produced chemicals may also be implicated in depression, and at some time in the near future drugs are likely to be developed that target these molecules.

TYPES OF TREATMENT

Treatments for depression can be divided into two classes: medical and nonmedical. We will briefly describe nonmedical approaches (covered in more detail in Chapter 12) and then focus on medical treatments in detail.

For many years, people were treated for depression with psychotherapy. More recently, two specialized forms of psychotherapy have been developed that now have fairly extensive studies documenting their effectiveness: cognitive therapy and interpersonal therapy.

Psychotherapy is the treatment of choice for a mild to moderately severe depression, especially when its onset appears to be related to major life stresses. It is also an important part of treatment for more severe depressions, although in such cases antidepressant medications may be the first-line treatment. Even when it is clear that the depression is directly due to a biochemical disorder or disease, psychotherapy is often essential to help a person learn how to cope with the disorder. It can also play an important role in successful relapse prevention.

Psychiatrists, psychologists, clinical social workers, and other licensed counselors provide psychotherapy. Such providers can be found by asking your family physician for a referral checking with your insurance carrier, or contacting your local mental health association. Although most licensed psychotherapists treat depression, it is a good idea to call and ask specifically whether the therapist has experience or special training in treating this disorder.

Biomedical treatments for depression fall into three classes: antidepressant medication treatments, high-intensity light therapy, and electroconvulsive therapy (ECT). Let's start with antidepressant medication treatment.

ANTIDEPRESSANTS:
WHAT THEY ARE AND HOW THEY WORK

Antidepressants are a specific class of psychiatric medications. They are neither tranquilizers nor stimulants. Antidepressants are believed to have their main effects on the aforementioned nerve cells: serotonin, norepinephrine, and/or dopamine. As a rule, after several weeks of continued treatment, antidepressant medications restore these nerve cells to a state of normal functioning. This point is worth emphasizing.

Some other drugs, like alcohol or tranquilizers, also can produce rather quick changes in one's feelings. However, such changes are truly drug-induced effects, and typically people feel drugged or at least know that "This feeling is not me—it's the drug."

This is not the case with antidepressants. The changes experienced by those who respond to these drugs occur because the medication has actually restored particular nerve cells to a state of normal functioning. One effect in particular is to activate the production of the brain protein BDNF, which plays an important role in the protection and repair of the nervous system. In fact, it is referred to as a neuroprotective protein. As the medications gradually take effect, normal brain function is restored and the experience generally does not feel like a drug effect. As mentioned earlier, in fact, most people report that they begin to feel like themselves again.

When brain functioning is restored, the most notable symptomatic changes are seen in the biological symptoms of depression (e.g., sleep, energy). Feelings of sadness, irritability, negative thinking, low self-esteem, and other core symptoms also lessen.

Unfortunately, antidepressants do not work rapidly. In almost every case in which the drugs eventually resolve the depression, somewhere between two and four weeks of treatment are needed before relief begins. Furthermore, for these medications to work, they must be taken as prescribed and on a regular daily basis. Much in the same way that antibiotics need some time to knock out an infection, antidepressants require time to gradually restore the brain to a state of normal functioning.

EFFECTIVENESS OF ANTIDEPRESSANTS

The National Institute of Mental Health (NIMH) has determined that 80 percent or more of people with depression can be successfully treated, including those suffering from very serious cases of depression. The treatments to which the NIMH refers generally involve a combination of antidepressant medications and psychotherapy. We, too, strongly encourage this combined approach. This high response rate, however, can be misleading.

In NIMH studies, patients are treated aggressively and are very closely followed up. Under real-life circumstances, many people either do not respond or experience only partial symptom reduction when treated with medication. The most common reasons are inadequate doses of antidepressants (primary care medical settings tend to use doses that are too low to be effective) and poor compliance with medication treatments (many people stay on the drugs for only a few days or a few weeks and stop taking them before the drug is likely to begin working). The latter may be due to side effects or feelings of pessimism and hopelessness that might lead a patient to give up too soon. The absence of close follow-up with the treating doctor is another factor. Finally, many depressed people just take medications without psychotherapy.

Currently, more than twenty antidepressants are on the market in the United States. They share some qualities in common, but each has particular effects and side effects, and works somewhat differently on the nervous system. In studies of large groups of depressed people where head-to-head comparisons between antidepressants have been made, it has generally been found that all are equally effective. However, these drugs differ considerably with regard to their side effects.

When you or a family member is being treated with antidepressants, it is essential to choose a medication that will work for that individual with minimal or no side effects. Depressed people are already suffering, and if they encounter new additional discomforts or health concerns, many stop taking the medication altogether and thus never experience symptom relief. So, although all antidepressants are equally effective, the reality is that those that are better tolerated are more likely to be taken as prescribed and ultimately to be more successful. And, as we will explain, some people respond well to one class of antidepressants but not to another class; thus, changes must often be made to achieve the best results.

From the late 1950s until the mid-1980s, most prescribed antidepressants were the tricyclic type. These first-generation drugs were effective in treating depression but had many problematic side effects. The development of newer antidepressants that are significantly more user-friendly (i.e., having fewer side effects and judged to be safer than earlier antidepressants) has been a major breakthrough of the past two decades.

CLASSES OF ANTIDEPRESSANTS

As noted above, not all antidepressants are alike. They all treat depression, but they differ considerably in their chemical makeup and particular side effects. We will look first at two broad classes: MAO inhibitors and standard antidepressants.

MAO INHIBITORS

First developed in the 1950s, MAO inhibitors are a specific class of antidepressants that work by inhibiting the action of a particular enzyme, monoamine oxidase, in the brain. This enzyme metabolizes (or chemically degrades) the neurotransmitters serotonin, dopamine, and norepinephrine, which are important brain chemicals. Thus, MAO inhibitors are able to prevent the monoamine oxidase enzyme from lowering the level of these neurotransmitters. This particular method used by MAO inhibitors to normalize brain chemical levels is different from the way standard antidepressants work.

MAO Inhibitors "No No" List

MAO inhibitors are very effective antidepressants, but unfortunately they may have some potentially dangerous drug–drug interactions. If combined with certain other medications, for instance, they can cause life-threatening reactions. Also, these drugs may have adverse interactions with various foods and alcoholic drinks, and some of these interactions can be fatal. For this reason, when people are prescribed an MAO inhibitor, they are advised about the potential risks and given a list of drugs and foods to avoid (see below). Because of these potential problems, MAO inhibitors are no longer widely prescribed. However, for some individuals they are the primary treatment of choice. Especially for those suffering from some very treatment-resistant depressions, MAO inhibitors are effective when other drugs have failed.

Foods to Avoid Completely with MAO Inhibitors

Cheese (except for Philadelphia cream cheese, ricotta, and cottage cheese), chicken and beef liver, sourdough bread, canned yams, yeast preparations (avoid brewer's yeast, powdered and caked yeast as sold in health food stores; Baker's yeast is OK), fava or broad beans, Chinese pea pods, sauerkraut, herring (pickled or kippered), smoked salmon, lox, beer, sherry, ale, red wine, liqueurs, cognac, vermouth, nonalcoholic beers and wines, canned figs, banana peel, protein extracts (found in some dried soups, soup cubes, and commercial gravies), tofu hot dogs, some meat products (bologna, salami, pepperoni, Spam, some types of sausage, hot dogs, jerky, corned beef, liverwurst), sour cream.

Avoid Excessive Amounts of These Foods

Yogurt, buttermilk, ripe avocados and guacamole, chocolate and/or caffeine, white wine and liquors, fresh bacon or ham (smoked bacon and ham are OK), pate, caviar, peanuts.

Medications to Avoid

Stimulant drugs (cocaine, crack, amphetamines, Dexedrine, Benzedrine, methedrine, methylphenidate—Ritalin, Concerta, Metadate, and others, diet pills), cold preparations, including over-the-counter products that contain decongestants (e.g., Sudafed, Contac; antihistamines and aspirin are OK), nasal sprays (saline and steroid nasal sprays are OK), adrenaline (make sure that your dentist knows you are taking MAO inhibitors because many local anesthetics contain adrenaline), tricyclic antidepressants, SSRI antidepressants (Prozac, Zoloft, and others), buspirone (BuSpar), dextromethorphan, levodopa, Demerol and other pain medications, certain antihypertensive medications (for high blood pressure or migraine headaches). Before taking any new medications (prescription or over-the-counter), be sure to talk to your physician or pharmacist about the medication's interactions with other drugs and food.

STANDARD ANTIDEPRESSANTS

The second broad class of antidepressants is referred to as standard antidepressants and includes all non–MAO-inhibitor antidepressants. This group is composed of the earliest generation of antidepressants (tricyclics, as noted above) and several newer agents commonly referred to as second-generation antidepressants (developed since the late 1980s).

The currently available antidepressants are listed below:

STANDARD ANTIDEPRESSANTS	
GENERIC NAME	TRADE NAME
imipramine	Tofranil
desipramine	Norpramin
amitriptyline	Elavil
nortriptyline	Aventyl, Pamelor
protriptyline	Vivactil
trimipramine	Surmontil
doxepin	Sinequan, Adapin
clomipramine	Anafranil
maprotiline	Ludiomil
amoxapine	Asendin
trazodone	Desyrel
fluoxetine	Prozac, Sarafem
bupropion	Wellbutrin
sertraline	Zoloft
paroxetine	Paxil
venlafaxine	Effexor
desvenlafaxine	Pristiq
fluvoxamine	Luvox
mirtazapine	Remeron
citalopram	Celexa
escitalopram	Lexapro
duloxetine	Cymbalta
atomoxetine	Strattera

MAO INHIBITORS	
GENERIC NAME	**TRADE NAME**
phenelzine	Nardil
tranylcypromine	Parnate
selegiline	Emsam (patch)

Note: In Part Two of this book we provide detailed information about each psychiatric medication.

The standard antidepressants differ from one another in two ways. First, each has its own particular side effect profile. Second, each has a somewhat different effect on the various key neurotransmitters: serotonin, dopamine, and norepinephrine. Some of these medications, such as Prozac and Zoloft, specifically target serotonin (5-HT) nerve cells. These antidepressants are often referred to as SSRIs (Selective Serotonin Reuptake Inhibitors). The term "reuptake" refers to the reabsorption of the neurotransmitter by the neuron that originally produced it.

Other standard antidepressants, such as Norpramin and Ludiomil, focus their actions exclusively on norepinephrine (NE) nerve cells. Still others have an impact on two groups of nerve cells and are often referred to as dual-action antidepressants. For instance, Wellbutrin targets NE and dopamine (DA); Effexor, Pristiq, Cymbalta, and Remeron focus on NE and 5-HT.

How do these actions on various nerve cells relate to the treatment of depression and the choice of medications? The research to date indicates that some people with depression have a malfunction primarily in the serotonin system in the brain, while in others, depression may be traceable to a disorder in the norepinephrine system. Furthermore, some depressed people may have biological disturbances in their dopamine system, or combined disturbances in any of the three nerve cell systems. This is important to remember because some patients are treated initially with an antidepressant that targets serotonin, let's say, and they may exhibit either no response or only a partial response. In these cases it does not mean that antidepressants in general will be ineffective. These patients may need to switch to another class of antidepressants (e.g., one targeting norepinephrine or a combination) and they then will go on to have a very good response.

It is often difficult for doctors to know initially which group of antidepressants will ultimately prove effective; thus, initial treatment must be trial and error. Guidelines are outlined below that can aid the physician in first choosing a medication, but often he or she will start treatment with one medication and is prepared to switch to another should the patient fail to show a good response.

WHAT TO EXPECT FROM MEDICATION TREATMENT

It is very important for patients about to undergo treatment to be well informed regarding the effects of the medication and, in particular, what to expect.

CHOOSING AN ANTIDEPRESSANT

Once the diagnosis and the decision to use antidepressants have been made, the physician will recommend a particular drug. Since the newer generation antidepressants are much better in terms of their side-effect profiles, typically one of these will be chosen as a first-line medication.

FIRST-LINE CHOICES

Several factors influence the particular choice of a first-line medication. Of course, these factors vary considerably from one prescriber to another. Several common guidelines that may influence this decision are listed as follows.

- Generally, if there have been previous depressive episodes and a particular medication was used successfully, then the doctor will recommend using that same drug again.

- Side-effect considerations. The physician will take careful note of each patient's medical history, age, gender, and other factors and, based on this information, will choose a medication that seems best suited to the particular patient with regard to its side effects. For example, if the patient is overweight, the doctor will be careful not to choose a medication that typically has weight gain as a side effect. Or, if the patient is experiencing significant fatigue and daytime drowsiness, the doctor is likely to choose an antidepressant that has minimal or no sedating side effects.

- A review of other medications currently taken by the patient will help the physician choose an antidepressant that is not likely to cause dangerous drug–drug interactions.

- The particular pattern of depressive symptoms can sometimes be a factor in medication choices. For example, people suffering from depression and obsessive-compulsive disorder (OCD) or those who have anxiety as a prominent symptom (see Chapter 7) often respond best to antidepressants that target serotonin (e.g., SSRIs like Prozac, Zoloft, or Lexapro). If the depression is accompanied by significant apathy and anhedonia, the more stimulating drug Wellbutrin is often the treatment of choice. Finally, individuals who suffer from very severe, recurrent depressions have been shown to respond somewhat more favorably to drugs that have dual actions (e.g., Effexor, Pristiq, Cymbalta, or Remeron).

These are the primary factors influencing the initial choice. Whether an individual continues to be treated with a specific antidepressant will depend on two factors: first, whether it is well tolerated (has no or minimal side effects), and second, how well the medication works to alleviate depressive symptoms.

ANTIDEPRESSANT DOSES

For any antidepressant medication to be effective, it must be taken at an adequate dose. One of the more common reasons why people fail to respond to treatment is inadequate dosage. This may be caused either by patients taking the medication on an irregular basis or by the medication having been prescribed at a subtherapeutic dose. To work properly, it is essential that these medications be taken on a regular daily basis, as prescribed.

Initially, many antidepressants are prescribed at a low dose, which is taken for a few days to see if it is well tolerated. Then the dosage is gradually increased to a level that is likely to be therapeutic. Some of the newer medications such as Prozac or Paxil may be started at the full dosage level. The precise dosage for any individual patient will depend on several factors that must be determined by the treating physician. For specific doses and side effects, please see the Quick Reference to Psychiatric Medication, pages 57–64, or specific drug information in Part Two of this book.

Note: Doses for people over the age of sixty are generally lower. Children normally have a high rate of liver metabolism since young bodies break down and excrete medications at a faster pace and thus must often take doses similar to adults in order to achieve adequate blood levels of the medication.

PHASES OF TREATMENT

Recently, several psychiatric groups have made specific recommendations regarding the medical treatment of depression. The following sections outline the generally agreed-upon treatment guidelines and focus on three specific phases of medical treatment.

PHASE ONE: ACUTE TREATMENT

This phase begins with the first dose of an antidepressant and continues until most or all of the depressive symptoms have disappeared. As noted earlier, in most cases (with all antidepressants) it is necessary to take the medication each day as directed. Typically it will take from two to four weeks of treatment before the first signs of improvement are noted. In some cases it may require six or more weeks to notice a response. For those suffering from depression, this waiting period often seems incredibly long, but it is absolutely necessary. The antidepressant must have a continuous effect on the malfunctioning nerve cells for this length of time in order to begin the process of normalizing brain functioning. If the correct medication has been selected and it is taken as prescribed, then the first signs of improvement will likely be noticed some time in this two- to four-week period.

Generally, the first signs of improvement include better quality sleep, decreased fatigue, decreased agitation, and a better sense of emotional control. Patients will still feel such emotions as sadness or irritability, but they often report an enhanced sense of control over these feelings. Other symptoms of depression usually take longer to respond. In successful treatments, many if not most depressive symptoms will be resolved within six to eight weeks after the beginning of treatment. In other cases, the response may not be as positive, and different measures must be used to produce a positive response. This will involve either a switch to another antidepressant or the addition of another drug—a strategy is referred to as augmentation.

The acute phase of treatment ends when the person is no longer suffering from the major symptoms of depression. When they begin to feel "normal" again, many people naturally assume that they can stop taking medication. But even though they feel fully recovered, many patients will relapse quickly if they stop taking antidepressants. It is strongly advised that they continue for an additional period of time.

PHASE TWO: CONTINUATION TREATMENT

This phase of treatment begins where the acute phase leaves off. The general guideline is for a patient to continue taking the antidepressant at the same dosage as during Phase One for a minimum of six months. This has been shown to play an important role in preventing acute relapse. After this additional six months of treatment, many people can then discontinue treatment without having a sudden relapse. Discontinuation should always be done gradually, over a period of several weeks. Sudden "cold turkey" discontinuation can result in withdrawal symptoms such as nausea, achiness, or flulike symptoms.

As mentioned earlier, however, in many instances depression will reoccur. This can take place several years after the first episode. Thus, treatment with antidepressants can be effective in resolving the current episode, and the extra six months of treatment often prevents an acute or sudden return of depressive symptoms. It will not, however, provide long-lasting protection from future episodes.

PHASE THREE: MAINTENANCE TREATMENT

If someone has been treated successfully for a first episode of clinical depression and has completed Phase Two, as a rule the physician will recommend discontinuation of the medications. Typically, as noted above, this will involve a gradual reduction of the dosage over a few weeks. When this is completed—and assuming that depressive symptoms do not reappear—then treatment is considered to have ended. All patients who have gone through an episode of depression should be made aware that depression can recur, and they should be taught to watch for any signs of reemerging symptoms. Should these reoccur, it is important to see a therapist or physician as soon as possible, because rapid treatment may prevent another full-blown episode.

If the depressive episode being treated is a second, third, or subsequent episode, many if not most psychiatrists will recommend ongoing antidepressant treatment, possibly indefinitely. Some people, however, may be reluctant to consider long-term medication use, even though it has been clearly established that this can be an effective approach to relapse prevention. In cases of recurring depression, it is not uncommon for later episodes to become even more severe and difficult to treat; thus, the prevention of additional episodes becomes crucial. Furthermore, to date there is little evidence to suggest that very-long-term treatment is dangerous. Many patients have been treated with antidepressants continuously for more than two decades without any evidence of harmful effects to their major organ systems. Additionally, the alternative to long-term treatment—uncontrolled and increasingly severe episodes—can carry grave consequences.

SIDE EFFECTS

All medications, prescription or over-the-counter, have side effects. It is important for patients to know about their particular prescription and its unique side effect profile. Many people treated with antidepressants notice no side effects at all. For those who do encounter side effects, they are generally minimal and not dangerous. This is especially the case with the newer generation of antidepressants. The Quick Reference, pages 58–59, provides an overview of common side effects of antidepressants. Part Two of this book, A Guide to Psychiatric Drugs, can help you locate your particular antidepressant and review a fairly complete list of possible side effects.

In almost all cases, side effects can be managed, either by a dosage adjustment or by a switch to another medication. Thus, it is very important to notify your treating therapist or physician if you encounter any significant side effects. Unfortunately, many depressed people who encounter them simply stop taking the medication and continue to suffer. But solutions to side-effect problems can almost always be found.

PRECAUTIONS AND CONTRAINDICATIONS

Antidepressant medications, especially the newer generation of drugs, have been found to be very safe. However, as with all medical treatments, some precautions are in order. First, it is important to know that several groups of people should either not take antidepressants or do so only under careful medical observation. These groups include people with seizure disorders, people with known allergies to antidepressants, people with narrow-angle glaucoma, and those who have recently experienced a heart attack. Most pregnant women can safely take antidepressants, but it is important to consult with your physician regarding this decision.

Some patients with these disorders or conditions may be

treated with antidepressants, but they must be monitored very carefully.

Caution: If taken at very high doses (for example, in an intentional or accidental overdose), some types of antidepressants can cause grave consequences. The newer antidepressants, fortunately, are much safer in this regard, but they can present serious medical complications if taken in inappropriately high doses. Thus, it is extremely important to take medications only as prescribed. If you or a loved one has ingested an excessive amount of an antidepressant, consider it a medical emergency and seek medical treatment immediately.

It is also important not to drink a great deal of alcohol while taking antidepressants. Typically, consuming one drink is not dangerous. However, ingesting a moderate to heavy amount of alcohol can be very risky and is extremely ill advised.

Finally, it is important to know that there are some potentially dangerous drug–drug interactions, not only with MAO inhibitors but also with standard antidepressants. A list of the more common potential drug–drug interactions can be found for each specific medication in Part Two. Also, be sure to discuss the safety of combining antidepressants with any prescription or over-the-counter drugs (including herbal products) with your physician or pharmacist.

KIDS AND ANTIDEPRESSANTS: THE FEAR AND THE FACTS

Media reports of increased suicidality among children and teenagers treated with antidepressants have understandably caused great concern, especially among parents of youngsters being treated for major depression. Suicide rates among adolescents increased 400 percent between 1950 and 1980, and currently suicide is the third leading cause of death for teenagers. Obviously, the specter of suicide is of great concern to all parents whose children suffer from severe depression.

DEPRESSION IN CHILDREN AND ADOLESCENTS
It has been established that yearly prevalence rates of major depression in young people are significant (2 percent for children and 10 percent for teenagers). Of great concern is that very serious depressive episodes in children and young adolescents may herald the onset of either severe and highly recurrent unipolar depression, as is true in 35 percent of cases, or bipolar disorder, as is seen in 48 percent of cases. This is based on a ten-year follow-up study after a first episode of depression (Geller et al. 2002, Geller and Del Bello 2003).

EFFICACY OF ANTIDEPRESSANTS WITH YOUNG PEOPLE
A large-scale federally funded research project, *Treatments for Adolescents with Depression Study* (TADS), evaluated the effectiveness of antidepressants in teenagers suffering with severe depression. The sample included 432 adolescents (ages 12–17). The subjects were randomly assigned to one of four groups. After twelve weeks of treatment, the percentages of responders were as follows:

- Placebo: 35 percent
- Cognitive-behavioral psychotherapy (CBT): 43 percent
- Prozac: 61 percent
- Combination CBT and Prozac: 71 percent

Here, drug treatments were significantly better than placebo or psychotherapy alone. These results are similar to the outcomes in studies of depressed adults. However, it is important to note that children younger than 12 were not included in this study. Studies of the effectiveness of antidepressant use in young children are inconclusive.

ANTIDEPRESSANTS AND SUICIDALITY

The initial concern over suicidality came from studies in England that raised fears about its increase in young patients treated with the antidepressant Paxil. In this study, which included 1300 patients, Paxil was compared with a placebo, and reports of increased suicidality were seen in 1.2 percent of patients taking placebo and 3.4 percent of those taking Paxil. This difference is statistically significant. It is important to note that there were no actual suicides in this group of youngsters, and some so-called suicidal events occurred in the Paxil group after the adolescents stopped taking the medication.

In trying to understand and address this issue, one significant problem is that the concept of suicidality has been very loosely defined in this and other studies. Most times it includes reports of increased thoughts about suicide, suicide gestures, self-mutilation without lethal intent, and in one instance even a report of a child slapping herself (Brown University 2004). Of course actual suicides and lethal attempts are also included under this umbrella of suicidality.

In the United States, the FDA has responded to concerns about increased suicidality by requiring drug companies to issue warnings about the use of these drugs with younger clients. Potentially dangerous side effects or reactions are now placed in a "black box" in the medication package insert and in the official drug guide, the *Physicians' Desk Reference*. The FDA also initiated a study to investigate the data. Currently, a database of 4400 teenagers treated with antidepressants is being evaluated. In this large group of studies of adolescents treated with SSRIs, there were also no actual suicides.

It has also been documented that in geographic areas where

antidepressants are in widespread use, suicide rates have dropped among adolescents (Mahler 2004). From 1957 to 1985, the suicide rate in the United States increased by 31 percent among all age groups. Yet, between 1986 and 1999, it dropped by 13.5 percent. During this same time period, the new generation of antidepressants came on the market, and a fourfold increase nationwide in prescriptions occurred for antidepressant medications (Grunebaum et al. 2004). It is important to note the vast majority of people who commit suicide have received no treatment at all. Finally, since the media coverage regarding potential suicidal risks with antidepressants began in 2003, there has been a decrease of 30 to 40 percent in prescriptions for antidepressants for children and teens, and since that time an 8 percent increase in actual suicides among youngsters (Centers for Disease Control and Prevention: Lubell et al. 2007).

Even though the likelihood of increased suicidality may be low according to large group studies, it is very important to be on the lookout for the emergence of suicidal tendencies in all patients who suffer from major depression. It is certainly possible that in some cases the drug can contribute to this problem. The following may account for the increased suicidality seen in some individuals treated with antidepressants.

RISK FACTORS FOR SUICIDE

- Antidepressants can provoke mania in some youngsters who have bipolar disorder (this will be discussed in more detail in the next chapter). Bipolar children typically experience what is called dysphoric mania. This is accompanied by symptoms of agitation, intense irritability, depression, and suicidal ideas. It is likely that the majority of children and teenagers who take antidepressants and then develop suicidal tendencies actually have bipolar disorder. This is why it is so important to screen for bipolar disorder and rule it out before considering the use of an antidepressant.

- Increased energy may occur before a decrease in depressed mood. The person then has the energy to carry out a suicide attempt. Clearly, untreated major depression carries significant risks of potential suicide, and antidepressants take several weeks of treatment before the first signs of clinical improvement appear. Depression can worsen during this start-up period of treatment.

It must always be strongly emphasized that suicidal behavior is extraordinarily common in depression, and parents, physicians, and therapists alike must be alert to potential increases in suicidality, regardless of the treatment received. The National Institute of Mental Health Web site www.nimh .nih.gov. has valuable information for parents concerned about this issue.

ARE ANTIDEPRESSANTS ADDICTIVE OR HABIT FORMING?

The question about addiction is common, and it is completely understandable. The answer is that antidepressants are absolutely *not* addictive. There is no evidence either from animal or human studies or from clinical findings that antidepressants are addictive or habit forming. However, it must be emphasized that some people may be treated for depression with other classes of drugs that can be habit forming. These medications are not antidepressants; rather, they are stimulants (Dexedrine, Ritalin, Adderall, and others) or minor tranquilizers (Ativan, Xanax, Valium, Klonopin, and others). There are appropriate medical uses of stimulants and tranquilizers, and in some cases they may be used appropriately as a part of treatment for depression. In this chapter, however, the focus is exclusively on the use of antidepressants, and these medications are neither addictive nor habit forming.

IS LONG-TERM USE OF ANTIDEPRESSANTS SAFE?

Because many people are treated with antidepressants for a prolonged period of time, the question of the safety of long-term use is important. Some individuals have been treated continuously for more than three decades with the early generation of antidepressants (tricyclic antidepressants such as imipramine and nortriptyline) without demonstrating any evidence of adverse impact on their major organ systems. These drugs appear to be quite safe for very long-term use. The newer medications have not been available long enough to enable us to be certain about their long-term effect on the human body. Some people, for example, have been treated with Prozac and some of the other newer antidepressants for more than fifteen years but not for longer periods of time. At this time, there are no indications of serious adverse effects in those individuals. However, in the absence of data collected over many years, the question of safety is difficult to determine in an absolute way.

In addressing the issue of long-term safety, one very important question emerges, "What are the risks of not using the medication?" For depression, this can be answered with some assurance. The lifetime mortality rate for death by suicide in people with recurrent depression is approximately 10 percent. Furthermore, if the disorder goes untreated, chronic depression has been associated with significantly higher rates of physical illness.

Finally, the toll taken on the quality of an individual's life when depression is not treated must be addressed. Thus, on the basis of available data, it seems clear that the decision not to treat results in significant risk, while long-term medication treatment appears to be accompanied by little risk to physical health.

WHAT IF THE FIRST TREATMENT IS NOT SUCCESSFUL?

In the medical treatment of most cases of clinical depression, the hoped-for effect will be some noticeable symptom reduction within the first two to four weeks. When this occurs, it is generally the case that additional improvement will be seen over the next few weeks. However, two classes of difficulties can arise: partial response to the medication or no response at all. The first difficulty occurs when the patient demonstrates only a partial response by week four. Before increasing the dosage or prescribing another medication, the physician must first determine that the diagnosis of depression is correct, that the patient is in fact taking the medication as prescribed, and that there is no ongoing alcohol or other substance abuse.

Once these issues have been evaluated, then the standard approach is to increase the dose of the antidepressant (always with careful monitoring to be sure that significant side effects do not emerge). It is not unusual that an increase in dose will yield good results. Should the first dose adjustment not be successful, the dose can continue to be increased as long as side effects do not interfere. This has been demonstrated to be the best first-step strategy for those with partial or no responses.

Should these attempts fail to result in significant improvement, then two standard strategies are often employed. One high-yield approach is to add a second medicine to the one already being taken. This approach, as mentioned earlier, is referred to as augmentation. Common augmentation choices include the addition of lithium, BuSpar (a non–habit-forming tranquilizer), small doses of thyroid hormone to the antidepressant, or the addition of an another drug from a different class of antidepressants (for example, adding Wellbutrin to an SSRI). Drug augmentation is very effective in about 30 percent of patients who have had only marginal responses to the initial antidepressant.

The second kind of difficulty occurs when the initial drug produces no symptom reduction during the first four to six weeks, despite dosage increases. In such cases, a common strategy is to stop the antidepressant and start treatment anew with a different medication, generally from another class (for example, switching from an SSRI like Prozac to a medication that targets norepinephrine and dopamine, like Wellbutrin).

Medication adjustments and augmentation strategies can be complex and very individualized, and thus it is beyond the scope of this book to discuss all the possibilities here. However, it is important for those who do not experience a good response to their first medication to know that many options exist. These people should not give up and conclude that antidepressants do not work for them. The majority of people with clinical depression *do* respond, and they respond well once the right medication or combination of medications is found.

INEFFECTIVE TREATMENTS FOR CLINICAL DEPRESSION

One very common mistake with clinical depression is to treat it only with antianxiety medications (also referred to as minor tranquilizers). Many people who suffer from depression also experience anxiety and agitation. For this reason they are sometimes misdiagnosed, are assumed to have an anxiety disorder or some form of generic "stress," and are prescribed only tranquilizers. This is often a significant mistake. Some people who experience severe depression accompanied by anxiety may be treated during the first month with tranquilizers along with an antidepressant. Generally, by week four the antidepressant itself will alleviate the anxiety, and the tranquilizer will no longer be needed. As a rule, minor tranquilizers alone are not effective for treating depression; in fact, they often increase depression over time.

In the 1950s and 1960s, physicians also tried using stimulants to treat depression. Not only were these attempts unsuccessful; in some cases there were disastrous consequences, including drug addiction. Stimulants include prescription drugs such as Dexedrine, Ritalin, Adderall, and others, and street drugs such as amphetamines and cocaine. Antidepressants are not stimulants. They are chemically different, and they operate in quite different ways than stimulants do. Most notably, antidepressants are not addictive, while stimulants can be. Sometimes stimulants can be added to antidepressants to treat depressions that present with extreme fatigue. But they should never be given alone, without an antidepressant.

Various herbal and so-called "natural" treatments have also been recommended for treating depression. Some of these include tyrosine, tryptophan, or ginseng. These products do not appear to be effective for treating major depression.

OVER-THE-COUNTER PRODUCTS
THAT CAN TREAT DEPRESSION

Three over-the-counter drugs have been shown in some studies to be effective in treating depression, especially mild depressions. These are St. John's wort and SAM-e. Two cautions in the use of these medications: First, both have been shown to cause mania in individuals who have bipolar disorder. Additionally, St. John's wort, which if taken alone is generally safe and well tolerated, is notorious for causing adverse interactions when combined with some types of prescription drugs. It is very important to check with your pharmacist to see if St. John's wort may interact negatively with prescription medications that you are already taking.

Recently several studies have shown omega-3 fatty acids to be effective in treating depression whether taken alone or in combination with antidepressants. See Chapter 12 for more details.

DIET AND DEPRESSION

What about diet? It is clear that the basic neurotransmitters implicated in depression are manufactured in the brain and rely on some essential amino acids derived through diet as their chemical building blocks.

Consequently, it is no surprise that there has been much speculation about the role of diet in emotional illness, especially depression. It is also true that many if not most people in the throes of depression do not practice good health habits. They tend to avoid exercise, drink too much alcohol, smoke too much, and eat a poor diet. Certainly establishing healthy habits—including a good diet—is important, especially when recovering from depression. However, research to date has failed to demonstrate that dietary approaches to treat clinical depression are successful.

NONMEDICAL TREATMENTS FOR DEPRESSION

As noted earlier, psychotherapy is the primary nonmedical treatment for depression, with a well-documented track record of effectiveness. Beyond therapy, a few other nonmedical approaches are worth noting. At the top of the list is exercise. Regular exercise has clearly been shown to improve the quality of sleep. There is also mounting evidence that regular exercise can successfully treat depression. Most studies recommend twenty minutes of exercise three or four times per week. Another popular approach is to exercise twice a day for ten minutes. The intensity of exercise need not be strenuous but can depend on your level of fitness. Thus, for those who are not fit, brisk walking is effective. For those who are more fit, jogging, running, or swimming is helpful. Finally, since antidepressants can take several weeks to begin working, we strongly recommend exercise to all people experiencing depression.

But let's face it—the most common problem is finding the motivation to exercise. The most practical solution is to have a coach, such as a spouse or friend, who can encourage you or even exercise with you. Almost without exception, ten to fifteen minutes of exercise will lift a depressed mood, and generally the impact of this will usually last for an hour. After several weeks of exercise, more potent antidepressant effects can be noticed.

HIGH-INTENSITY LIGHT THERAPY

High-intensity light therapy is another nonmedical approach. In the past two decades, a great deal has been learned about the need for daylight. When one's exposure to daylight is inadequate, it can have a dramatic effect on sleep patterns, hormone levels, and mood. This effect is most pronounced in those who suffer from what is now called seasonal affective disorder (SAD). Such people have a strong tendency to become quite depressed each year during the fall and winter months. Worldwide, the incidence of SAD is consistently higher during the fall and winter in geographic locations farther away from the equator and closer to the poles.

For instance, although the incidence of people in Florida who experience SAD is about 1.5 percent, the incidence in New England is about 9.5 percent (Rosenthal 2006). After years of careful study, it has been determined that the decrease in exposure to bright light is the culprit. So it should come as no surprise that SAD is also common in those who work night shifts (about 20 percent of working adults in the United States), who sleep during the day and thus get little exposure to bright light.

The current theory holds that humans, like most animals, evolved and developed biological systems that respond to, and are in sync with, their natural environment. One aspect of the environment is the amount of daily light exposure. Bright light enters the eye and activates a nerve pathway, the retinal–hypothalamic nerve, that strongly affects brain chemistry. Human beings evolved for 5 million years in equatorial Africa, where there are twelve hours of sunlight every day of the year. The human brain evolved and came to rely on a good deal of light stimulation each day in order to regulate and maintain certain aspects of brain chemistry.

Light therapy has been found to be very effective for patients with SAD. Recent studies have also shown this treatment to be helpful for people with nonseasonal depressions. This treatment involves daily exposure to a source of bright light, either from commercially available light boxes or by making a point of going outside each day and receiving a certain amount of exposure to sunlight. It is light entering the eye that matters, not exposure to the skin, so be sure to use sunscreen.

The details of high-intensity light therapy for SAD are beyond the scope of this book. The interested readers referred to Dr. Norman Rosenthal's excellent book *Winter Blues.*

Caution: For those with a history of bipolar disorder, light therapy should be done only under medical supervision because it can sometimes cause such an individual to shift into a manic state.

TREATING OTHER TYPES OF DEPRESSION

DYSTHYMIA

As described above, episodes of major depression are often extremely intense. If not treated, they typically last for several months. In addition to these kinds of episodic depressions, some people also suffer from a very long-lasting type of low-grade depression, referred to as dysthymia. It is believed that this disorder affects about 5 percent of the population (Kessler et al. 1994). Typically, it begins in childhood or adolescence and continues for many years—often for a lifetime. With dysthymia, the depression does not reach the depths of major depression, and most dysthymic people continue to function; they can carry out the tasks of daily life. However, their lives are burdened by an almost constant low-grade depression. This usually manifests in the following symptoms: feelings of inadequacy or low self-esteem, persistent lack of enthusiasm, fatigue, no zest for life, irritability, and a strong tendency for negative, pessimistic thinking.

People with dysthymia can be treated by psychotherapy, and some studies have shown that many of them also respond to antidepressant medications. The response rate to medication treatments is about 65 percent. This is somewhat less than the response rates seen when treating major depression, but for those who do have a good response, medication treatment can be a godsend.

When medication treatments are successful for people with dysthymia, these patients often make comments like "I have never felt this good in my entire life." This kind of very positive result has led many investigators to conclude that probably some forms of dysthymia are caused by a chronic, subtle neurochemical malfunction. What remains unclear—assuming that patients have demonstrated a good response to antidepressants—is how long they must be treated.

PREMENSTRUAL DYSPHORIA

About 70 percent of all women notice some changes in their emotions when they are premenstrual. For most, the changes are slight. However, it has been estimated that about 3 to 5 percent of women experience very intense mood symptoms during this part of their menstrual cycle, referred to as premenstrual dysphoria. The emotional changes can include depression, anxiety, and/or irritability. Many psychiatric specialists have noted that the serotonin antidepressants (SSRIs) appear to be effective in reducing these mood symptoms and are more effective in accomplishing this than other classes of antidepressants. The emotional brain is packed with estrogen-sensitive receptors, and it makes sense that significant fluctuations in female hormones, especially estrogen, may destabilize the chemical functioning in the limbic system.

There are two main strategies for using SSRIs to treat premenstrual mood changes. The first is treatment in which the woman takes antidepressants continuously, not just premenstrually. This is the case for women who are experiencing a major depression and encounter increased depressive symptoms premenstrually. When this occurs, the treating doctor will often instruct the patient to increase the dose of her SSRI slightly on days when symptoms are more intense. A second strategy is for women who are depressed only for the few days they are premenstrual, and they do not experience intense mood changes at any other time of the month. This approach involves using SSRIs only on those days during which she experiences symptoms. While antidepressants take several weeks to begin reducing symptoms in all other forms of depression, in premenstrual dysphoria symptoms often improve within a few hours after the first dose is taken.

It should be noted that exercise, exposure to bright light, and some dietary changes (decreased salt and caffeine) may also play an important role in the treatment of premenstrual dysphoria.

PSYCHOTIC DEPRESSION

Some types of major depression can become so severe that there is a significant breakdown of the personality. When this occurs, patients begin to suffer from psychotic symptoms.

The most common psychotic symptoms seen in severe major depression include the following:

- Delusions (extremely unrealistic and even bizarre beliefs, e.g., "I am the devil," "I am dead," "My internal organs are rotten")
- Hallucinations (such as hearing voices)
- Confusion and gross disorganization of thinking
- Extreme neglect of hygiene
- Refusal to eat (which can become life threatening)
- Profoundly impaired judgment (such people may not be able to appreciate the seriousness of their condition and may refuse to cooperate with treatment)

It is also important to know that during periods of psychotic depression, the risk of suicide can be very high. In every instance of psychotic depression, immediate treatment should be sought.

Psychotherapy alone is rarely helpful for those in the midst of a psychotic depression. Medical treatment, which may include psychiatric hospitalization, is always warranted. Two medical treatments have proved to be effective with psychotic depression. The first is the combined use of antidepressants and antipsychotic medications. Either class of medication alone is not very effective. It is clear that appropriate treatment must include both (see also Chapter 8).

The second-line treatment is electroconvulsive therapy (ECT), commonly referred to as shock therapy. Electroconvulsive therapy was first developed in the late 1930s. Initially, it was inappropriately used to treat a wide variety of mental illnesses. The early procedures were crude, and some resulted in dangerous consequences for patients. The treatment took on an ominous appearance, especially as it was depicted in the press. However, ECT was found to be tremendously effective for a particular subgroup of psychiatric patients: those suffering from extremely severe depression, especially psychotic depression.

Fortunately, significant changes have taken place in recent times. The technique has been refined and now can be conducted in a safe and effective manner. Today, ECT is administered with the patient under general anesthesia, and the patient is monitored by a team of physicians and nurses. ECT is always accompanied by the use of psychiatric medication treatment.

Note: As effective as ECT is for initial treatment of severe depression, without ongoing medication treatment, relapses are common.

CHAPTER 6

Bipolar Disorders

INTRODUCTION

In the most general sense, bipolar disorder, also known as manic depression, is characterized by wide swings in mood that alternate between mania and depression. These two emotional states can be viewed as opposite ends, or "poles," of a continuum, hence the term "bipolar" (*bi* is the Latin term for two). During an episode of mania, a person's mood is abnormally elevated, or euphoric. The depression associated with bipolar disorder can be equal in severity to major depression (see Chapter 5) and is recognized by feelings of intense sadness and hopelessness. Although several different types of bipolar disorder exist, central to all are the swings between an elevated mood and a depressed mood.

On average, 4 to 5 percent of the adult population in the United States is afflicted with bipolar disorder (Akiskal et al. 2000) It often appears first in adolescence or early adulthood, but it can begin in childhood. Bipolar disorder is considered a long-term illness, characterized by patterns of multiple episodes. The average number of episodes of either mania or depression in a lifetime is approximately ten. Some people experience considerably more episodes. The interval between episodes, called cycles, can vary from person to person. It is not uncommon for five or more years to pass between the first and second episodes. However, over a lifetime, the periods between subsequent episodes become shorter. The average episode lasts between four and twelve months, manic phases being somewhat shorter. It is important to emphasize that in spite of the general estimates of cycling frequency and length described above, bipolar disorder is extremely variable in its course.

Effective treatments exist for bipolar disorder,* but it is important to recognize that the consequences of this disease can be devastating. There are significant negative effects on marital and family relationships, on occupational or school functioning, and on quality of life. In comparison with the general population, divorce rates are two to three times higher, and job performance is twice as likely to be impaired. Substance abuse, recklessness, and inflicting harm on oneself or others are commonly associated with bipolar disorder, as is a high risk of suicide. At least 15 to 20 percent of people with bipolar disorder will commit suicide, according to the American Psychiatric Association.

For most people with the disorder, the symptoms can be treated effectively. However, for about 20 to 30 percent, the course of their illness will be more difficult. For some people,

---

* Treatment guidelines are drawn largely from the following sources:
American Psychiatric Association:
www.psychiatryonline.com/pracGuide/pracGuideHome.aspx

Texas Department of Mental Health: Texas Medication Algorithm Project
www.dshs.state.tx.us/mhprograms/TMAPover.shtm

Systematic Treatment Enhancement Program for Bipolar Disorder: National Institute of Mental Health
www.nimh.nih.gov/health/trials/practical/step-bd/index.shtml

the core symptoms will not respond adequately to treatment. Others may experience some degree of mood swings on a chronic basis, even if their most intense symptoms have been relieved.

MAKING THE DIAGNOSIS

As with any psychological or medical diagnosis, a clear understanding of the core symptoms of bipolar disorder is essential. Mania is considered to be an abnormally elevated mood that persists for one week or more. This state is often described as a "natural high," and someone who is manic may deny that this mood is abnormal and will resist attempts at help or treatment. Even though mania can exist in mild, moderate, or severe forms, generally it causes significant impairment in daily functioning.

In addition to the elevated mood, it is very important that the associated behaviors be recognized. These behaviors, such as spending sprees, intense irritability, and inappropriate sexual activity can cause significant difficulty and distress in the lives of all involved. Hospitalization is often required during a manic episode to ensure the safety of the individual and to start treatment that would otherwise not be adhered to or be refused.

At the most extreme, during a manic episode a person can suffer from psychotic symptoms such as hallucinations (hearing voices or seeing images that do not exist in reality) or delusions (bizarre and unrealistic beliefs). These psychotic symptoms clearly indicate a loss of contact with reality. There is often an observable disorganization in speech and an inability to carry out normal daily activities, such as eating or bathing.

HYPOMANIA

Hypomania is another important term to understand. A hypomanic episode differs from a manic episode in that social or occupational functioning is not appreciably impaired. As in mania, the mood is abnormally elevated, and many of the associated behaviors are present. However, hypomania does not involve psychotic symptoms, and most daily functioning is maintained. Hospitalization is not required to treat a hypomanic episode. A small percentage of people with bipolar illness experience chronic hypomania, referred to as hyperthymia.

In both mania and hypomania, there can be a strong desire by the individual to continue in this state. Patients often say that they are at their most creative or productive when in a manic or hypomanic state. There may be a tendency to achieve this "high" and maintain it. This often translates into a refusal to seek help or adhere to treatment that has been prescribed previously. However, it must be emphasized that all people suffering such an episode are unable to function as mania becomes more severe. The high turns into an out-of-control roller coaster of intense emotions and severely impaired judgment.

CORE SYMPTOMS OF MANIA

- Excessive euphoric or high feelings
- Extreme irritability
- Distractibility
- Unrealistic and inflated beliefs in one's abilities, grandiosity
- Dramatic mannerisms
- Racing thoughts, called flight of ideas
- Loud, pressured, and rapid speech that is difficult to interrupt and subject to changing topics, often unrelated

- Increased energy, activity, restlessness
- Decreased need for sleep
- Increased sex drive or provocative behavior, which can be aggressive or promiscuous
- Poor judgment
- Abuse of substances, particularly stimulants, alcohol, and caffeine
- Spending or gambling sprees

Note: The biological symptoms of depression, as well as the core symptoms of depression mentioned in Chapter 5, are also characteristic of the depressed phase of bipolar disorder.

CORE SYMPTOMS OF DEPRESSION
- Mood of sadness, despair, emptiness
- Anhedonia, the loss of ability to experience pleasure
- Low self-esteem
- Apathy, low motivation, social withdrawal
- Excessive emotional sensitivity
- Negative, pessimistic thinking
- Irritability
- Suicidal thoughts

BIOLOGICAL SYMPTOMS OF DEPRESSION
- Fatigue
- Appetite disturbance, either decreased or increased, with accompanying weight loss or gain
- Decreased sex drive
- Restlessness, agitation, or psychomotor retardation
- Very unpleasant moods that usually include feeling worse in the morning
- Impaired concentration and forgetfulness

- Pronounced anhedonia, the total loss of ability to experience pleasure
- Sleep disturbances, such as waking very early in the morning, frequently waking throughout the night, sleeping excessively

The most frequent cluster of symptoms seen in bipolar depression is referred to as atypical symptoms. They include sleeping a lot, increased appetite and weight gain, and extreme fatigue.

THE SUBTYPES OF BIPOLAR DISORDER

Three common subtypes of bipolar disorder exist: bipolar I, bipolar II, and cyclothymia. Although a full diagnostic discussion is beyond the scope of this book, it is worth noting that there can be accompanying features to a bipolar diagnosis. For instance, sometimes bipolar disorder is associated with a seasonal pattern or occurs shortly after childbirth.

It is important to know that childhood-onset bipolar disorder is significantly different in several ways from bipolar disorder that begins first in adolescence or early adulthood. The diagnosis and treatment of childhood bipolar disorder is currently a topic of great interest and some controversy. Thus, we will talk about it in a separate section, and address the medication treatment of children later in this chapter.

BIPOLAR I

The diagnosis of bipolar I is generally made when there has been at least one major depressive episode and at least one episode of mania. The diagnosis also may be made on the basis of a single manic episode, with no past depressive episodes. This diagnosis comes closest to the historical concept of classic bipolar disorder. The lifetime prevalence of bipolar I is 1 percent. It is equally common in women and men. Manias with euphoria are sometimes referred to as classic mania. At times, feelings of mania and depression can occur concurrently within the same twenty-four-hour period. If such a pattern persists, this is called the mixed type of bipolar I disorder, or sometimes dysphoric mania.

BIPOLAR II

Bipolar II is diagnosed when there has been at least one episode of major depression and at least one episode of hypomania. Because hypomanic symptoms may be more subtle than those of mania, this diagnosis is sometimes difficult to establish. Hypomania is not always experienced as euphoria. Rather, some people will describe "being extremely irritable" or "having a low frustration tolerance." Most forms of hypomania are accompanied by increased energy and a decreased need for sleep. The lifetime prevalence rate of bipolar II is 4 percent, and more women than men have bipolar II disorder, according to the American Psychiatric Association (2000).

For both bipolar I and bipolar II, an especially difficult-to-treat cycling pattern may develop, called rapid cycling. This means that a person has four or more episodes of depression, or mania, or hypomania, in a twelve-month period. Approximately 20 percent of people with bipolar disorder will experience episodes of rapid cycling. In most cases, it lasts for a period of several months and rarely becomes chronic. Rapid cycling is often caused by substance abuse, thyroid disease, and/or the use of antidepressant drugs. As we'll see later in this chapter, antidepressants are risky drugs to use in bipolar disorder. More women than men also experience rapid cycling, according to the American Psychiatric Association (2000).

CYCLOTHYMIA

Cyclothymia involves a long-term cyclic pattern of both hypomanic and depressive symptoms. The depressive symptoms are not severe enough or long enough to be considered a major depression. However, over a period of years, some people suffering with cyclothymia will begin to develop more severe manias and depressions (and, in a sense, convert to bipolar I or bipolar II).

OTHER DIAGNOSTIC ISSUES

Mania may occur as a consequence of certain medical conditions, or it may be induced by medication treatment or recreational drugs. The following sections show examples of each. These causes of mania do not contribute to large numbers of cases of bipolar disorder.

Depression also can be caused by various medical conditions. These were discussed in detail in Chapter 5.

MEDICAL CONDITIONS THAT CAN INDUCE MANIA
- Injury or trauma to the brain (e.g., stroke)
- Hyperthyroidism
- Brain infections (e.g., encephalitis)
- Seizure disorders
- Brain tumors

DRUGS THAT CAN INDUCE MANIA
- Stimulants (e.g., cocaine or amphetamines)
- Antidepressants
- Some medications used to lower blood pressure
- Steroid anti-inflammatory medications (e.g., prednisone) in higher doses

- Anticholinergic medications (e.g., benztropine)
- Thyroid hormones (e.g., levothyroxine)

IS A MEDICAL OR PSYCHIATRIC EXAM NECESSARY?

Evaluation by a medical doctor, psychologist, or psychiatrist, is often necessary to diagnose bipolar disorder. Medical causes of the symptoms may need to be identified and treated. If medications are implicated, they will have to be changed and the underlying medical condition stabilized. This is especially true if the first episode of mania emerges in someone forty years of age or older, according to the American Psychiatric Association (2000). Most mood-stabilizing medications used to treat bipolar disorder necessitate laboratory measurements that require a physician's monitoring.

BIPOLAR DISORDER AND THE BRAIN

Bipolar disorder was first described in the early 1920s. Much research is still needed to yield a more complete understanding of what occurs in the brain during manic or depressed states. Proposed theories focus primarily on biological and genetic causes and less on environmental influences, although the latter have great importance. Many of the same neurotransmitter systems implicated in depression and anxiety—serotonin, norepinephrine, dopamine, gamma-amino butyric acid (GABA), and glutamate—are assumed to be dysregulated in bipolar disorder, most likely in some combination. However, the manner in which these neurotransmitter systems are dysregulated varies between disorders. Consider a metaphor: the thermostat in your house regulates a fairly stable temperature. If it gets too cold, the heater turns on. If it gets too hot, the air conditioner turns on. Somewhat similar emotion regulators exist in the brain, and they appear to malfunction in bipolar disorder.

Because bipolar disorder is characterized by its cyclic nature, attempts have been made to determine whether mania and depression can be explained by an interruption in normal biological rhythms. In particular, the circadian cycle may be disrupted and become unpredictable (American Psychiatric Association 1994b). Because some of the medications used to treat bipolar disorder are anticonvulsants, researchers have looked for a link between the brain activity patterns of people with seizure disorders and have compared them to people with bipolar disorder.

The particular mechanism in question is called kindling. Kindling is a process in which the brain becomes progressively more sensitive to various stimuli, both normal and stressful. Over time, the sensitization increases to a point where the brain spontaneously begins to show abnormal activity, even when there are no stressful triggering events. Although such a connection makes intuitive sense, this area of research has not yet provided conclusive evidence. At the same time, lifestyle adjustments that have been shown to stabilize the circadian rhythm are often very successful, along with medical treatment, in helping people maintain stability.

RESEARCH LIMITATIONS

Research efforts are extensive in the area of bipolar disorder. However, there are certain limits that impede progress. For instance, carrying out studies in those who are acutely manic is difficult because of their hyperactivity and tendency to be uncooperative. Sometimes genetic studies are carried out initially with just a small group of subjects, but when these same studies are repeated with more people, the original conclusions are not supported.

There is fairly strong evidence that bipolar disorder often runs in families. Currently, researchers have not identified a particular genetic means of transmission, but it is known that the occurrence of bipolar disorder increases if close relatives also have the disorder. Drawing any conclusions about a genetic predisposition must be done cautiously, since the role of environmental factors in the disorder is also thought to be of major importance (American Psychiatric Association 2000). In sum, it is thought that there is a strong inherited vulnerability for bipolar disorder. However, the degree of this vulnerability is not uniform and varies greatly from person to person.

TREATMENTS FOR BIPOLAR DISORDER

Bipolar disorder is predominantly treated with medication. Two other components of treatment are also extremely important. The first is education and adjustment of lifestyle to minimize future episodes. Family members and significant others who participate in this education and modification of lifestyle can greatly help a person deal effectively with bipolar disorder.

Psychotherapy also has a place in the treatment of bipolar disorder. It is most effective when provided in a supportive manner and aimed at helping clients recognize the impact that the symptoms of bipolar disorder have on their lives. This type of therapy helps people gain insight into their behavior and learn how to avoid painful repetitions. Three forms of psychotherapy have been shown in research to be very effective as an adjunct to medication. They are interpersonal and social rhythm therapy, cognitive-behavioral therapy, and family-focused psychoeducation.

Psychotherapy can make a significant difference in relapse prevention. Thus, if you or a family member seeks out psychotherapy, please be sure to inquire if the potential therapist uses one of these models. Other forms of psychotherapy have not been shown to be effective in treating bipolar disorder.

When interviewing a therapist, be sure to look for someone who is skilled in treating bipolar disorder. It is also important that the therapist have an established relationship with a psychiatrist, so that medications can be managed successfully and compliance enhanced. In practice, most primary care physicians will refer a person with bipolar disorder to a psychiatrist because of the specialized care required. We agree with this practice and recommend that bipolar disorder should be treated by a psychiatrist rather than a primary care provider in most cases.

EDUCATION AND LIFESTYLE MANAGEMENT

Education is most effective when provided on an ongoing basis. The ability for someone who is manic to retain information may be compromised. Sharing factual information repeatedly over time in different ways is more effective than providing the information only once. Informed people will also be more confident in their ability to manage their lives. With that confidence comes the ability to implement the recommended lifestyle changes.

KEY ELEMENTS OF EDUCATION AND LIFESTYLE FACTORS
- Learn as much as you can about bipolar disorder.
- Learn as much as you can about your medications.
- Adhere to prescribed treatment, because not doing so will *always* lead to relapse.

- Be patient with your treatment regimen, as it may take some time for the proper medications or dosages to be found.
- Accept that sometimes hospitalization may be necessary if symptoms are particularly severe.
- Report symptoms early so that treatment can be started or changed as soon as possible.
- Establish regular sleeping and eating cycles, and keep a written record if necessary to help establish a consistent daily schedule. Waking up at the same time each day (regardless of whether it is on a weekday or weekend) is a potent measure that helps to stabilize the circadian rhythm. This is a very high-yield strategy.
- Keep an accurate chronological record of when episodes occur, how severe they are, what might have triggered them, and how long they last.
- Recognize that even though this is a biological disorder, stressful life events can trigger manic or depressed episodes.
- Ask for feedback from others about how you are doing. It is especially helpful to ask relatives or close friends to let you know if they see any behavioral changes that might be the first sign of a new episode.
- Avoid substance abuse, including caffeine. Caffeine can significantly disrupt sleep, and sleep deprivation is a very common trigger for episodes—especially manic episodes. Keep your caffeine intake at or below 250 mg per day, and only use it in the morning. You can easily calculate the amount of caffeine you ingest by filling out the caffeine questionnaire in the Appendix of this book.

MEDICATION TREATMENT OF BIPOLAR DISORDER

Medications used in bipolar disorder are intended to treat acute episodes of mania or depression and also to prevent future episodes from occurring. These medications are referred to by various terms: mood stabilizers, antimanic agents, bipolar medications, or anticycling agents. Additionally, all antipsychotic medications have been shown to be effective antimanic agents, even when there are no psychotic symptoms, and thus these drugs are used frequently to treat bipolar disorder.

MEDICATIONS USED TO TREAT MANIA AND BIPOLAR DEPRESSION
MEDICATIONS USED TO TREAT MANIA
(ANTIMANIC MEDICATIONS)
- Lithium
- Valproate (Depakote, Depakene)
- Carbamazepine (Tegretol, Equetro)
- Oxcarbazepine (Trileptal)
- All antipsychotic medications also treat mania (See Chapter 8)

MEDICATIONS USED TO TREAT BIPOLAR DEPRESSION
- Lithium
- Olanzapine/fluoxetine combination (Symbyax)
- Lamotrigine (Lamictal)
- Quetiapine (Seroquel, which is also an antimanic and antipsychotic agent; see Chapter 8)

Antidepressants are occasionally used to treat the depressive episodes in bipolar disorder. However, antidepressants, effective with unipolar depression, generally are not effective in treating bipolar depression and are often associated with cycle acceleration (a worsening of the disorder, causing more frequent episodes) and switching (where the antidepressant causes the depressed person to switch to a manic episode).

Antidepressants should never be used as a single medication in the treatment of bipolar disorder. Even if combined with antimanic drugs, they carry the risks mentioned above. If psychotic symptoms are present, antipsychotics may also be necessary (see Chapter 8). If the person is extremely anxious or agitated, an antianxiety medicine may also be prescribed (see Chapter 7).

ANTIMANIC MEDICATIONS AND HOW THEY WORK

The five most widely used medications used to treat manic episodes and prevent recurrence of mania are lithium, carbamazepine (Tegretol, Equetro), oxcarbazepine (Trileptal), valproate (Depakote), and antipsychotics (a list of antipsychotics appears in Chapter 8).

Carbamazepine, oxcarbazepine, and valproate are anticonvulsants: drugs originally developed to treat epilepsy. Three additional anticonvulsants—gabapentin, topiramate, and lamotrigine—are often used to treat bipolar disorder, but they do not treat manic episodes (the uses of these agents are described later in this chapter).

All these medications work differently from one another. This means that for some people it will be necessary to try different medicines until the best one can be determined. It can also mean that if one antimanic drug does not work well, there is a good chance that another one will. The antimanic medications generally begin to take effect within the first week of treatment. However, full stabilization of mood and behaviors can take up to eight weeks.

It is also important to note that most people with bipolar disorder are treated with several medications simultaneously (in the United States the average number of medications taken in treating bipolar disorder is three). This is often necessary to achieve the most effective control over mood episodes and sometimes is helpful in reducing side effects.

RESEARCH ON EFFECTIVENESS

Most people experience some symptom relief with antimanic drugs. In the United States, lithium is the medication that has been most widely used since the early 1970s. Its effectiveness has been studied much more than other antimanic medications. In general, about 60 to 80 percent of all people taking lithium experience a significant reduction in symptoms. Lithium has two other positive benefits. First, it can prevent relapse of both mania and depression and is thus a true mood stabilizer. Second, several recent studies have clearly demonstrated that people being treated with lithium have an incredibly low rate of suicide attempts—lower than that seen with any other bipolar medication.

Of the anticonvulsants, valproate and carbamazepine have been used for a much longer period of time and have been studied more intensively than gabapentin, topiramate, oxcarbazepine, and lamotrigine. Valproate and carbamazepine are very effective medications, not only for classic mania but also for the treatment of rapid cycling bipolar disorder and other difficult-to-treat cases.

Finally, as noted above, all antipsychotic medications have robust antimanic effects. There is increasing evidence that the effectiveness of an antimanic medication, or a combination of medications, may change over the course of the disease for a given person. A medication that previously worked well for someone may begin to lose effectiveness for reasons that are not clearly understood. On the other hand, many people with bipolar disorder, once they have found the right medication or medication combination, can maintain mood stability over a very long period of time.

As with all medications, the side effects, drug interactions, or effects of the particular drug on an existing medical condition must be considered. With the antimanic medications, these factors often determine which medication will work best for a given individual. Because the antimanic agents differ so much from one another, we will discuss each one individually.

LITHIUM

Lithium is a basic element found on the periodic chart of elements in the same chemical family as sodium and potassium. Lithium shares some, but not all, of the properties of the other elements in its family. Although it is widely found in nature, a physiological function for lithium has not been discovered.

The exact way in which lithium works is not completely understood. Current research suggests that it works inside the nerve cells in the brain to stabilize overactive systems that regulate mood. These overactive circuits can lead to either mania or depression, depending on which system is affected. It appears that lithium can interrupt several overactive pathways, which may explain its effectiveness in treating both mania and depression. It also appears to be neuroprotective. Chronic bipolar disorder, if untreated or inadequately treated, can eventually result in particular forms of brain damage, and lithium helps prevent this from happening.

WHAT TO EXPECT FROM LITHIUM TREATMENT

When lithium is initiated, the starting dose will be in the range of 600 to 900 mg per day. The dose will be gradually increased over the first seven to ten days. During and immediately following the acute manic phase, the dose will be kept at about

1200 to 2400 mg daily. After the acute episode has resolved, many patients will not need as much lithium. The dose during the maintenance phase will be between 600 and 1800 mg per day.

The best way to ensure that the correct dosage of lithium is being taken is to measure the amount of lithium in the blood. This is necessary because lithium can have some very serious side effects, which are often related to its level in the bloodstream. The amount of lithium required to produce symptom relief is very close to the amount that can be dangerously high, or toxic. To avoid problems with a high blood level of lithium, laboratory tests are performed periodically to make sure the range is both safe and effective. It is important to discuss the frequency of these laboratory tests with the doctor who is prescribing lithium. The dosages and blood level values for lithium are summarized below:

- Acute mania: dosage 1200–2400 mg/day; blood level 0.8–1.5 mEq/l
- Maintenance: dosage 600–1800 mg/day; blood level 0.6–1.2 mEq/l

SIDE EFFECTS

To get the most benefit from treatment with lithium, it is extremely important to have an understanding of the side effects. Many side effects are not serious and can be effectively managed. Others can be more serious. All side effects should be reported to the doctor. If the side effects are severe, they should be reported immediately. The following information is not inclusive and is intended to give only a general idea of what to watch for.

- Nausea, vomiting, or diarrhea: These can occur to varying degrees and at any time during treatment. These side effects can be minimized by taking lithium with food or meals. However, if these symptoms are severe, or arise suddenly after someone has been taking lithium for some time and who has not previously been bothered by these side effects, the doctor should be notified immediately.

- Tremor of the hands: Many people will experience a slight tremor in the hands when lithium is first started. This usually goes away with time. If this hand tremor becomes more noticeable or appears suddenly, the doctor should be notified.

- Drowsiness, fatigue: When people first start taking lithium, they may experience some degree of drowsiness or sedation. Usually this is not severe and goes away with time. However, if a person is noticeably sedated, appears confused, or has slurred speech or difficulty walking, the doctor should be notified immediately. People often report feeling "slowed down" while taking lithium. This is different from the drowsiness described above. Sometimes this just means that the symptoms of mania or hypomania are responding to treatment. As mentioned earlier, some people do not like to lose the manic high and will use this effect as a reason to stop taking lithium.

- Kidney function: Lithium relies on the kidneys to be removed from the body. Keeping the kidneys functioning well by drinking lots of fluids helps to ensure that lithium is removed from the body properly. Lithium can cause increased urination and thirst, which with time will go away for most people. Anytime a person becomes dehydrated, or loses sodium from the body, there is a potential for lithium levels to increase. People can become dehydrated from food poisoning or having the flu, especially if they experience excessive nausea or vomiting, run a fever, sweat excessively, or take certain medications. The doctor prescribing lithium should be informed of any of the above-mentioned situations.

- Effects on the thyroid gland: Lithium can cause a change in the results of some laboratory tests that are used to measure thyroid function. For most people, this is not significant. The doctor may decide that supplementing lithium with a thyroid medication is the best approach, or may try another mood stabilizer.
- Weight gain: Weight gain, from five to twenty pounds, may occur while a person is taking lithium. This side effect will cause some people to want to stop the medication.
- Rash or acne: Either or both can result from taking lithium. If the rash and/or acne are severe enough, the lithium may need to be stopped.

CARBAMAZEPINE

Carbamazepine (brand names Tegretol and Equetro) has been used for more than thirty-five years to treat bipolar disorder. This medicine is chemically related to the tricyclic antidepressants. The exact way in which carbamazepine works has not been identified. It has been widely studied, without yielding conclusive results, to support the theory that it works by reducing the kindling process. As described previously, kindling is a process by which the brain becomes increasingly sensitized to various stimuli, and eventually spontaneous abnormal brain activity occurs. Carbamazepine also affects the regulation of the movement of sodium and potassium in and out of nerve cells. And, like lithium, it can stabilize malfunctioning neurotransmitter circuits inside cells.

WHAT TO EXPECT FROM CARBAMAZEPINE TREATMENT

When carbamazepine is initiated, the starting dose will be in the range of 200 to 400 mg per day. Over the first two to three weeks, the dose will be increased to a range of 600 to 1600 mg daily. Smaller, more gradual increases in dosage can help keep side effects to a minimum. The amount of carbamazepine in the bloodstream must be measured periodically. The blood level that is safe and effective for most people is 4 to 10 mcg/ml.

SIDE EFFECTS

- Stomach upset: Nausea, vomiting, diarrhea, and stomach cramps can occur. These side effects can be minimized by taking the dose with food or milk.
- Sedation and drowsiness: Most noticeable when the drug is first started, these side effects go away for most people. Dizziness and blurred vision are also possible.
- Red, itching rash, or hives: Sometimes those skin irritations do not go away and the drug must be stopped. Carbamazepine also can increase the skin's sensitivity to sunlight, leading to sunburn or discoloration. The use of sunscreen is recommended.
- Heart rate: The heart rate can become slowed with carbamazepine. This is most likely to be a problem for older people.
- Effects on blood: Although it is rare in adults, carbamazepine can cause anemia, or lower the red blood cell or white blood cell count.
- Effects on the liver: Carbamazepine can cause damage to the liver, but this is rare. Laboratory tests can monitor for this effect.

VALPROATE

Valproate, also called valproic acid and known by the brand-names Depakote and Depakene, has been used for about twenty years in the treatment of bipolar disorder. The precise manner in which valproate works has not been determined. One of its strongest effects is on a neurotransmitter called GABA. It is thought that valproate increases the GABA levels in the brain, which leads to a decrease in manic symptoms.

WHAT TO EXPECT FROM VALPROATE TREATMENT

When valproate treatment is initiated, the starting dose will be in the range of 500 to 750 mg per day. Sometimes the starting dose can be higher, as long as the person does not experience serious side effects, especially stomach upset. The dose will be increased over the first one or two weeks to 750 to 1500 mg daily. The amount of valproate in the bloodstream will be measured periodically. The level that is safe and effective for most people is 50 to 100 mcg/ml.

SIDE EFFECTS

- Stomach upset: Nausea, vomiting, and indigestion are common, although usually not severe, and diminish with time. The delayed-release tablet form is less likely to cause stomach upset than are the capsules. Rarely, valproate can cause pain and inflammation in the pancreas; the sign that this may be occurring is severe abdominal pain. Notify your physician immediately if you experience sudden, very intense abdominal pain.
- Dizziness, moderate drowsiness, hand tremor: These side effects are usually not significant and will go away with time. However, if a person is noticeably sedated, appears confused, or has slurred speech or difficulty walking, the doctor should be notified immediately.

- Tremor of the hands: Many people experience a slight tremor in the hands when valproate is first started. This usually goes away with time. Limiting or avoiding caffeine will help lessen this tremor. Other medications sometimes can be added to help reduce a tremor.
- Weight gain or loss: This is usually accompanied by an increase or decrease in appetite.
- Hair loss: This may be a short-term effect.
- Interference with blood clotting: Although rare, sometimes the normal manner in which blood clots may be inhibited. The result can be increased bleeding and/or bruising.
- Liver damage: Rarely, valproate can cause damage to the liver. Laboratory tests should be done to monitor for this possibility.

OTHER ANTICONVULSANTS USED TO TREAT ASPECTS OF BIPOLAR DISORDER

A brief discussion of three additional drugs follows.

GABAPENTIN

This medication, marketed under the brand name of Neurontin, is thought to have an effect on the GABA neurotransmitter system. It is not clear whether this action explains how it might be helpful in bipolar disorder. It does not treat mania but is often an "add-on" drug used to reduce anxiety. The dose of gabapentin is usually 300 to 2400 mg per day. Blood level monitoring is not necessary for this drug. Common side effects are drowsiness, tremor, and blurred vision.

LAMOTRIGINE

This medication, whose brand name is Lamictal, is assumed to work by decreasing the effects of an excitatory neurotransmitter called glutamate. This may or may not explain how it works in treating bipolar disorder. Lamotrigine is one of the most effective medications in treating bipolar depression. The dose of lamotrigine is 200 to 500 mg daily. To avoid serious side effects, this drug is started at very low doses (e.g., 25 mg per day) and gradually increased. Blood level monitoring is recommended. The common side effects are drowsiness, headache, blurred vision, stomach upset, and skin rash. A very serious rash or immunological condition, Stevens-Johnson syndrome, has also been reported. Since the standard practice has recently been to start with very low doses and gradually increase the amount of drug, the risk of developing this syndrome is now considered to be extraordinarily rare. The exception is that Stevens-Johnson syndrome is more common in children, and thus this drug is used only rarely to treat children.

TOPIRAMATE

This medication does not appear to be effective in treating mania but often is an "add-on" drug. Generally it is given because of one of its side effects: weight loss. Since many bipolar medications can cause weight gain, taking topiramate along with the other medications may prevent weight gain. Daily doses of topiramate are 50 to 300 mg. The most troublesome side effect is short-term memory loss. When the medication is stopped, this adverse effect goes away.

GENERAL PRECAUTIONS AND CONTRAINDICATIONS

Some general precautions apply to bipolar medications. None is considered absolutely safe during pregnancy. All carry particular risks to the fetus, and their use in pregnancy should be avoided if possible, particularly in the first three months of gestation. However, if a pregnant woman's bipolar illness is extremely serious, and no other alternative exists, it may be necessary for her to take a bipolar medication. This should be done only under very close management by a doctor.

Lithium is generally not recommended for people who have kidney disease. The anticonvulsants should be used cautiously if there is liver damage or kidney disease.

Caution: There can be serious consequences if these medications are taken in very high doses, as in accidental or intentional overdoses. An overdose of lithium is especially dangerous and can be fatal if levels are extremely high. There is no known antidote for a serious lithium overdose. There are severe consequences to overdoses of all the anticonvulsant medicines, as well. Serious overdoses can lead to death.

Because antidepressants are frequently prescribed for the depressed phase of bipolar disorder, it is important, again, to be aware that antidepressants can be associated with triggering manic or hypomanic episodes. This is why treatment guidelines increasingly recommend that antidepressants not be used unless absolutely necessary.

There are important drug–drug interactions to be aware of with bipolar medications. These are outlined in Part Two of this book. If you are seeing more than one doctor, make sure each physician is aware of all the medications you are taking. Checking with a doctor or pharmacist before using any over-the-counter medication is strongly advised.

Alcohol should also be avoided by anyone taking any bipolar medication. Even moderate use is not recommended, and long-term or heavy use is potentially dangerous. Additional sedative effects can occur when many of these drugs are combined with alcohol. Also, because alcohol can cause mood changes, the effectiveness of the bipolar medications may be significantly decreased. Potentially, alcoholism can damage the liver, which also means that the body will have more difficulty metabolizing the anticonvulsant bipolar medications.

ARE BIPOLAR MEDICATIONS ADDICTIVE OR HABIT FORMING?

None of the bipolar medications mentioned in this chapter are known to cause tolerance, dependence, or addiction. There is one exception: Some of the antianxiety medications (e.g., Valium, Xanax, Ativan, Klonopin) that are used in conjunction with the bipolar medications do have that potential. These medicines should be used with caution if the patient has a history of alcohol or drug abuse.

Another area for concern arises when someone in a manic episode uses prescribed medications inappropriately in an attempt to maintain the "high" of mania. Even if these medicines do not have the properties of abusable substances, the poor judgment characteristic of a manic episode can lead a person to take doses or combinations of medications in ways not intended, under the mistaken assumption that the high can be achieved. Sometimes the result can be that a person ingests dangerously high doses or unsafe combinations of a variety of medications.

WHAT IF THE FIRST-LINE TREATMENT IS NOT SUCCESSFUL?

For most people, antimanic medications will begin to work within the first week. Medications used to treat bipolar depression generally take at least three to four weeks to begin working. Over the next six to eight weeks there should be noticeable and progressive improvement in symptoms. If this expected progression does not happen, there are several steps to follow:

- Verify the diagnosis of bipolar disorder.
- Determine that the medication regimen is being followed.
- Identify current medications that might be causing persisting symptoms.
- Rule out any substance or alcohol abuse.

Once these issues have been satisfactorily addressed, if the dose of any of the medications can be safely increased, such an increase, may be prescribed—but with careful monitoring. Because increasing the dose can lead to more side effects, another strategy, called augmentation, may be used.

With augmentation, usually a second bipolar medication is added (e.g., Seroquel plus lithium). An antidepressant also can be used, with caution, if the persisting symptoms are depressive in nature. If there are persistent manic or hypomanic symptoms, an evaluation of the current medications may reveal that it is prudent to stop one of the medications. This can be a very frustrating time for those who have a hard time controlling symptoms in spite of many medication changes. It is important to evaluate where the patient is located in the lifetime course of the disorder. There is some evidence that medications may lose their effectiveness as the course of bipolar disorder worsens over time.

ELECTROCONVULSIVE THERAPY

If repeated medication trials fail or are contraindicated, electroconvulsive therapy (ECT) is an alternative treatment. For both manic and depressed phases, ECT can be extremely effective and provide prompt results. The modern methods by which ECT is administered are very safe.

OTHER TREATMENTS FOR BIPOLAR DISORDER

Following are brief accounts of other treatments that are sometimes used or discussed for bipolar disorder. The results of most of these treatments have not been widely studied, and they may or may not hold strong hope as potential treatments. We think it is important to mention them in case other references to them surface. They are almost always reserved for very difficult cases of bipolar disorder. It is important to reiterate that these therapies do not have an established place among standard treatments. They may be a reasonable choice to consider if other alternatives have failed.

CALCIUM CHANNEL BLOCKERS

Usually, these medications are used to treat cardiac conditions and high blood pressure. There has been some interest in their role in treating bipolar disorder. The two medicines most often discussed are verapamil and nimodipine. Verapamil is the one medication for treating bipolar disorder that is considered the safest drug to use during pregnancy.

OMEGA-3 FATTY ACIDS

Omega-3 fatty acids are usually available in the form of fish oil capsules or oil derived from flax or walnut seed. Studies have shown that omega-3 fatty acids, when taken along with regular bipolar medications, can help some people achieve greater stability and reduce the risk of relapse. The dose generally recommended is 2 grams per day (typically they are sold as 500-mg capsules; thus, you would need to take four capsules per day). Omega-3 does not become effective right away. Typically, the results are realized after three months of daily use. At the recommended dose, there are little if any side effects. Additionally, omega-3 fatty acids have been shown to significantly improve the heart and vascular system.

BIPOLAR DISORDER IN CHILDREN AND YOUNG ADOLESCENTS

Bipolar disorder may first occur in childhood (it is now thought that possibly as many as 25 percent of cases begin that early). We consider early-onset bipolar to mean an onset in prepubertal children. After puberty, bipolar disorder in teenagers generally resembles that seen in adults. The age at onset is unclear, but it appears that most occur after the age of six years. As noted earlier, childhood bipolar disorder has some specific features that are dissimilar to the type of bipolar disorder that occurs after puberty and in adulthood. It too has both manic and depressive episodes.

In almost half of preadolescent children experiencing a very severe episode of depression, the episode ultimately turns out to the first manifestation of bipolar illness. In children with bipolar disorder, 70 percent initially present with depression, and on average they have had between two and four depressive episodes prior to their first manic episode (Geller and DelBello 2003). It is very important to determine if these first episodes are associated with an underlying bipolar disorder. This is especially critical, since, as we have mentioned, there has been growing concern that the use of antidepressants may in the long run be risky in bipolar patients, potentially exacerbating a manic episode or causing cycle acceleration. Thus, any therapist or physician who is evaluating a seriously depressed child, in addition to making a diagnosis of major depression, must also conduct a comprehensive evaluation to rule out potential bipolar disorder (of course, this is true for adults and adolescents also). The following history and clinical features should alert the therapist or physician to a higher risk of bipolar disorder in a depressed youngster.

RED FLAGS FOR POSSIBLE BIPOLAR DISORDER IN CHILDREN AND YOUNG ADOLESCENTS

- Atypical depressive symptoms (e.g., hypersomnia, or excessive sleeping; severe fatigue; increased appetite; carbohydrate craving; weight gain).
- Seasonal (late fall and winter) depressions.
- Psychotic symptoms (e.g., hallucinations or delusions).
- History of ADHD (attention deficit hyperactivity disorder) or ADHD-like symptoms. *Note:* most children with a history of ADHD do not develop bipolar disorder, but some children with early-onset bipolar disorders do show a history of behaviors during infancy and early childhood that resemble ADHD (e.g., hyperactivity, impulsivity, difficulty staying on task at school and with homework).
- Positive family history of bipolar disorder (most children with bipolar disorder have parents or grandparents who have suffered from bipolar disorder).

DIAGNOSTIC ISSUES

The signs and symptoms of childhood-onset mania (see below) differ from those in the adult and adolescent versions of the disorder.

SIGNS AND SYMPTOMS OF EARLY-ONSET BIPOLAR DISORDER:

- Nonepisodic (more continuous); may last for years if untreated
- Mixed mania is most typical with marked depression and irritability
- Intense rage episodes
- Severe oppositional behavior
- Rapid cycling mood swings and severe emotional instability

MEDICATION TREATMENT

Currently, no medications are FDA approved for the treatment of bipolar disorder in children. However, the same medications used to treat adult-onset bipolar disorder are in widespread use with children. Only time will tell if these same agents are truly effective for treating this disorder in children. The choice of treatment will depend on the current clinical presentation.

MAJOR DEPRESSION WHEN BIPOLAR DISORDER IS SUSPECTED

- Since antidepressants may provoke switching or cycle acceleration, they should be avoided as a monotherapy.
- Bipolar medications that have some antidepressant actions should be used first (e.g., lithium, Seroquel, or Symbyax). *Note*: lamotrigine (Lamictal) is an effective

treatment for bipolar depression, but owing to an increased risk of Stevens-Johnson syndrome, it should be used with extreme caution in children.

MANIA

- If there is very severe agitation, generally the child has to be hospitalized. Tranquilizers or antipsychotic medications are used to quell severe agitation. Lithium and anticonvulsant antimanic medications often take seven to fourteen days to begin reducing symptoms. Tranquilizers and atypical antipsychotics may begin to work in several hours.
- Head-to-head comparisons of antimanic drugs fail to show that any one is superior, at least in group studies. Thus, the choice of treatment is often based on the side effect profile of the medication. Ultimately, the majority of children with mania must be treated with two or more antimanic medications in combination to achieve a good outcome (Kowatch 2000, Emslie and Mayes 2001, Geller 2003).

TREATMENT EFFECTIVENESS

Unfortunately, the treatment of childhood-onset bipolar disorder is enormously challenging. Outcomes are much less positive than in adolescents and adults. Most of the time, children are treated with a host of medications in an attempt to find drugs that can be tolerated and are effective. Multiple medication trials can be very frustrating for both children and their parents. Systematic trials of medications not uncommonly require months of trial and error. Generally, very severe symptoms can be addressed in a few weeks, but many bipolar symptoms linger and are difficult to treat.

The most critical factors remain treating the disorder early (e.g., early recognition and treatment) and avoiding the use of antidepressants in children when bipolar is suspected.

For a more detailed discussion of the diagnosis and treatment of childhood-onset bipolar, the reader is referred to an excellent book, *The Bipolar Child* by Demitri Papolos, M.D. and Janice Papolos (third edition, 2007).

CHAPTER 7

Anxiety Disorders

INTRODUCTION

Anxiety is a part of life. Indeed, in many respects it is hard-wired into our brains. When people feel anxious or threatened, they are likely to respond with an increase in tension and the physiological arousal that has been called the fight-or-flight response. This is an automatic biological response that prepares us for action. The basic paradigm of the fight-or-flight response is that of prehistoric hunters confronted by a saber-toothed tiger. They must act quickly either by attacking the tiger or by fleeing—both actions requiring rapid mobilization of energy and alertness. This is a life-saving response; that is why it evolved and continues to exist some 30,000 years after the extinction of saber-toothed tigers.

In modern life, however, this fight-or-flight response can go awry. For example, people with anxiety disorders can experience the full set of these biological reactions without an actual threat being present. That is, their hearts beat faster, their lungs breathe more oxygen, they sweat more, their pupils dilate, their hands and feet tingle and go numb from decreased blood flow, and they produce and secrete adrenaline and other stress hormones in larger amounts. In today's world many of us are rarely faced with real physical danger. But we are biologically programmed to react to stress itself.

This means that our bodies react to the many stresses of modern life as if they were physical threats, like tigers, instead of financial woes, marital problems, or deadline pressures. In addition, many people have an exaggerated physiological and psychological response even to minor stresses. People suffering from some anxiety disorders often experience the complete physiological fight-or-flight response even in the absence of any stressful event.

ANXIETY DISORDERS

There are several types of anxiety disorders, including situational anxiety, phobias, social anxiety, panic disorder, generalized anxiety disorder, and obsessive-compulsive disorder. (*Note:* post-traumatic stress disorder or PTSD, is often considered to also be an anxiety disorder. PTSD, however, results in several other symptoms in addition to anxiety and thus is covered separately in Chapter 10).

The distinctions between these various types of anxiety depend on whether the anxiety is brief or constant, and whether it is generalized (experienced in almost all situations) or specific to a particular situation.

Situational anxiety refers to what is often simply called stress. It is an overly anxious reaction to a situation. Phobias refer to an exaggerated fear of a particular thing, such as spiders or flying in an airplane. Social anxiety refers to intense anxiety about social situations. Panic disorder is distinguished by sudden attacks of very severe anxiety that last for only a few minutes. Generalized anxiety disorder manifests as a near-constant anxiety. Obsessive-compulsive disorder is distinguished by compulsive, ritualistic behaviors and/or frightening thoughts (e.g., fears regarding dirt, germs, and contamination).

Altogether these disorders affect between 10 and 20 percent of the population at any given time, and some 25 percent of people over their lifespans (Kessler et al. 1994). In their more severe forms, anxiety disorders cause tremendous suffering, are very disabling, and are sometimes associated with suicide. Often some of the symptoms begin in childhood, so that the person has a lifelong struggle with anxiety. In this chapter we will take a separate look at each type of anxiety disorder and its medical treatment.

MEDICAL CAUSES OF ANXIETY

Sometimes anxiety is attributable to underlying medical conditions and certain drugs. Hyperthyroidism, for instance, is one of the more common physical causes of anxiety. When the thyroid gland is overactive, it can produce symptoms that mimic an anxiety disorder, such as tremulousness, feelings of anxiety, and rapid heart rate.

MEDICAL DISORDERS THAT MAY CAUSE ANXIETY
- Hyperthyroidism
- Meniere's disease (early stages)
- Parathyroid disease
- Partial-complex seizures
- Postconcussion syndrome
- Premenstrual syndrome
- Pulmonary embolism
- Adrenal tumor
- Mitral valve prolapse[1]

1. Mitral valve prolapse (MVP) does not cause anxiety, but MVP and anxiety disorders often coexist. This may be due to some common underlying genetic factor.

- Alcoholism
- Angina pectoris
- Cardiac arrhythmia
- Cushing's disease
- Coronary insufficiency
- Degenerative diseases of the central nervous system
- Delirium[1]

In addition, many drugs can cause anxiety. Among them are amphetamines, asthma medications, caffeine, central nervous system depressants such as alcohol (withdrawal from), cocaine, nasal decongestants, steroids, and appetite suppressants.

In the initial evaluation of an anxiety disorder, it is always good to have a physical examination, including appropriate laboratory tests, and to give a thorough drug history, including prescription, over-the-counter, and street drugs. If a medical condition or drug use is found, it is important to first treat the underlying disorder that may be causing the anxiety or to address the drug use. Then, if necessary, treatment targeted specifically at anxiety can begin.

SITUATIONAL ANXIETY AND ADJUSTMENT DISORDER WITH ANXIETY

DIAGNOSIS

To understand this type of anxiety disorder better, we need to examine the fight-or-flight response more closely. As stated earlier, our brains are hard wired to react to stress in a particular way.

---

1. Delirium can occur as a result of many toxic and metabolic conditions and often produces anxiety and agitation.

A stressful event evokes both a thinking response in the cortex (e.g., perceiving potential danger in the environment) and an emotional response in the limbic system. The limbic system, with input from the cortex, then induces a multitude of physiological changes, as described above, including a release of stress hormones, which prepares us for action. People experience these physiological changes as anxiety.

At mild or moderate levels, situational anxiety is usually well tolerated and prepares us to perform better. However, when an event is particularly stressful, we may experience severe or overwhelming anxiety. The same event may be more stressful to some people than to others. One's previous experiences color the way in which the event is viewed. Also, some people may become alarmed by their reaction and thereby compound their anxiety.

For example, when interviewing for a job, most people tend to be somewhat anxious. If, however, they react to this anxiety with alarm, thinking they are sure to do poorly in the interview, this anticipation or belief will increase their anxiety, and they are more likely to appear anxious and to stumble over their words. This type of situational anxiety is usually self limiting and eventually dissipates as the stressful event recedes into the past.

MEDICAL TREATMENT

In most cases it is not necessary or appropriate to use psychiatric medications for situational anxiety unless symptoms become severe. The usual medical treatment for situational anxiety is the use of antianxiety medications, also called minor tranquilizers. These medications have been used since the mid-1950s to treat anxiety. They are usually very effective at relieving the symptoms of anxiety, and they have few side effects, mainly sedation and a tendency to increase the effects of other drugs, such as alcohol. They also can be habit-forming if used for more than a few weeks.

Antianxiety drugs are commonly divided into two groups: those that treat daytime anxiety, and those that target nighttime anxiety, which can interfere with the ability to go to sleep. The latter are sleeping pills (insomnia is covered in detail in Chapter 9.) The table below shows a list of antianxiety drugs class.

ANTIANXIETY DRUGS	
GENERIC NAME	BRAND NAME
Benzodiazepines	
diazepam	Valium
chlordiazepoxide	Librium
prazepam	Centrax
clorazepate	Tranxene
cionazepam	Klonopin
lorazepam	Ativan
alprazolam	Xanax
oxazepam	Serax
Other Antianxiety Medications	
buspirone	BuSpar
gabapentin	Neurontin
hydroxyzine	Atarax, Vistaril
propranolol	Inderal
atenolol	Tenormin
guanfacine	Tenex
clonidine	Catapres
prazosin	Minipress

Often someone will be prescribed a minor tranquilizer to be taken when the anxiety is particularly severe. Thus, several doses may be taken on some days and none on others. Usually these antianxiety medications can be used safely for two to five months without risk of significant dependency. However, when they are used for more than six months, dependency is likely. Over time, as the anxiety gradually diminishes, the medication can be used less frequently and eventually discontinued.

MINOR TRANQUILIZERS

Minor tranquilizers are the most commonly prescribed antianxiety medications. In fact, at times they have been the most commonly prescribed of all prescription medications. Their widespread use is due to their safety and effectiveness and to the ubiquity of anxiety disorders. These medications approach 100 percent effectiveness. They work by binding to certain receptor sites in the brain associated with the neurotransmitter GABA. When they bind to this receptor, they reduce the reactiveness of the limbic system.

Caution: If these medications have been taken daily for several weeks or more, they should never be stopped abruptly because of the risk of serious withdrawal symptoms.

TREATMENT CONSIDERATIONS: WHAT TO EXPECT

In cases of situational anxiety, initially a low dose of medication may be prescribed. Typically, 0.5 to 1 mg of lorazepam, or the equivalent, is an effective starting dose, taken up to two to three times daily. For situational anxiety, however, it is usually not necessary to take the medication routinely. It can be taken when anxiety increases or when an increase is anticipated. This reduction in anxiety helps people to function better and allows time to address the causal situation. The medication can be gradually tapered off. The average length of treatment is a few weeks to a few months. In situational anxiety, insomnia, especially a difficulty in falling asleep, is often a problem. These medications have proved useful for dealing with this problem on a short-term basis.

SIDE EFFECTS

As a rule, minor tranquilizers are relatively free of side effects if they are taken in the correct dose. However, the correct dose varies from person to person. If the dose is too low, the anxiety will still be noticeable. If the dose is too high, the person may feel drowsy or even drunk, talk with slurred speech, and walk unsteadily. Obviously, driving a car or operating machinery should not be attempted under these circumstances. If the dose is correct, however, people are usually able to drive and to do all of their customary activities. As with all medications, other reactions are possible. Some people may develop a rash. On very rare occasions some people react "paradoxically" and become more agitated instead of calmer.

ADDICTION POTENTIAL

Minor tranquilizers have an addiction potential similar to that of alcohol. When taken, they can create feelings that are like those experienced when drinking alcohol. They also have a withdrawal syndrome similar to alcohol. (Contrary to popular belief, alcohol can be habit forming, but not everyone becomes dependent on it.) Most people can use minor tranquilizers in a controlled fashion, but some tend to become hooked on them. Generally they are people who are genetically predisposed to substance abuse and/or those with a prior history of alcoholism or other forms of drug abuse. Fortunately, minor tranquilizers are not toxic to the brain, liver, and other organs, as alcohol is. In general, they are very helpful for reducing suffering, and they are safe but must be used with caution and for short-term treatment.

OTHER TREATMENTS

As noted above, minor tranquilizers are the mainstay of the treatment of situational anxiety, but other medications can be considered. These include the antihistamines and beta blockers. The main antihistamine used for anxiety is hydroxyzine (Vistaril or Atarax). It is sedating and has some antianxiety effect. It is not habit forming. The main problem with it is that often, a dose large enough to reduce anxiety may produce significant drowsiness. The usual starting dose is 10 to 25 mg three to four times daily.

Beta blockers are blood pressure medications that block the effects of adrenaline. They are better at reducing the physical symptoms of anxiety (rapid heart rate, trembling, and perspiration) than the emotional feeling of anxiety. They can cause low blood pressure and light-headedness. The usual starting dose is 20 to 40 mg of propranolol, or the equivalent. They are not habit forming but should not be stopped abruptly because of the possibility of temporarily raising the person's blood pressure. Also, long-term use has occasionally been associated with causing depression.

PSYCHOLOGICAL TREATMENTS

Psychotherapy is often very helpful for treating situational anxiety. Discussing the stressful situation helps reduce the anxiety response, and different anxiety management strategies can be used to reduce the severity of the anxiety symptoms. Problem-solving discussions and learning how to use effective coping techniques can guide the anxiety sufferer to correct or alter stress-producing situations.

ARE MEDICATIONS HABIT FORMING?

DRUG DEPENDENCE

When some medications are taken on a regular basis, they may cause dependence. However, dependence is not the same as drug abuse (addiction). Dependence simply means that the body adapts to the medication—that is, the body gets used to the medication. When this occurs, if the medication is abruptly discontinued, there may be withdrawal symptoms (the body's reaction to a sudden chemical change). Depending on the medication, withdrawal symptoms can be fairly mild (e.g., a slight headache or nausea) or very severe (e.g., seizures). Technically, drug dependence does not mean abuse or addiction.

DRUG ABUSE

Some medications have the potential for addiction, especially if the patient has a history of prior substance abuse. With addiction there is dependence and withdrawal symptoms upon sudden discontinuation, as well as three additional important features:

- There may be drug craving—a strong desire to use the drug to experience pleasure or euphoria.
- There is a need to use higher and higher doses to achieve euphoria.
- The drug use continues even when it is apparent that it is causing health problems, occupational or academic failure, serious interpersonal difficulties, or legal problems.

MEDICATIONS AND ABUSE POTENTIAL

MEDICATION CLASS	DEPENDENCE	ADDICTION
Antidepressants	Yes[1]	No
Antianxiety medications	Yes[2]	Yes[2]
Lithium	No	No
Antipsychotics	No	No
Stimulants	Yes[2]	Yes[2]

1. Antidepressants can have withdrawal symptoms (all except Prozac), but withdrawal symptoms can be largely avoided by gradually discontinuing the medication over a period of several weeks. Do not discontinue "cold turkey" without your doctor's advice
2. Generally these drugs are addictive only for those who are prone to addiction (e.g., have a personal or family history of drug addiction and/or alcoholism)

PHOBIAS

DIAGNOSIS

Phobias are characterized by a fear of a particular object or situation. When someone who has a phobia is faced with the feared object or situation, this leads to increased anxiety and frequently to avoidance of the feared object or situation. Often this causes only minimal disruption, but it can be significant when a person's job requires exposure to the object of the phobia. For example, someone who has a phobia of flying in airplanes, but whose job involves a lot of travel, will be severely affected by such a phobia.

MEDICAL TREATMENT

Antianxiety medication can be prescribed to reduce anxiety when the phobic person is exposed to the object of the phobia, thereby making the anxiety easier to tolerate. For example, someone with a fear of flying can take a minor tranquilizer just before boarding the plane (one hour before the flight). Once the flight has begun, the anxiety usually diminishes, and the rest of the flight can be completed without excessive anxiety.

Beta blockers are another class of medication used to treat phobias. They can be used for example, to treat a phobia of public speaking. As a rule, propranolol (10–20 mg) or atenolol (25–50 mg), taken thirty minutes before speaking, will significantly reduce the jitters associated with public speaking. Beta blockers have the effect of lowering blood pressure, but they are not habit forming, and in these low doses they usually do not have side effects.

PSYCHOLOGICAL TREATMENT

Psychological treatment is very important in the treatment of simple phobias. It usually involves a type of treatment referred to as exposure and systematic desensitization, in which the phobic person is repeatedly exposed to the phobic stimulus and gradually becomes more and more comfortable with it. Basically, it is impossible to truly overcome a phobia without facing the fear. The key is to do it gradually so that the anxiety is not severe, and to experience success in facing the feared situation a little at a time.

SOCIAL ANXIETY DISORDER

DIAGNOSIS

Social anxiety refers to an exaggerated fear of social situations. People with social phobia are very anxious about being in social situations and will often avoid them as much as possible. When in a social situation, they experience severe anxiety and are plagued with thoughts about how the other people present are probably judging them in very negative ways. They often fear embarrassment or humiliation. Sometimes people with social phobia may have occasional panic attacks in reaction to social situations. It is not uncommon for people with social phobia to use alcohol or antianxiety medications to control their anxiety. Studies suggest that between 5 and 10 percent of all people will experience social anxiety at some time during their life (Kessler et al. 1994). This disorder causes significant degrees of distress and at times leads to social isolation, depression, alcoholism, or drug abuse.

MEDICAL TREATMENTS

Two types of medication have shown promise in the treatment of social phobia: antidepressant and antianxiety drugs. The MAO inhibitor antidepressants are most effective. These medications, however, have significant serious side effects and therefore are not usually the first-line choice (discussed in Chapter 5). Some studies have shown a benefit from the SSRI antidepressants (also discussed in Chapter 5). These medications are safer than MAO inhibitors and are usually well tolerated. Antianxiety medications frequently are helpful, but they must be used with caution because social phobia is usually a chronic condition, and continued use of these medications may lead to dependency and at times to abuse.

PSYCHOLOGICAL TREATMENTS

The most effective treatment for social phobia is group psychotherapy. In a group, the phobic person is faced with his or her specific social anxiety and has the opportunity within the group structure to develop more effective social skills. The group provides a chance to practice interacting in a supportive setting. However, this often necessitates long-term group treatment.

PANIC DISORDER

DIAGNOSIS

Panic disorder is characterized by acute attacks of anxiety so severe that sufferers often fear they will go crazy or die. These attacks come on very suddenly, are very intense, and last from a few minutes to twenty minutes. The attacks are accompanied by any of the following physical symptoms:

- Shortness of breath
- Tremulousness or restless
- Fear of losing control or going crazy
- Rapid heartbeat or palpitations
- Tingling (usually of the hands)
- Light-headedness and dizziness
- Feeling of choking
- Nausea or abdominal distress
- Chills or hot flushes
- Chest pain or discomfort
- Sweating
- Feelings of unreality
- Fear of dying

Typically, panic disorder begins with a single isolated panic attack. (See "Jill's Story" in Chapter 1.) This attack is so frightening that the person often becomes anxious and fearful about experiencing another one. Significant anticipatory anxiety can lead to periodic full-blown panic attacks.

Such people often come to feel more secure at home and develop phobias about traveling any distance away from home. They are especially uncomfortable when they feel trapped and are unable to go home immediately, as in heavy traffic, in line at the supermarket, or in a crowd. Thus, people with panic disorder go from having discrete anxiety attacks to having near-constant anxiety and phobias of specific activities, with periodic full-blown panic attacks. This can progress to agoraphobia, a condition in which the fears are so pervasive and intense that the person essentially becomes housebound.

PANIC DISORDER AND THE BRAIN

Panic disorder is probably caused by a dysregulation of the neurochemical norepinephrine, such that a large amount of norepinephrine is released very suddenly. Norepinephrine is an adrenaline-like compound that is released in the brain and body during the flight-or-fight response. It produces increased heart rate, elevated blood pressure, and other physical symptoms of anxiety. Evidence suggests that in panic disorder, there is an abnormality in the part of the brain called the locus coeruleus. The locus coeruleus (LC) stimulates the release of norepinephrine in other parts of the brain. It appears that in people with panic disorder, the LC overreacts to even minor stimuli. It is as if the LC has a hair trigger so delicate that a small stimulus produces a strong reaction. In addition, people with panic disorder tend to have higher than normal resting levels of anxiety or norepinephrine, so that they tend to be always on the verge of a panic attack.

MEDICAL TREATMENT

Panic disorder is usually treated with minor tranquilizers and/or antidepressants. Minor tranquilizers, or antianxiety medications, offer the advantage of working quickly and having few side effects. Unfortunately, they can be habit forming. Antidepressants, on the other hand, are slow to work and often have multiple side effects, but they are not habit forming. It should be noted that all antidepressants can be effective in treating panic disorder, with one exception: Wellbutrin is ineffective and may actually increase panic symptoms. Other medications, such beta blockers and buspirone (BuSpar), may be helpful as adjuncts to the treatment of panic disorder, but they are not first-line treatments. They may treat anticipatory anxiety, but are ineffective in treating panic attacks.

Initially, minor tranquilizers often are used to gain quick control over the panic attacks, which are frequently intolerable and debilitating. Then, an antidepressant may be added. The antidepressant must be started at a very low dose, because this often increases anxiety at the start. The starting dose may be as low as 5 mg or less of fluoxetine (Prozac). (See the table Antidepressants in Chapter 5.) They may take up to six weeks to begin to have a significant benefit. Then the dose of the minor tranquilizer can be reduced gradually and, it is hoped, soon discontinued. As a rule, medication must be continued for one to three years, but some people must take it indefinitely because they experience a return of symptoms whenever the dosage is reduced.

It is important to note that some patients are erroneously told to take a minor tranquilizer if they feel a panic attack coming on. This is ineffective, since tranquilizers take thirty to forty-five minutes to reach the brain, and most panic attacks are over in a matter of minutes. Thus, if someone is being treated only with tranquilizers, that person must take them continuously. The advantage of antidepressants is that they are active twenty-four hours a day.

PSYCHOLOGICAL TREATMENT

Psychotherapy, particularly cognitive-behavioral therapy, can be very helpful in treating panic disorder. Treatment for panic disorder can be seen as having two phases: first, medication and/or cognitive-behavioral treatment for the panic attacks per se, and second, cognitive-behavioral treatment for the associated phobias. Once the frequency and severity of the panic attacks have been reduced, gradually panic disorder sufferers will experience less anticipatory anxiety about having a panic attack.

They can then begin to confront some of their phobias, secure in the knowledge that they are not likely to have a panic attack. Often, however, panic attacks cannot be entirely eliminated, although almost always they can be reduced in intensity. These less severe waves of anxiety are referred to as limited symptom attacks, which also last only a few minutes and are much easier to tolerate. Cognitive therapy and/or relaxation training is often helpful for this.

Although strenuous exercise infrequently can precipitate a panic attack, in the long run exercise is extremely helpful in reducing the frequency of the attacks. It is also important to avoid drugs that have stimulant properties, as they may induce panic attacks. These drugs include caffeine and decongestants such as pseudoephedrine.

GENERALIZED ANXIETY DISORDER

DIAGNOSIS

Generalized anxiety disorder (GAD) is characterized by almost constant anxiety. People suffering from this disorder are nervous most of the time regardless of the situation. They tend to be preoccupied about things that might go wrong. This makes any situation that is the least challenging much more difficult because of the associated anxiety and worry. This anxiety is accompanied by the following symptoms:

- Restlessness or feeling keyed up or on edge
- Easily fatigued
- Difficulty concentrating or mind going blank

- Irritability
- Muscle tension
- Sleep disturbance, especially difficulty in falling asleep

GENERALIZED ANXIETY DISORDER AND THE BRAIN

The cause of generalized anxiety disorder is not well under-stood at this time. One significant observation is that many people with GAD go on to develop clinical depression. There is likely some imbalance involving the serotonin and/or nor-epinephrine systems. It is as though, physiologically, these people are in a perpetual state of the fight-or-flight response.

MEDICAL TREATMENT

Psychological factors are often important in GAD, and psy-chotherapy is often helpful for reducing symptoms. Three types of medication are most frequently used in the treatment of GAD: minor tranquilizers, buspirone, and antidepressants. As noted earlier, minor tranquilizers are antianxiety medica-tions that reduce anxiety within thirty minutes of ingestion. They can be habit forming, so that their use in a chronic dis-order is controversial. However, some people are able to take a stable dose daily for many years with significant benefit and no apparent adverse effects (Hollister 1993). Other people tend to use higher and higher doses and are prone to abusing these medications. Clearly in such cases the use of minor tran-quilizers is not indicated. Those who are particularly prone to abuse usually have a history of alcohol or drug abuse, or they have blood relatives with such a history.

Buspirone (BuSpar) is a first-line medication treatment used particularly for GAD. It is an antianxiety medication, but one that is quite different from the minor tranquilizers. Bus-pirone is not habit forming. It requires one to two weeks (or longer) of daily use before results are seen. The most common side effects are nausea, dizziness, headache, and, paradoxically, occasional anxiety. These side effects tend to subside after two to three weeks. The usual starting dose for buspirone is 5 to 10 mg twice daily.

Antidepressants, except for Wellbutrin, may also be helpful in GAD. Beta blockers and hydroxyzine, too, are helpful for some.

PSYCHOLOGICAL TREATMENT

Various types of therapy are often useful in treating GAD. These include the more traditional "talk therapy" and cognitive-behavioral therapy. Treatment is often slow and may last many months.

OBSESSIVE-COMPULSIVE DISORDER

DIAGNOSIS

Obsessive-compulsive disorder (OCD) is characterized by ob- sessional thoughts and/or compulsive behaviors. Obsessional thoughts are intrusive thoughts that are very distressing to the person thinking them. They evoke a great deal of fearful anxi- ety (e.g., fears about oneself or loved ones becoming ill, in- fected with deadly viruses, or dying).

Compulsive behaviors are ritualistic behaviors that the per- son feels compelled to perform to ward off some impending calamity or to reduce the feeling of intense anxiety. Examples include checking locks, compulsive counting, tapping a cer- tain number of times, positioning objects in specific ways, or excessive hand washing.

When the disorder is severe, much of the OCD person's time is occupied by the symptoms, so that performing even a simple task can become very time-consuming.

OBSESSIVE-COMPULSIVE DISORDER AND THE BRAIN

Obsessive-compulsive disorder appears to be caused by a serotonin imbalance. PET scans show increased metabolic activity in the prefrontal cortex of the brain. Interestingly, these abnormalities tend to normalize during treatment, whether the treatment is cognitive-behavioral, pharmacological, or a combination of both.

MEDICAL TREATMENT

Serotonin antidepressants are the most effective treatment for OCD. These include the SSRIs and clomipramine (see the table that follows). Other medications, such as minor tranquilizers and buspirone, may be helpful as adjuncts to first-line treatments. Treatment for anxiety with these antidepressants is similar to the treatment for depression. However, higher doses often may be required to control the symptoms, (e.g., 60–80 mg per day of fluoxetine, or the equivalent).

It is important to note that most anxiety disorders that are treated with antidepressants tend to respond within four to six weeks. The first signs of improvement may similarly be seen in the treatment of OCD. However, continued improvement often occurs gradually during the first year of treatment. Thus, the amount of symptomatic relief experienced at three months is generally only a partial response, and it is wise to keep taking the medication, as the additional improvement will unfold gradually over several weeks. When people are successfully treated for OCD with antidepressants, they will almost always experience a full return of symptoms if the medication is discontinued. Many will choose to stay on medications for the rest of their lives. Another option is to begin psychological treatment in the hope of being able to eventually reduce the use of medications.

ANTIDEPRESSANTS USED TO TREAT OCD	
GENERIC NAME	BRAND NAME
clomipramine	Anafranil
fluoxetine	Prozac
sertraline	Zoloft
paroxetine	Paxil
fluvoxamine	Luvox
citalopram	Celexa
escitalopram	Lexapro

PSYCHOLOGICAL TREATMENT

Cognitive-behavioral therapy is also very effective in treating OCD. In this form of treatment, the patient begins with exposure (e.g., if there is a fear of dirt, germs, and contamination, the exposure might be to touch a garbage can). This is then followed by a strategy called response prevention, which means not doing the rituals, such as hand washing. For exposure therapy to work, this response prevention must continue for a minimum of fifteen minutes. During the next few weeks of treatment, this time is gradually increased to an hour. Although the initial experience of this treatment is very anxiety provoking, within a few weeks patients find that they can tolerate the anxiety better than they ever have before. Positive outcomes are seen in 75 percent of people treated with this approach, with little relapse.

CHAPTER 8

Schizophrenia and Other Psychotic Disorders

INTRODUCTION

Psychotic disorders are among the most serious mental illnesses. The term "psychosis" refers to a condition in which there is a significant loss of being in touch with consensual reality and the creation of a new personal reality. Thus, people who are psychotic not only have lost touch with what is actually happening but often develop very surreal or bizarre thoughts about what is occurring (e.g., "Aliens have installed hidden cameras in my home").

There are several different forms of psychosis, or psychotic disorders. These include schizophrenia, psychotic depression, manic psychosis, atypical psychosis, and the organic psychoses. (When the psychosis is caused by a medical condition, such as Alzheimer's disease or a stroke, it is called an organic psychosis.) Many medical conditions can cause psychotic symptoms—for example, brain tumors, dementia, and hormone problems—can also cause psychosis. The focus in this chapter is on schizophrenia and similar psychoses.

Schizophrenia is considered a prototypical psychotic disorder. The name does not mean "split personality" or "multiple personality disorder," as is sometimes thought. "Schizophrenia" means "split mind" and refers to a disorder characterized by hallucinations, delusions, and disorganized thinking. It affects approximately 1 percent of the population (APA 1994a). Schizophrenia is found in all countries and all cultures, and it has been recognized since the time of Hippocrates. It often, but not always, leads to a chronic disabling condition. New medication treatments, however, offer renewed hope for the treatment of this condition.

DIAGNOSIS

The diagnosis of schizophrenia is made more on the basis of the course of the illness than on the person's condition at any one point in time. The course includes the initial (prodromal) phase, when the person tends to become more withdrawn and has difficulties concentrating and performing daily activities. Often during this phase, schizophrenia may be misdiagnosed as depression. If this happens, the next phase—the acute phase—reveals the true nature of the illness.

In the acute phase, the person becomes floridly psychotic, behaving in a markedly different manner from his or her usual way of functioning—a way that is usually judged by others as bizarre or crazy. He or she may talk in a very irrational manner and say things that are clearly unbelievable. Later, usually after some type of treatment, people with schizophrenia enter what is called the residual phase, where symptoms are less severe. As in the prodromal phase, sufferers in the residual phase may seem quiet, subdued, or depressed.

MAKING THE DIAGNOSIS

Some of the important markers of schizophrenia are as follows: The course of the illness, including the prodromal, active, and residual phases, must last longer than six months. In cases where the person recovers in less than six months, the diagnosis is schizophreniform disorder.

During the acute phase, certain key symptoms must be present for a diagnosis of schizophrenia to be made correctly. The acute phase is the phase that must be distinguished from other types of psychosis. Manic psychosis and psychotic depression may appear to be similar to schizophrenia. The key differences between these illnesses are seen in the differences in mood changes.

Manic psychosis is accompanied by a strong elevation of mood, such as euphoria or anger, but it may be indistinguishable from the acute phase of schizophrenia. Psychotic depression includes the full array of clinical depression symptoms, which precede the development of psychotic depression symptoms. In this disorder, a person first becomes depressed and then develops psychotic symptoms. These symptoms often involve guilt and/or medical concerns. For example, some people believe that they hear voices telling them that they deserve to die because they are so bad and worthless. Others might believe that they have developed undetected brain tumors or stomach cancers.

Atypical psychosis and delusional disorder are less severe than the disorders discussed above, involving little disorganization of thinking. Furthermore, they usually do not last as long. Certain drugs (stimulants and hallucinogens) and some medical diseases can cause syndromes that mimic schizophrenia.

SIGNS AND SYMPTOMS

The signs and symptoms of schizophrenia are grouped into four types: positive, negative, disorganization, and characterological.

Positive symptoms include hallucinations, delusions, agitation, floridly bizarre behavior, and "first-rank" symptoms, which can include the belief that one is broadcasting one's thoughts to the world and/or the belief that one's thoughts, feelings, and actions are being controlled by an external agent.

Negative symptoms include anhedonia (the inability to feel pleasure), apathy, blunted affect, poverty of thought, feelings of emptiness, and a complete lack of imagination.

Disorganization symptoms include behavioral disorganization, distractibility, and thought disorder (i.e., marked confusion).

Characterological symptoms include social isolation or alienation, marked feelings of inadequacy, and poorly developed social skills.

HALLUCINATIONS AND DELUSIONS

When a person hears, sees, or smells something that is not there, as in hearing voices or seeing visions, that is called a hallucination. Delusions are false beliefs, belief in something that is not true. These delusions might be something that could be true, such as "I am being followed by the FBI," but in schizophrenia they are often quite bizarre, such as "Martians have installed electromagnetic lasers in my apartment and are broadcasting information about Earth to their leaders."

Because schizophrenia so profoundly alters a person's thinking, the person often has a distorted view of what is happening to him or her. Friends and family are often more aware of these profound changes than the person with schizophrenia, and they may see the need for treatment much more clearly than the person does. Someone with schizophrenia may deny that he or she is ill or may tend to minimize the problem. When this occurs, the person may be quite resistant to treatment, thus making the process of obtaining treatment difficult. This can be especially hard on family members as they try to encourage the person to cooperate with treatment.

OTHER CONSIDERATIONS

Schizophrenia must be distinguished from a psychosis caused by a medical illness or drugs. Where drug use is suspected, a urine drug screen can be helpful. Usually, medical illnesses result in other symptoms that will show up in a physical examination or laboratory test. A century ago neurosyphilis was a common cause of psychosis. Today it has all but disappeared; nevertheless, it should be checked for by an easy laboratory test. And, as stated above, brain tumors, and hormone problems can also cause psychosis. The causes of organic psychoses are legion, but they can be grouped into the following types:

CAUSES OF ORGANIC PSYCHOSES
- Metabolic
- Organ failure, such as kidney failure
- Hypoxia (oxygen deficiency)
- Hypoglycemia (insufficient blood sugar)
- Vitamin deficiency
- Endocrinopathy, such as hyperthyroidism
- Fluid or electrolyte imbalance
- Porphyria (abnormalities of porphyrin metabolism)
- Drug or alcohol intoxication or withdrawal
- Infections
- Epilepsy

- Head injury
- Vascular diseases, such as lupus
- Intracranial tumor
- Cerebral degenerative diseases
- Dementias, such as Alzheimer's disease
- Multiple sclerosis
- Huntington's chorea
- Parkinson's disease

SCHIZOPHRENIA AND THE BRAIN

In recent years, an accumulating body of evidence has demonstrated important differences between the normal brain and the brains of people with schizophrenia. In the schizophrenic brain, several types of changes have been noted:

- Underdevelopment of particular parts of the brain associated with information processing
- Decreased metabolic activity in the prefrontal cortex, which correlates with the severity of negative symptoms
- Increased dopamine (a neurochemical) activity, which correlates with the severity of positive symptoms

How these changes produce the symptoms of schizophrenia is a matter of much theorizing at this point.

ANTIPSYCHOTIC MEDICATIONS: WHAT THEY ARE AND HOW THEY WORK

Antipsychotic medications help to reduce psychotic symptoms. They are often used in schizophrenia, but they will treat psychotic symptoms regardless of the cause of the psychosis. They are somewhat sedating, but that is not how they work. Antipsychotic medications specifically target psychotic symptoms, especially delusions, hallucinations, and disorganized thinking. Until recently they all worked by blocking dopamine in certain parts of the brain. Now there are newer agents, the atypical antipsychotics, which have a somewhat different mechanism of action. The atypical antipsychotics block dopamine in varying degrees, and also increase serotonin activity.

TYPES OF ANTIPSYCHOTICS

The older medications have traditionally been divided into high-potency and low-potency types. They all work basically the same way, but each type has a significantly different side effect profile.

The high-potency medications, such as haloperidol, require lower doses and produce less sedation. However, they have a greater tendency to produce extrapyramidal (neurological) side effects, such as Parkinsonian-like behavior (tremors, lack of facial expressions, stiff gait).

One problem with the older medications is that they tend to work very well for the positive symptoms of schizophrenia, but they often have little or no effect on negative symptoms. This has meant that although the floridly psychotic symptoms were controlled so that people with schizophrenia could function outside of hospital settings, they often continued to feel listless, be very isolative, and lead very restricted lives. The newer atypical agents help treat the negative symptoms as well as the positive ones, so that patients not only think better but may also feel better (e.g., they may experience more vitality and a greater sense of "aliveness"). Unfortunately, several of the atypical antipsychotics tend to cause metabolic effects, including weight gain and elevated cholesterol and blood sugar.

WHAT TO EXPECT FROM MEDICATION TREATMENT

Once the diagnosis of schizophrenia or schizophreniform disorder has been made, the physician will probably recommend treatment with an antipsychotic medication. A list of antipsychotic medications is given below, and doses are listed in the Quick Reference.

ANTIPSYCHOTIC MEDICATIONS	
GENERIC NAME	BRAND NAME
Low potency	
chlorpromazine	Thorazine
thioridazine	Mellaril
clozapine	Clozaril
mesoridazine	Serentil
quetiapine	Seroquel
High potency	
molindone	Moban
perphenazine	Trilafon
loxapine	Loxitane
trifluoperazine	Stelazine
fluphenazine	Prolixin
thiothixene	Navane
haloperidol	Haldol
pimozide	Orap
risperidone	Risperdal
paliperidone	Invega
olanzapine	Zyprexa
ziprasidone	Geodon
aripiprazole	Abilify

CHOICE OF MEDICATION

Antipsychotic medications often are started in a hospital setting because they can be prescribed more aggressively there, and high doses are often used. In this chapter, however, the focus is on use in the outpatient setting. From the many possible antipsychotics available, one will be chosen for an initial trial on the basis of these factors: previous response to medication; amount of agitation present; the patient's general health and well-being, including other illnesses; and other medications being taken.

Based on these and other considerations, a medication will be chosen. Generally, if a particular medication has worked well in the past, it will be used again. If a person is physically healthy and very agitated, a sedating antipsychotic may be chosen. Otherwise, one with fewer sedative and other side effects may be used. Another decision to be made is whether to use an atypical antipsychotic. Depending on the degree of withdrawal (negative) symptoms, this may be a good first-line choice. Some physicians recommend that atypical antipsychotics always be used first because of the better response of negative symptoms and the possibility of reduced risk of a particular side effect called tardive dyskinesia. Tardive dyskinesia, or TD, is a neurological condition which can develop during treatment with antipsychotic medication. It often does not appear until after months, or even years, of treatment. TD produces involuntary movements, usually of the face, lips and tongue, but sometimes limbs or torso. It is discussed further under side effects (see pages 178–79). However, atypical antipsychotics have the risk of metabolic effects (see pages 176–77). No one antipsychotic is always effective or always well tolerated. Once the medication has been chosen, treatment can be started with a low dose, typically the equivalent of 1 mg of haloperidol two or three times per day.

The decision whether or not to use an atypical antipsychotic is controversial. When the atypical antipsychotics were initially used, it was thought that their benefits of reduced risk of tardive dyskinesia, and improvement of negative symptoms and cognition, justified their much higher cost. However, now that they have been shown to have significant metabolic effects, the choice is less clear.

A large study funded by the National Institute of Mental Health, the CATIE study, compared the effectiveness and risk of a typical antipsychotic (perphenazine) with several of the atypical antipsychotics. The atypicals, except for olanzapine, did not show any increased effectiveness. But olanzapine also had increased side effects.

If a high-potency traditional antipsychotic is started, an anti-Parkinsonian medication (discussed below under "Extrapyramidal Side Effects") is often also begun. This second medication is given to prevent some possible unpleasant side effects from the antipsychotic medication, such as tremors or muscle spasms.

If there is only a small amount of benefit within a week, the medication can be increased, perhaps to the equivalent of 2 mg of haloperidol two to three times per day. It can then be stepped up gradually to an effective dose or until side effects become a problem. Outside of the hospital, it is unusual to go above 20 mg of haloperidol, or the equivalent, per day. And, as stated above, if the first medication does not work or has intolerable side effects, another medication should be tried.

The choice of the second medication will be based on what was wrong with the first. For example, if the first one was too sedating, a medication that causes less drowsiness will be tried next. Sometimes several medications must be tried before one is found that works and has minimal side effects.

PHASES OF TREATMENT

Treatment may be divided into the acute and maintenance phases. During the acute phase, medication treatment is initiated and the more prominent psychotic symptoms are controlled. This phase usually lasts from several days to several weeks. Often higher doses of medication are required during the acute phase.

During the maintenance phase, the medication is gradually reduced, and more attention is paid to negative symptoms and level of functioning. The maintenance phase is a lifelong process in schizophrenia. Involving family members is often important during the maintenance phase for helping a schizophrenia patient (or the family members) to recognize the early signs of a recurrence of the illness.

Often, increasing the dosage of the medication can prevent further worsening of the condition. Some of these medications also come in an injectable form that releases the medicine slowly over a period of two to four weeks. This can be very helpful for people who are careless about taking their medications in pill form. With long-term use of the medication, symptoms of tardive dyskinesia need to be checked for at least every six months.

SIDE EFFECTS

Treatment with medication usually involves starting with a low dose of a given medication and gradually raising the dosage until the symptoms are controlled. As the dose is raised, more and more side effects may appear. There are several common types of side effects. If they become intolerable, it is usually helpful to switch to another medication that produces less of that type of side effect. The most common side effects are grouped as follows:

EXTRAPYRAMIDAL SIDE EFFECTS

Extrapyramid side effects involve the neurological system. There are three types: Parkinsonian, dystonic, and akathisia. Parkinsonian side effects refer to a group of symptoms that mimic Parkinson's disease. The patient's movements are slowed, a tremor may be present, the face shows less expression, and the walk is slow, with only small steps possible.

Dystonia refers to a muscle spasm, usually of the neck. This can be very painful if not treated promptly.

Akathisia refers to a type of restlessness. The patient feels very uncomfortable and cannot sit still.

All these side effects can be treated with anti-Parkinsonian medications. With the use of such medications, higher and more effective doses of the antipsychotics can be used. The anti-Parkinsonian medications produce side effects of their own, but the dry mouth, blurred vision, and constipation they cause are usually not severe.

METABOLIC SIDE EFFECTS

Metabolic side effects are produced mainly by the atypical antipsychotics, although traditional antipsychotics can often cause weight gain. Metabolic effects besides weight gain include altered carbohydrate metabolism similar to diabetes, and altered lipid metabolism. In some cases, altered carbohydrate metabolism has not been discovered until a person goes into diabetic coma. Also, the weight gain and elevated cholesterol and triglyceride levels may increase the risk of heart disease. In general, these effects pose little risk in the short term. However, antipsychotic medications are often taken for years. Therefore, because of the potential seriousness of these side effects over the long term, all patients taking atypical antipsychotics should have their weight, blood sugar, and cholesterol monitored. The risk of metabolic effects varies between the atypicals, with clozapine and olanzapine having the highest risk, risperidone and quetiapine having moderate risk, and aripiprazole and ziprasidone having little to no risk.

ANTICHOLINERGIC SIDE EFFECTS

Antipsychotic medications can also inhibit a part of the nervous system called the cholinergic nervous system and can cause the same side effects as the anti-Parkinsonian medications described above, such as constipation and dry mouth. Some antipsychotic drugs, like haloperidol, produce very few anticholinergic side effects. Others, like chlorpromazine, produce significant amounts.

LIGHT-HEADEDNESS

Antipsychotic medications tend to interfere with the body's ability to maintain a stable blood pressure. Thus, when people taking this kind of medication stand up suddenly from a sitting position, they may experience a brief drop in blood pressure, causing light-headedness, which can lead to falls and possible injuries.

MISCELLANEOUS SIDE EFFECTS

Other side effects can be caused by antipsychotic medications: They tend to interfere with temperature regulation and may lead to heat stroke, especially if the person exercises during warm weather. They also raise prolactin (a hormone) levels and may cause lactation.

Neuroleptic malignant syndrome (NMS) is also a rare but potentially fatal reaction to antipsychotic medication. It is characterized by fever, confusion, and rigidity. If not recognized and treated promptly, it can lead to irreversible coma and death.

The medication clozapine occasionally can cause agranulocytosis, a potentially fatal decrease in the number of white blood cells. For this reason, weekly blood tests are required during the first six months of treatment. Your doctor may determine that after six months, twice a week is sufficient. As with all medications, some people may have allergic reactions. If any of the following side effects is experienced, the doctor should be notified promptly:

- Confusion
- Inability to urinate
- Rash
- Involuntary movements
- Severe sedation
- Prolonged or severe constipation
- Falls
- Muscle spasms
- High fever
- Jaundice
- Severe restlessness

TARDIVE DYSKINESIA

Most of the side effects of antipsychotics appear in the first days or weeks of treatment, but tardive dyskinesia—which involves involuntary movements of the face or limbs—may not appear until many months, even years of treatment. Usually it manifests as twitches in some of the facial muscles. It is of serious concern because no really effective treatment exists for tardive dyskinesia and because it may be irreversible, or only very slowly reversible.

Thus unlike the antianxiety and antidepressant medications, antipsychotic medication can have severe, long-lasting side effects. For this reason, their use must be approached with more caution.

One reason for the increased use of the atypical antipsychotics is that they have much less risk (about one tenth) of causing tardive dyskinesia. On the other hand, because the psychoses usually are severely debilitating, the use of these medications may be justified, even lifesaving. When a doctor is choosing to use these medications, the potential hazards of not treating (e.g., institutionalization, disability, and suicide) must be weighed against the possible side effects.

ANTIPSYCHOTIC MEDICATIONS ARE NOT HABIT FORMING

Antipsychotic medications are definitely not addictive. As a rule, these medications are mildly or moderately unpleasant to take. People take them because they can function much better and because psychosis is so much worse. Even though the medications are not addictive, they do have other potential risks when prescribed long-term, as described above.

OTHER TREATMENT CONSIDERATIONS

What if several medications are tried and none works? One important strategy is to reevaluate the diagnosis. For example, is some other type of medical problem contributing to the psychosis? If the diagnosis is certain, there are other medications that may help. The most likely are mood stabilizers, anticonvulsants, and lithium (see Chapter 6). Adding one of these to the antipsychotic may be helpful. Sometimes, antianxiety or antidepressant medication may also be helpful.

CHAPTER 9

Sleep Disorders

SLEEP

Although we do not yet understand the precise way in which sleep is restorative, we do know that it is very important to our health and functioning. Sleep helps us consolidate memory and process emotionally charged experience. Many studies have shown that inadequate sleep leads to impaired functioning. In fact, it is estimated that almost half of all heavy truck accidents can be traced to driver fatigue.

Dr. William Dement, a preeminent sleep researcher at the Stanford University sleep lab found that the average person needs eight to nine hours of sleep to be fully rested. Dr. Dement concluded that most people are in a chronically sleep-deprived state. Sleep deprivation has these effects:

- Fatigue (of course)
- Reduced ability to think clearly and maintain attention
- Impaired memory
- Reduced emotional control leading to increased irritability and reactivity
- Paradoxically, sleep deprivation can lead to increased insomnia

There are different patterns of sleep disturbance:

- Difficulty falling asleep (initial insomnia)
- Restless sleep: tossing and turning all night, with frequent awakening
- Early morning awakening: waking several hours before morning (e.g., 3 or 4 a.m.) and having difficulty falling back to sleep
- Hypersomnia: sleeping excessively

CAUSES OF INSOMNIA

All sleep problems can be caused by stress, tension, anxiety, depression, or other psychiatric disorders. If this is the case, the sleep disorder is called a secondary insomnia, since it is due to another condition. There are also primary insomnias in which the sleep disturbance is the main symptom of the disorder.

The main causes of insomnia are these:

- Situational stress and worry
- Anxiety, depression, and other emotional disorders
- Medications, drugs, and alcohol
- Medical illness

Situational stress and worry is a common cause of sleep disturbance. Probably everyone has experienced it at one time or another. It usually causes difficulty falling asleep or restless sleep. Fortunately, it usually resolves within a few days or when the stress is reduced. Sometimes stress leads to disturbing dreams or nightmares that interfere with sleep. Improved sleep hygiene often helps.

Most psychiatric disorders can affect sleep. When this is the case, the best approach is to treat the primary disorder (for example, treat the depression). Unfortunately, sleep does not always get better even when the symptoms of the disorder are greatly improved. Sometimes treatment with an antidepressant will lead to significant improvement in mood, but the person may still have difficulty falling asleep. In this case, sleeping pills or other sedative medications are often used.

Many medications and other drugs adversely affect sleep. The most common offenders are these:

- Caffeine
- Decongestants (e.g., pseudoephedrine, often found in cold medications)
- Alcohol
- Tranquilizers (e.g., Xanax, Ativan, Valium)
- Sleeping pills (no kidding . . . see below)
- Steroids
- Bronchodilators (used to treat asthma)

Everyone knows that caffeine taken later in the day or in the evening can make it difficult to fall asleep. But caffeine also can have a huge impact on interfering with the ability to get restorative sleep. Amounts ingested in excess of 250 mg, even when taken before noon, can reduce the amount of time a person spends in deep sleep. The consequence is more fatigue the next day and escalating amounts of caffeine to combat the fatigue.

You can make sure that your caffeine level is not too high by taking the simple caffeine questionnaire in the Appendix. For people suffering from anxiety disorders, the goal should be to completely eliminate caffeine, which often increases symptoms of anxiety and can contribute to destabilizing people with bipolar disorder. For others, the goal should be to keep caffeine consumption below 250 mg—and none after noon.

It may be surprising to see alcohol, tranquilizers, and sleeping pills on this list. Indeed, they are often effective in helping people fall asleep. But then two things happen. First, there is often a rebound when the drug or alcohol wears off, so the person awakens in the middle of the night and has difficulty falling back to sleep. In addition, some sleeping pills (but not all) and most tranquilizers disturb the quality of sleep by reducing the amount of time spent in deep sleep.

Sleep has five stages, which can be divided into light sleep, deep sleep, and REM (rapid eye movement) or dream sleep. During sleep we cycle through these different stages of sleep, beginning with light sleep, then deep sleep, and then dream sleep. Each cycle takes 75 to 90 minutes, so we have five to six cycles in a good night's sleep.

Studies have shown that people feel more rested and function better on tests when they have had more deep sleep. By reducing the amount of deep sleep, sedatives can interfere with restorative sleep even though the person may be sedated or asleep for over eight hours.

Many if not most medical illnesses can cause sleep disturbance. Medical conditions that commonly cause insomnia include:

- Chronic pain conditions
- Congestive heart failure
- Respiratory diseases, including chronic lung disease
- Acid reflux (GERD)
- Hot flashes associated with perimenopause
- Hyperthyroidism

SLEEP HYGIENE

Sleep hygiene refers to steps one can take to prepare the body and mind for sleep and thereby improve the quality of sleep. Here are helpful activities to establish good sleep hygiene.

- Avoid emotionally intense experiences prior to retiring to bed as they always generate the release of stress hormones that interfere with the ability to go to sleep. This includes arguments with your spouse or even action-packed movies.
- Use the bed for only two activities: sleeping and love-making.
- Turn down the lights about one-half hour before retiring. The brain is programmed to respond chemically to environmental cues, one of which is light. As light levels decrease, activating neurotransmitters shut down, and certain brain chemicals such as melatonin are secreted, lowering arousal levels in the brain and making the transition to sleep easier.
- Sleep cool. Turn off the electric blanket and sleep at a cool temperature. This has been shown to increase the ability to enter into deep sleep.
- A hot bath or shower (followed by a few minutes of cool-down before getting into bed), gentle stretches, and relaxation exercises will also improve sleep. Muscle tension sends nerve impulses up the spinal cord and keeps the brain in a state of excitation. For this reason, any activity that results in decreased muscle tension can help improve the ability to fall asleep.
- Avoid alcohol. Although it may relax and cause drowsiness, it can also interfere with sleep. In particular, as the alcohol is being metabolized by the body it is chemically

altered. Several hours after you drink alcohol, some of these metabolic by-products actually stimulate the brain and cause a person either to wake up in the middle of the night or to enter into only the lightest stages of sleep. Alcohol destroys deep sleep.

- Reduce worry. This is a lot easier said than done! But, ongoing thinking and anxiety over troublesome matters late in the evening can keep the brain in a state of excitation. This may explain why monotonous thinking such as counting sheep sometimes can be soothing and helps people fall sleep. With the mind focused on sheep, it won't be attending to worries. Plus, it is pretty boring to watch sheep jump over a fence. Reading a book is probably even more effective.

- Engage in regular exercise. Exercise has many benefits, among them is its powerful ability to yield significantly better quality sleep, especially deep sleep. How much exercise and what kind? It is hard to know for sure, but the indications are that both aerobic and less strenuous exercise help. Twenty minutes three times a week seems to be adequate, although most experts recommend at least some exercise each day. *Note:* It is important that you not perform strenuous exercise in the two hours just prior to retiring. Exercise before bedtime can actually interfere with the ability to go to sleep. So plan to exercise earlier in the day.

- Resetting your biological clock will enhance sleep. Early-morning bright-light exposure is believed to recalibrate the circadian rhythm, which plays an important role in regulating brain chemistry in general and in influencing sleep patterns in particular. First establish a regular time to wake up. Biological systems and rhythms organize around a predictable cycles. Also get early-morning exposure to bright light at the same time each morning: Upon awakening, open the blinds and let the sunshine in. In winter months, spend the first thirty minutes of the morning in a well-lighted place.

SLEEP DISORDERS

Sleep apnea and restless legs syndrome, also referred to as periodic limb movements in sleep, or PLMS, are primary sleep disorders. The main symptom of both is fatigue caused by disturbed sleep. Other primary sleep disorders, including narcolepsy and circadian rhythm disorders, will not be discussed.

SLEEP APNEA

Sleep apnea is characterized by transient periods of breathing cessation, or apnea, during sleep. These periods last only a few seconds, but they are serious enough to cause partial awakening and thus disturb sleep. They may occur several hundred times each night. Diagnosis can be made by a polysomnogram taken during a sleep study wherein breathing, EEG (electroencephalogram), and other vital signs are monitored. The main symptom of sleep apnea is daytime fatigue, but it is also often associated with loud snoring, or gasping for breath during the night. Often the person is unaware of the apneic episodes and only notices the fatigue.

Sleep apnea can be caused by the collapse of the muscles of the throat during sleep (obstructive type) and/or by the failure of the respiratory center in the brain to instruct the lungs to breathe during sleep (central type). Both types may be present. Generally, obstructive sleep apnea is treated with a CPAP (breathing) machine or by a tracheostomy. But they are of less benefit in central apnea. In addition to CPAP, central sleep apnea may improve through treatment of underlying medical conditions, such as congestive heart failure. Many people have a combination of both central and obstructive sleep apnea. Evaluation and treatment of sleep apnea is best done by a sleep specialist.

RESTLESS LEGS SYNDROME

Restless legs syndrome (RLS), as the name suggests, involves a sensation that one's leg are moving. Most people with RLS also have periodic limb movements in sleep (PLMS), meaning that they move their arms and legs frequently during sleep. RLS also results in fatigue. It is usually diagnosed by a person's history, but the diagnosis can be confirmed by polysomnography. RLS or PLMS is usually treated with a medication that increases the activity of dopamine, such as pramipexole (Mirapex) or ropinirole (Requip). Other medications sometimes used include tranquilizers (e.g., clonazepam), opiates, or anticonvulsants (e.g., gabapentin). RLS is worsened by some antidepressants and caffeine. Thus, treatment often involves reducing the offending medications and caffeine.

MEDICATIONS FOR RESTLESS LEGS SYNDROME (AND PLMS)

MEDICATIONS FOR RESTLESS LEGS SYNDROME (AND PLMS)		
GENERIC	BRAND	DOSAGE
pramipexole	Mirapex	0.125–2.0 mg
ropinirole	Requip	0.25–4 mg

SLEEPING MEDICATIONS

Sleep medications, referred to as hypnotics, are used to treat insomnia regardless of the cause. Because of this, and because they are very effective and have few side effects, they have become immensely popular. As reported by the *New York Times*,

IMS America (IMS, or Intercontinental Marketing Services, tracks pharmaceutical data) found that Americans received over 40 million prescriptions for sleeping pills in 2005. The National Sleep Foundation survey (Sleep in America, 1997) found that 25 percent of Americans take such medications every year. Thus, insomnia is a very common problem, and Americans spend millions of dollars every year on sleeping pills to treat it. But despite their effectiveness and relative safety, several important considerations should be noted about their use.

- When a sleep disorder is due to another condition such as depression, sleep apnea, or congestive heart failure, the most important thing is to treat the primary condition.
- Most sleep medications, except zolpidem (Ambien), zaleplon (Sonata), eszopiclone (Lunesta), and ramelteon (Rozerem), reduce the amount of deep sleep and therefore may contribute to daytime fatigue.
- Sometimes sleeping pills cause sedation that continues into the next morning.
- Sometimes sleeping pills cause amnesia, so that people do not remember what they have done. A classic example is the person who wakes up in the morning to find cracker crumbs in the bed and does not remember having eaten crackers during the night. Of greater concern is someone who drives their car in this condition. This has been most reported with triazolam (Halcion) and zolpidem (Ambien) and appears to be associated with the short half-life of the drug.
- Most sleeping pills are habit forming. This means they usually should be used only for a short time. With continued use, tolerance often develops, requiring an increase in dose, and then dependence. Thus, instead of sleeping with the medication, you soon can no longer

sleep without it. If the medication is to be used for more than several weeks, it is best to take it no more than three nights per week. Ramelteon (Rozemem) is the only sleeping pill that is not habit forming. This is because it works at the melatonin receptor.

Other medications that produce sedation but are not sleeping pills are often used for sleep because they are not addictive. These include trazodone (Desyrel), quetiapine (Seroquel), mirtazapine (Remeron), and diphenhydramine (Benadryl). But because these medications have more serious side effects, they are generally reserved for more severe and/or chronic forms of insomnia. The benzodiazepine antianxiety medications such as Ativan or Xanax are also used sometimes for sleep and have the same problems as the benzodiazepine hypnotics: they are habit forming and suppress deep sleep.

The following is a list of the most frequently prescribed sleep medications:

SLEEP MEDICATIONS	
GENERIC NAME	BRAND NAME
flurazepam	Dalmane
temazepam	Restoril
triazolam	Halcion
estazolam	ProSom
quazepam	Doral
zolpidem	Ambien
zaleplon	Sonata
eszopiclone	Lunesta
ramelteon	Rozerem
diphenhydramine	Benadryl

CHAPTER 10

ADHD, Eating Disorders, Dementia, and Other Disorders

INTRODUCTION

In this chapter, we will discuss several types of disorders that are generally less common and about which less is known. These include attention deficit disorder, eating disorders, borderline personality disorder, post-traumatic stress disorder, aggression, and dementia. Since medications usually prescribed for these disorders are also used to treat psychiatric disorders discussed in previous chapters, they will only be outlined here. For example, since antidepressants are used to treat several of these disorders, detailed discussions of these drugs can be found in Chapter 5.

ATTENTION DEFICIT HYPERACTIVITY DISORDER (ADHD)

Attention deficit/hyperactivity disorder (ADHD) is characterized by the inability to focus and sustain one's attention on activities. This disorder begins in early childhood and if untreated, often results in poor school performance and sometimes in behavioral problems. Approximately two thirds of those who develop ADHD in childhood will continue to have these problems into adulthood (Hill and Schoener 1996). Untreated ADHD in adults usually results in poor work performance and relationship difficulties. People with ADHD are easily bored and find it difficult to focus on a task long enough to complete it. Thus, they frequently fail to complete many tasks and if left untreated may get into trouble for not doing better. They also may seek alternative stimulation, and, as a result, get into trouble for their activities. Often anxiety and depression develop as a result of these focus difficulties, and low self-esteem is almost always a consequence.

DIAGNOSIS

The diagnosis of ADHD is based on family history, behavioral history, and current symptoms. During childhood, the most common symptoms are hyperactivity, impulsivity, impaired self-control, difficulty staying on task, inattention to detail, and limited ability for internal motivation (e.g., to continue to work at a boring task). ADHD always begins in childhood. If the disorder continues into late adolescence, the hyperactivity symptoms almost always subside, but the core symptoms of impaired attention, impulsivity, and difficulties staying on task continue. Classic ADHD in late adolescence and adulthood respond well to stimulants.

In childhood there are two primary forms of attentional problems. The first is full spectrum ADHD (attention problems, impulsivity, troubles staying on task, behavioral problems, and hyperactivity). Another disorder has been referred to solely as the "inattentive subtype." Recent studies have revealed that the inattentive form is unrelated to actual ADHD. The underlying biology and the response to medications is quite different than ADHD. In addition, the strictly inattentive type does not have impulsivity or hyperactivity. Rather, its main features are information processing deficits. This is seen as difficulties maintaining focused concentration and what parents and teachers often describe as "spacyness." Many of these children also are prone to daydreaming. This disorder occurs more often in girls than in boys and usually is identified later.

While most cases of ADHD are diagnosed at ages 4 or 5, children with the inattentive type are typically not recognized until second, third, or fourth grade. This is also a disorder that is often accompanied by a good deal of anxiety. Although many children with the inattentive type are treated with stimulants (e.g., Ritalin), these medications are generally not effective and may increase anxiety. A trial on low doses of stimulants may be appropriate since a small percent of children may benefit slightly. However, unfortunately most do not benefit and to date there are not good medical treatments for this type of attentional problem.

The diagnosis of ADHD can be somewhat controversial, as it is sometimes difficult to diagnose precisely what degree of attentional problems is normal at a certain age, or what may be caused by situational factors, anxiety, or depression. It is important to note that ADHD symptoms are context dependent and may not be present when the person is doing something inherently exciting and stimulating, such as playing a video game. The symptoms are much more noticeable when the person is doing something still and quiet, such as reading.

When six of the following symptoms of inattention or impulsivity have been present for at least six months, ADHD can be diagnosed with a fair measure of accuracy:

- Carelessness
- Difficulty sustaining attention

- Inattentive listening
- Failure to follow through on tasks
- Difficulty with organizing activities
- Avoidance of activities requiring prolonged mental effort
- Forgetfulness
- Frequent distraction
- Frequent loss of materials required for activities
- Fidgeting or squirming
- Difficulty staying seated in class
- Inappropriate activity (running, climbing)
- Difficulty playing quietly
- Answering questions before they have been completely stated
- Difficulty waiting for turn

ADHD AND THE BRAIN

Many theories have been advanced to explain ADHD. In the past, it was called minimal brain dysfunction because it was thought that some neurological dysfunction of the brain was interfering with the ability to pay attention. Neurological abnormalities can sometimes be demonstrated, but most of the time none can be found. It has been shown, however, that ADHD tends to be inherited, which implies a biological basis. Positive emission tomography (PET), fMRI, and SPECT brain scans of people with ADHD have demonstrated an area of decreased metabolic activity in the prefrontal cortex (Zametkin et al. 1990).

MEDICAL TREATMENTS

Several types of medication are helpful in the treatment of ADHD. These include stimulants, alpha-2 adrenergic agonists, and antidepressants. Stimulants are the most effective form of treatment, but because they can be habit forming, they have been the subject of much controversy. It must be noted, however, that properly diagnosed and treated children and adolescents rarely abuse the prescribed medications. Also, many people are reluctant to give psychiatric medication to children, since studies about the effects on long-term use in children, especially under the age of six, have not been done. Certainly, no one wants to prescribe psychoactive medication for children unless it is absolutely necessary, but the cost of not treating ADHD can be high.

When ADHD is not treated, children can face difficulty socially and academically. They can also develop long-lasting psychological problems related to impulsivity, having adults angry with them often, and being unable to complete tasks successfully. These experiences can lead to low self-esteem and feeling that they are "bad" and "failures." These same issues arise for adults with ADHD who go untreated as well. People with mild ADHD may get through childhood despite their attentional deficit with few noticeable problems. But, as adolescents or adults they may begin to have very significant problems.

STIMULANTS

Stimulants are considered the mainstay of ADHD treatment. They are highly effective (approaching 90 per cent), and are generally well tolerated. Stimulants usually start to work about thirty minutes after ingestion. They may be taken two or three times per day, although the more recent long-acting formulations, taken once daily are often preferred. Individuals vary in their response to classes of stimulants. Some people respond well to methylphenidate (Ritalin and others), and others respond preferentially to amphetamines (Adderall and others) (see the table that follows). If one type of stimulant is not effective or has significant side effects, it is best to try another type. The most common side effects include the following, along with preventive measures:

- Initial insomnia (take earlier or use shorter-acting medication)
- Anorexia (or loss of appetite may require dose adjustment)
- Stomachache (take with food)
- Mild dysphoria (switch to another medication)
- Lethargy (reduce dose)

GENERIC AND BRAND-NAME STIMULANTS	
GENERIC NAME	BRAND NAME
methylphenidate	Ritalin
methylphenidate	Concerta
methylphenidate	Metadate
methylphenidate	Methylin
methylphenidate	Daytrana (patch)
dexmethylphenidate	Focalin
dextroamphetamine	Dexedrine
lisdexamfetamine	Vyvanse
pemoline	Cylert
l & d amphetamine	Adderall
modafinil	Provigil

ALPHA-2 ADRENERGIC AGONISTS

Clonidine (Catapres) and guanfacine (Tenex) may be used to treat core ADHD symptoms, but they are most effective in reducing restlessness, impulsivity, irritability, and aggression, and are often added to a stimulant to aid in sleep.

ANTIDEPRESSANTS

Antidepressants such as atomoxetine (Strattera) are not as effective as stimulants and tend to have more side effects, but they are especially helpful when the person is also depressed or cannot tolerate the side effects of stimulants since every individual's body chemical may react slightly differently. Two antidepressants are commonly prescribed for the treatment of ADHD: Strattera and Wellbutrin. Wellbutrin is not FDA approved for use with children, although it has been shown to be effective for some children, adolescents, and adults. Strattera, FDA approved for treating ADHD, is technically an antidepressant, but it is marketed only for the treatment of ADHD. Dosing for children with Strattera is based on the person's weight: 1.2–1.8 mg per kilogram (to figure kilograms take weight in pounds and divide by 2.2).

They have several other advantages:

- Once-a-day dosing
- No need for special prescription
- No addiction potential
- Clinical effects typically last around the clock. This may be one of the biggest advantages to using one of these antidepressants. Stimulants wear off during the day and cannot be given in the evening or late afternoon. Wellbutrin and Strattera are effective during the day and into the evening.

Please note: while stimulants begin working within an hour after taking the first dose, antidepressants require a more prolonged time before positive effects are seen (anywhere from 5 days to a month).

ALPHA-2 ADRENERGIC AGONISTS	
GENERIC NAME	BRAND NAME
clonidine	Catapres
guanfacine	Tenex

ANTIDEPRESSANTS USED TO TREAT ADHD	
GENERIC NAME	BRAND NAME
atomoxetine	Strattera
bupropion	Wellbutrin

TREATMENT CONSIDERATIONS: WHAT TO EXPECT

Treatment for ADHD is begun with a low dose of medication, such as 5 mg of Ritalin or Dexedrine two to three times a day or a low dose of an extended-release version of the medication. If full benefit is not achieved, the dose is gradually increased. Benefit should be noticeable virtually with the first dose, but several days or weeks may be needed for a full ion. If the child demonstrates excessive nervousness, extreme loss of appetite, or occasional drowsiness, the dosage should be decreased. If one stimulant does not work, another one can be tried. These medications come in slow-release (SR) and extended-release (XR) forms because the standard preparations may work for only three to four hours. This necessitates several doses per day (leading to missed doses) and may result in several periods of rebound hyperactivity between doses. Thus, the longer-acting preparations generally produce a smoother, sustained benefit lasting all day. The more common side effects include anxiety, nervousness, appetite suppression, and insomnia.

These side effects can usually be controlled by adjusting the amount and timing of the doses.

Antidepressants may also be used. These may be tried initially, in cases where the patients (usually adolescents or adults) have a history of stimulant abuse, or after the stimulants have failed to work. These medications offer the advantage of not being habit forming, but they have more side effects than the stimulants. Again, it is usual to start with a low dose and gradually increase the level until an effective one is reached. Benefits usually take two weeks or more to appear. (See Chapter 5 for a more complete discussion of antidepressants.) It is important to note that the FDA has issued a warning that antidepressants can cause increased thoughts of suicide in children and adolescents (this issue is discussed in detail in Chapter 5).

Clonidine, normally prescribed to treat high blood pressure, is another medication sometime used for ADHD. It also has some antianxiety properties that can be helpful and is usually used in combination with other medications. Again, one starts with a low dose, usually 0.1 mg, which increases gradually. Typical side effects include low blood pressure (which may cause dizziness) and fatigue or low energy. Other medications, such as antianxiety, antipsychotic, lithium, or anticonvulsant medication may be added to clonidine to gain further benefit. The choice of another medication depends on other features; for example, someone with ADHD who also has mood swings might be treated with a mood stabilizer such as lithium.

STIMULANTS BY TYPICAL DOSAGE

IMMEDIATE-RELEASE	TYPICAL DAILY DOSE
Methylphenidate	
Ritalin	10–60 mg
Metadate	10–60 mg
Methylin	10–60 mg
Concerta	18–54 mg
Dexmethylphenidate (Focalin)	5–20 mg
Dextroamphetamine	
Dexedrine	5–40 mg
Amphetamines	
Amphetamine salts (Adderall)	5–40 mg
Methamphetamine (Desoxyn)	5–25 mg
EXTENDED-RELEASE	**TYPICAL DAILY DOSE**
Methylphenidate	
Ritalin SR	20–60 mg
Ritalin LA	20–60 mg
Metadate ER	10–60 mg
Metadate CD	20–60 mg
Methylin ER	20–60 mg
Concerta	18–54 mg
Daytrana (transdermal patch)	10–30 mg
Dextroamphetamine	
Dexedrine spansules	5–40 mg
Amphetamine	
Adderall XR	5–40 mg
Lisdexamfetamine	
Vyvanse	30–70 mg

ALPHA-2 ADRENERGIC AGENTS TYPICAL DOSAGE		
GENERIC	BRAND NAME	TYPICAL DOSE
Clonidine	Catapres	0.15–0.4 mg
Guanfacine	Tenex	0.25–1.0 mg

ANTIDEPRESSANTS USED TO TREAT ADHD TYPICAL DOSAGE		
GENERIC	BRAND NAME	TYPICAL DAILY DOSE
Buproprion	Wellbutrin SR/XL	150–300 mg
Atomoxetine	Strattera	1.2–1.8 mg/kg

ARE STIMULANTS SAFE FOR LONG-TERM USE?

As with any potentially habit-forming medication, stimulants must be used with caution. In children, stimulants can cause growth suppression, which maybe temporary but needs to be monitored. But keep in mind these medications have been used for decades without any major demonstrable ill effects. *Note:* Children with heart disease may experience potentially dangerous side effects, such as sudden death. All children should have a physical examination to see if further cardiac evaluation, such as an EKG, is indicated.

Interestingly, children with ADHD who are treated show a 50 percent decreased risk for substance abuse as they age, compared with those with who go untreated.

EATING DISORDERS

There are two main types of eating disorders: anorexia and bulimia. Anorexia involves severe weight loss and maintenance of low body weight by restricting food intake and/or purging (vomiting immediately after eating). People with anorexia are obsessed with their weight and see themselves as fat, even though they are below normal body weight. People with bulimia overeat in binges and then purge after eating. They may consume huge amounts of food and then spend hours purging to avoid gaining weight. They are often slightly overweight.

DIAGNOSIS

The diagnosis of anorexia depends on the maintenance of an abnormally low body weight (less than 85 percent of the ideal weight) and a distortion of body image. No matter how thin anorexics are, they see themselves as fat. Often they do excessive amounts of exercising to maintain their low weight, and they may also use laxatives for purging. Anorexia can lead to severe malnutrition, which can be life-threatening and always warrants treatment.

The diagnosis of bulimia depends on frequent binge eating followed by efforts to get rid of the food, either by vomiting or by taking laxatives or diuretics. Bulimia, too, can cause serious medical problems, such as bleeding from a tear in the stomach or teeth and gum disease.

EATING DISORDERS AND BIOLOGY

The cause of eating disorders is not fully understood. Twin studies have shown a significant genetic/biological basis for anorexia. Some evidence suggests that anorexia has an addictive aspect. It has been demonstrated that fasting causes the release of endorphins in the brain. These are the brain's own morphine-like substances, which are also released by strenuous exercise. When endorphins are released, they give the person a sense of feeling good, or a "high." Thus, it is thought that people with anorexia are essentially addicted to fasting. Anorexia often begins when people experience a significant unintentional weight loss—from an illness, for example. They then may feel a need to maintain the reduced weight, and feel fat if they gain any weight, so they take the necessary steps to keep their weight down by restricting their food intake and increasing their exercise.

Bulimia appears to be related to depression. Often people with bulimia engage in binge eating when they are upset or when they feel emotionally out of control. After bingeing, they panic and do something like inducing vomiting to get rid of the food.

MEDICAL TREATMENT

No medication has demonstrated great success in the treatment of anorexia, although several kinds have sometimes been helpful. The most important treatment is weight gain. This is accomplished with a behavioral program that rewards eating and increased weight. With prolonged fasting, the stomach loses its ability to handle food easily. Sometimes medication is used to help the stomach work properly; one such drug is cisapride (one brand name is Propulsid). Medication like naltrexone, which blocks the "high" of fasting, can be helpful. Naltrexone blocks the effects of opiates and is used to treat heroin addiction and alcoholism.

Other types of medication that may be helpful in selected cases include antianxiety, antidepressant, antipsychotic, and anticonvulsant medications and lithium (which are discussed in the chapter on bipolar disorders).

Bulimia, on the other hand, has been shown to respond well to antidepressants. An antiseizure medication, Topamax, has recently shown promise in treating bulimia.

Caution: Buproprion (Wellbutrin) cannot be used in the

treatment of eating disorders because of the risk of seizures in this group of patients. Any other antidepressant may be used. Usually an SSRI is prescribed, with good benefit. Sometimes higher doses are required to treat bulimia than are used with depression (e.g., 60 to 80 mg of fluoxetine). Otherwise, treatment with these medications is the same as when they are used to treat depression.

BORDERLINE PERSONALITY DISORDERS

The term "borderline personality disorder" refers to a rather heterogeneous group of disorders. At times this group has seemed so heterogeneous that the very concept of the diagnosis has been questioned. The term originally referred to people whose disorder was on the "borderline" between neurosis and psychosis. Over time it has become more refined, but it still retains this association.

Today, the term refers to people whose emotional disorder is more severe than is usually seen in a neurosis, but they are not psychotic, or only transiently so. Studies suggest that this disorder occurs in about 2 to 4 percent of the general population and in 10 to 25 percent of those who are treated in outpatient mental health clinics. Because of their very intense symptomatology, these people tend to be conspicuous. Their intensely volatile relationships often lead them into legal difficulties and attract the attention of the police, friends, and neighbors.

DIAGNOSIS

In the *Diagnostic and Statistical Manual of Mental Disorders* (DSM-IV-TR), the diagnosis by borderline personality is made by the symptomatology. The following symptoms are the criteria:

- Frantic efforts to avoid abandonment
- Unstable and intense relationships
- Persistently unstable self-image
- Impulsive behavior that is potentially dangerous
- Suicidal or self-mutilating behavior
- Mood swings
- Chronic feelings of emptiness
- Poorly controlled outbursts of anger
- Transient paranoia or dissociative spells

Five of these nine criteria must be present for a diagnosis of borderline personality disorder to be made.

CAUSES OF BORDERLINE PERSONALITY DISORDER

Many of the writings on borderline personality disorder focus either on the role of severe neglect or traumatic events during childhood or on the failure of the parents to help a child develop a sturdy sense of self. Other studies look at inborn temperamental factors (Mahler 1975, Gunderson 1984, Hartocollis 1977, Silver 1992). At present there is no definitive answer about the cause. It appears that people with borderline personality disorder have a combination of psychological and constitutional factors, in varying degrees.

MEDICAL TREATMENT

No medication is specific for the treatment of borderline personality disorder, but several medication types may help in reducing the symptoms. At the heart of this disorder is a tendency for intense emotional reactivity or sensitivity to rejection or threat of abandonment. Several kinds of antidepressants, particularly the MAO inhibitors and SSRIs, can be helpful in reducing this sensitivity to rejection or abandonment (Norden 1989a, 1989, 1995).

Mood stabilizers, including lithium, anticonvulsants, and atypical antipsychotics, can be helpful in reducing mood swings and controlling anger. Antidepressants can be helpful in treating associated depression and anxiety. Antipsychotic medications can be helpful with paranoia or during periods of disorganization.

Caution: Because of the borderline person's tendency to engage in self-harming behavior, caution must be used when prescribing any medication. It is safest to use only medications that are not likely to be toxic in overdose and to avoid medications such as the minor tranquilizers, which are habit forming.

PSYCHOTHERAPY

Long-term psychotherapy is an important, if not essential, part of the treatment of borderline personality disorder. A good relationship with a therapist can have a very stabilizing effect and can help the person weather the ups and downs of other relationships. One issue that must be addressed is how to handle crises. The borderline person may tend to behave self-destructively in a crisis. Constructive ways of handling inevitable crises must be explored and reinforced. These include turning to supportive friends and using crisis hot lines and emergency rooms. Some studies show that certain types of group therapy and educational groups, such as dialectical behavior therapy can also be very helpful in learning new coping skills (Linehan 1993). See *Integrative Treatment for Borderline Personality Disorders* (Preston 2006) and *I Hate You—Don't Leave Me* (Kreisman 1989) for more complete discussions of this disorder.

POST-TRAUMATIC STRESS DISORDER

Post-traumatic stress disorder (PTSD) refers to a set of specific types of reactions to an extremely stressful event. The term "PTSD" is relatively new. It came into use during the treatment of Vietnam War veterans, but the syndrome has been recognized for decades and has variously been called combat neurosis, shell shock, or traumatic neurosis.

Recently, post-traumatic stress disorder has become a somewhat controversial diagnosis because some individuals have used it to apply for disability payments and for damages in litigation. Nevertheless, it remains an important psychological disorder, with treatments and therapies directed toward the specific set of trauma reactions.

Post-traumatic stress disorder is often caused by a combination of exposure to violence and helplessness. For example, children who are physically or sexually abused, or who witness spousal abuse, are likely to suffer from PTSD. Adults who were victims of or witness to violent crimes, survivors of natural disasters like earthquakes and floods, and refugees and combatants from war have often been diagnosed with PTSD after the crime or the war has ended. It seems that as violence becomes more commonplace in our modern world, so too does the incidence of PTSD increase.

DIAGNOSIS

When people are exposed to a traumatic event, they go through several stages of emotional response. Initially, there is shock. The person is both horrified and numb. This may last for several hours to several days. Then the person goes through a period of alternating between overwhelming memories of the event and a state of numbness or emotional detachment. The traumatic memories may come as intrusive images, or flashbacks, or in nightmares. The person feels on edge and is easily startled. There may be intense anxiety, panic attacks, and/or depression. The following are the key symptoms of PTSD:

- Increased autonomic arousal (e.g., anxiety, tension, irritability, easily startled, easily overwhelmed by feelings)
- Persistent reliving of the trauma (intrusive memories, thoughts, and nightmares)
- Avoidance (social withdrawal and avoidance of any situation that might serve as a reminder of the traumatic event)
- Emotional numbing

Depression, panic attacks, or substance abuse may also develop as associated features.

With emotional support and therapy, over time most people are gradually able to reestablish a sense of security and to work through most of their feelings about the trauma. However, if the trauma was severe or took place in childhood, these symptoms may be very persistent.

MEDICATION TREATMENT

The use of medication in the treatment of PTSD is mostly directed at associated features, such as panic attacks. However, medication is also often used in the initial stage, immediately after the trauma, when the person is feeling very anxious and overwhelmed and having difficulty sleeping. At this time, minor tranquilizers are often used. However, some evidence suggests that minor tranquilizers may interfere with the emotional healing process. Beta blockers may be better for reducing the tension and hypervigilance that are present during the first few days. SSRI antidepressants are being used successfully to reduce overwhelming intrusive symptoms (e.g., flashbacks). If panic attacks, depression, or psychotic symptoms develop, they can be treated with the appropriate medications (as they would when PTSD is not present). The antihypertensive drug Minipress has been used in experimental studies to reduce or eliminate nightmares.

NONMEDICATION TREATMENT

Nonmedication forms of treatment are very important in PTSD. Experiencing intense trauma is a major assault on a person's sense of being in control of life. Reestablishing a sense of control and a feeling of safety is a crucial first step for healing to take place. A particular form of psychotherapy, cognitive-behavioral therapy, has the best track record in the treatment of PTSD; response rates are significantly higher than those seen when only medication is used. Additionally, ongoing support groups may be helpful in diminishing the emotional reactions over time. A number of support groups are organized around specific types of trauma, such as Vietnam War veterans, veterans of the Iraq War, victims of violent crime, and survivors of incest or rape. Despite the benefits of support groups, some people will be too uncomfortable in a group and will require individual treatment.

AGGRESSION

Aggression, including irritability, hostility, or violent behavior, can be associated with several mental disorder and it can occur in a number of contexts. When treating aggression, it is important to first treat any underlying condition. For example, aggression is fairly common in alcoholism, bipolar disorder, and psychosis. To control the aggression, it is first necessary to treat the primary disorder. These are the disorders that are frequently associated with aggression:

- Attention deficit hyperactivity disorder
- Antisocial personality disorder
- Borderline personality disorder
- Conduct disorder
- Delirium
- Dementia
- Depression
- Intermittent explosive disorder (sudden episodes of aggressive behavior)
- Medication-induced aggression
- Mania (bipolar disorder)
- Mental retardation
- Paranoid disorder
- Post-concussion syndrome (following brain trauma or head injury)
- Schizophrenia
- Substance use disorders
- Temporal lobe epilepsy

As stated above, quite often the aggression can be controlled by treating the primary disorder. For example, those suffering from paranoid psychosis may become violent because they think people are trying to kill them. When the psychosis is treated and they are no longer paranoid, the tendency toward violence usually subsides. Sometimes medications are used more specifically to try to control the aggression. Medications that may be helpful include anticonvulsants, antipsychotics, beta blockers, buspirone, clonidine, lithium, and SSRIs. The choice of medications is guided by the associated features. For example, a person with aggression associated with mood swings might be treated with a mood stabilizer, such as lithium, or valproate or an atypical antipsychotic. The following table shows which types of medication target specific associated features of various disorders.

MEDICATION TYPES FOR AGGRESSION DISORDERS	
MEDICATION TYPES	ASSOCIATED FEATURES/DISORDERS
Anticonvulsants	Labile mood, poor impulse control, (e.g., carbamazepine), organicity (damage to the brain)
Antipsychotics	Disorganized behavior
Atypical antipsychotics	Mood swings, disorganized behavior
Beta blockers (e.g., propranolol)	Organicity (e.g., dementia)
Buspirone	Organicity
Clonidine	Anxiety, agitation
Lithium	Labile mood, impulsivity
SSRIs	Anger "attacks," irritability

ALZHEIMER'S DISEASE AND DEMENTIA

Dementia refers to a significant impairment in cognitive functioning, especially memory. Alzheimer's disease is the most well-known type of dementia, but other types are fairly common. They include Lewy body dementia, Pick's disease (frontotemporal dementia), multi-infarct dementia, Parkinson's disease, and alcoholic dementia. Dementia is not caused by aging, but it does tend to become more common as people grow older. Approximately 10 percent of the population have dementia and/or significant memory impairment at age seventy, 20 percent at age eighty (APA 1989), and 80 percent at age ninety. In the evaluation of dementia, a thorough medical evaluation, including laboratory tests, is crucial to look for diseases that cause dementia. Often a brain scan is necessary as well. Some studies indicate that about 15 percent of those diagnosed with dementia illness have treatable medical conditions, which if treated might cure the dementia (APA 1989).

MEDICAL TREATMENT

New medications are being developed for the treatment of Alzheimer's disease. Tacrine (Cognex) was the first, but it can have significant liver toxicity and requires multiple doses per day; thus, it is rarely used these days. Two newer drugs—donepezil (Aricept) and memantine (Namenda)—avoid these problems. These medications do not cure Alzheimer's disease, but they can sometimes improve alertness and cognitive functioning in people who are in the early stage of the disease (i.e., in terms of mental functioning, often they can effectively roll back the clock for about one year for Alzheimer's patients but then the deterioration will progress). Their usefulness in other types of dementia is under study. Other medications are in development.

Other types of dementia are helped by treating the underlying cause whenever possible. Even when the dementia itself is not treatable, different aspects of the disorder may be treatable. For example, people who have dementia often become paranoid because they do not understand what is going on around them. Antipsychotic medication is usually effective for treating this disorder. (*Note:* The atypical antipsychotics have been shown to be associated with increased mortality in the elderly.) Agitation and depression are sometimes seen in those with dementia and may benefit from treatment with antidepressant or antianxiety medication.

CHAPTER 11

Medication During Childhood, Adolescence, Pregnancy, and Old Age

CHILDREN, ADOLESCENTS, AND PSYCHIATRIC MEDICATIONS

These days children and adolescents are often treated with psychiatric medicines. This practice has sparked a national debate. Some people argue that children do not suffer from "true" mental health problems because their problems are not biological and that most symptoms can be corrected by a change in environment or parenting style. Those who hold this belief contend that the real causes of emotional distress in children and adolescents are societal pressures and family lifestyle changes that have led to the emergence of emotional and behavioral problems in children.

On the other hand, those who have witnessed the benefits of medications also present some strong arguments. Seeing a child's self-esteem improve because of better school performance and social adjustment, or witnessing a child come back from the brink of suicide, constitute strong arguments in the opposite direction. Furthermore, there is increasing evidence that genetic influences can predispose a child or teenager to depression, bipolar disorder, or attention deficit hyperactivity disorder (ADHD).

Both sides present passionate and convincing arguments. As with most worthy debates, the answers will probably lie somewhere in the middle and incorporate elements of both sides' arguments. Until this complex issue is resolved, however, the reality is that children are receiving a variety of medicines, most commonly stimulants, antidepressants, and mood stabilizers. It is not the intention of this book to preferentially support either side. Rather, we want to provide you with as much information as possible so that medicines prescribed for your children will lead to a successful outcome.

If a child in your care is taking medicines, or if you are trying to decide whether to begin a medication regimen, you can take some steps to ensure the safest and most effective course of treatment. These measures are described below.

SAFETY ISSUES FOR YOUNGER PEOPLE

Make sure you understand your child's diagnosis and how it was made. The prescribing of psychiatric medications can be done by general practitioners, pediatricians, or psychiatrists. Ask for a detailed explanation as to why the doctor has decided that a particular medication is necessary—for example, a stimulant or antidepressant. Find out how often the doctor treats this particular condition. Ideally, the treatment is being provided by a highly trained child or adolescent psychiatrist who has obtained a complete psychological testing profile from a psychologist. Unfortunately, many areas of the country currently have a shortage of mental health professionals.

If your primary care doctor or pediatrician is prescribing psychiatric medication for your child, make sure you are comfortable with his or her expertise in the area. For instance, does the physician have specialized training in the field, as evidenced by his or her licensure? Does the local mental health association recommend the doctor? You could also get a second opinion on the doctor's qualifications. Talk to other parents and children being treated for the same condition.

SOCIAL ENVIRONMENT ISSUES

The parent or caregiver of a child who has been prescribed a course of psychiatric medication must understand that drugs are probably only a part of the required treatment. As with adults, but in a more complex manner, environmental factors may be contributing to the child's current difficulties. Be aware that some family therapy may need to take place or that some social factors may need to change. Be willing to participate actively in the complete treatment plan.

COMPLIANCE

You must also understand the necessity of compliance. It will be important to identify any barriers to ensuring that the medication is taken consistently. For example, some school systems will allow medications to be brought to, or stored on, school premise only with written permission of a doctor and then only in the original prescription bottle. This can create the need to time the doses very carefully so that none are missed.

A child may have multiple residences. You must make sure that a supply of medicine is available at each house. Are there members of the child's family or school system who are opposed to the medicine? It is essential to encourage everyone involved in your child's care to honestly discuss what reservations they may have. When family members or caregivers do not support the prescribed treatment, the child receives mixed signals and may become distressed and confused.

LEGAL ISSUES

For certain stimulants, special prescriptions are required every time the medicine is filled at a pharmacy. This is federal law, and there are no ways to get around it. The doctor has to write these prescriptions by hand, and they cannot be refilled in the traditional sense. This legal requirement can lead to frustration and, more importantly, to missed doses if careful planning is not done ahead of time. Do not get close to running out of medicine. Know when your doctor's office is open and closed. Find out if your doctor has a colleague or partner who could write a prescription in an emergency.

DOSAGES FOR YOUNGER PEOPLE

When the doctor prescribes a medication for a child or teenager, some general dosing considerations are taken into account. Younger children, especially, may be more sensitive to side effects. It is advisable to start out with a low dose, sometimes a small test dose, and increase the dosage slowly over time. Be sure you understand exactly the dosing range for the medicine your child is taking. Sometimes dosages are based on your child's weight. Make sure your doctor monitors and is made aware of any changes in your child's weight.

It is generally assumed that children are more efficient metabolizers of medication than adults and even adolescents. Therefore, the amount of medication in the bloodstream might be more susceptible to ups and downs. Sometimes a medicine that an adult can take on a once-a-day basis may need to be given two or three times a day to a child.

Children are susceptible to the full range of side effects from any given medication. Some side effects may be of greater concern. For example, the cardiac side effects of tricyclic antidepressants may be more serious in children than in adults. It is also necessary to take some special precautions if your child is receiving a tricyclic antidepressant. Be sure to ask your doctor about the safe use of tricyclics for your child.

To summarize, psychiatric medications can be a safe and effective part of your child's treatment. It is very likely, however, that medicine will not be all that is required to help your child get better. Learning as much as possible about the medicine and finding a qualified doctor to work with will greatly increase the chances of successful treatment.

Most psychiatric medications used in treatment of children and teenagers are not FDA approved for use with youngsters (although they are in widespread use). The specific dosing guidelines vary widely depending on the age, weight, and other factors for each individual child. The following list summarizes generally agreed-upon guidelines, but please keep in mind that dosing in youngsters is not as well defined as it is in adults. You will also note that this list only includes some psychiatric drugs. Newer medications that have not been on the market long enough are not listed since we do not yet have enough information to determine dosing guidelines.

PSYCHOTROPIC MEDICATION GUIDELINES: CHILDREN AND ADOLESCENTS		
MEDICATION	TOTAL DAILY DOSE	DAILY (WEIGHT ADJUSTED)
Antidepressants		
Prozac*	5–40 mg	0.25–0.75 mg/kg
Zoloft*	25–200 mg	1.5–3.0 mg/kg
Paxil*	10–30 mg	0.25–0.75 mg/kg
Celexa*	5–40 mg	0.25–0.75 mg/kg
Lexapro*	5–20 mg	0.125–0.375 mg/kg
Wellbutrin	50–300 mg	3–6 mg/kg

* SSRIs

MEDICATION	TOTAL DAILY DOSE	DAILY (WEIGHT ADJUSTED)
Antidepressants (continued)		
Effexor	37.5–150 mg	1–3 mg/kg
Strattera	60–120 mg	1.2–1.8 mg/kg
Anti-Obsessional/Anxiety		
SSRIs	above	above
Luvox	50–300 mg	1.5–4.5 mg/kg
Anafranil	25–300 mg	2–5 mg/kg
Antianxiety		
BuSpar	5–40 mg	0.5–1.0 mg/kg
Klonopin	0.5–6 mg	0.02–0.1 mg/kg
Xanax	0.5–6 mg	0.02–0.1 mg/kg
Ativan	0.5–6 mg	0.04–0.15 mg/kg
Antipsychotics		
Zyprexa	5–20 mg	1–3 mg/kg
Risperdal	0.5–6 mg	0.1–0.5 mg/kg
Seroquel	25–400 mg	3–6 mg/kg
Clozaril	25–400 mg	3–6 mg/kg
Mood Stabilizers		
Lithium	300–2100 mg	blood levels
Depakote	250–1500 mg	blood levels
Tegretol	200–1000 mg	blood levels
Lamictal	200–500 mg	1–10 mg/kg
Neurontin	300–1200 mg	10 mg/kg
Topamax	50–400 mg	3–6 mg/kg
Stimulants		
Dexedrine	5–40 mg	0.3–1.5 mg/kg
Ritalin, etc.	5–60 mg	1–2 mg/kg
Adderall	5–40 mg	0.5–1.5 mg/kg

PSYCHOTROPIC MEDICATION GUIDELINES: CHILDREN AND ADOLESCENTS *(continued)*		
MEDICATION	TOTAL DAILY DOSE	DAILY (WEIGHT ADJUSTED)
Other		
Clonidine	0.025–0.6 mg	0.001–0.01 mg/kg
Inderal	20–160 mg	2–4 mg/kg
Benadryl	10–25 mg	0.5 mg/kg
Weight Conversion		
Weight in pounds/2.2 = kg		

Note: This list includes only selected medications (those commonly used). It should serve as a reference only and not as a guide for prescribing. In addition, most of the aforementioned drugs, although commonly used in clinical practice, are not FDA approved for treatment with children.

PREGNANCY AND PSYCHOTROPIC MEDICATIONS

Some of the most frequently asked questions about psychotropic medications concern their safety if they are taken during pregnancy. However, before specific discussion about particular medications, it is important to explain how information regarding safe drug use during pregnancy is obtained, because there are limits on how research in this area can be carried out.

HOW SAFETY IS DETERMINED

Much of the information about safe use during pregnancy comes from studies on animals. Although these studies are extensive, it cannot be assumed that the findings will necessarily apply to humans. Even if human studies are available, they are often not conducted among large numbers of people, so applying the results to the general population must be done cautiously. Therefore, it may be very difficult for your doctor to give you an absolute answer about whether a particular drug has been shown to be safe.

Some drugs are safer than others during pregnancy, while some other drugs should be avoided entirely. Still others are considered safe only during the second and third trimester and should not be given in the first trimester. Because the first trimester is the period when fetal cells are rapidly growing, dividing, and forming into organs, it is considered the time of highest risk for damage from medicines. However, organs, including the brain, continue to develop during the second and third trimesters and even after birth. Thus, some medicines could be potentially harmful to the baby throughout an entire pregnancy. Furthermore, these effects might be such that they might not be noticed until later in the child's life; for example, behavioral problems would not be apparent during infancy.

Keep in mind that women often do not realize they are pregnant until after conception has taken place and fetal development has begun. Therefore, before starting a new medication, it is important that your doctor is aware of any plans you may have for becoming pregnant in the near future. In this situation, you and your doctor might have to decide whether this is the best time for you to have a baby, and take into account what would happen if you didn't start a particular medicine right now. Obviously, this is a personal and complex issue, but women who wish to become pregnant and who may also require medications to treat depression face it frequently.

PREGNANCY, BREAST FEEDING, AND DRUGS				
CLASS OF MEDICATION	COMMENTS	TERATO-GENICITY	EFFECTS ON NEWBORN FROM EXPOSURE DURING PREGNANCY	FOUND IN BREAST MILK
Antidepressants	There is inconclusive data on whether the rate of miscarriages is increased with antidepressants. MAOIs, bupropion, and venlafaxine have not been studied widely in humans.	Not established	For tricyclic antidepressants, effects on the newborn can include drowsiness and difficulty urinating. For serotonin-type antidepressants, effects on the newborn can include restlessness and difficulty sleeping.	Yes, to a degree
Antipsychotics	Antipsychotics may be preferred over lithium for bipolar disorder during the first trimester. The lowest possible dose is recommended.	Not suspected	Low motor activity	Yes

			Suspected risk of spinal bifida	Yes
Anticonvulsants (valproic acid and carbamazepine)		All are known or suspected teratogens (producing fetal malformations).	Suspected risk of spinal bifida	Yes
Lithium	Historically, lithium use has not been advised during pregnancy. However, your doctor might consider lithium safer than anticonvulsants in the second and third trimester—with very close monitoring.	Known	Possible malformation of heart valve	Yes, to a high degree
Benzodiazepines	Avoid in first trimester.	Some are known teratogens.	Low motor activity Possible drug withdrawal	Yes

COMPLICATIONS OF PREGNANCY AND MEDICATION

Here is a brief summary of possible types of complications that may occur with medications taken during pregnancy:

- Teratogenesis: malformation of the fetus or fetal organs (this risk is greatest during the first trimester when organs are being formed)
- Increased risk of miscarriage
- Drug effects on the growth and development of the fetus
- Drug effects on labor and delivery
- Residual drug effects on the newborn
- Impact of pregnancy on the way a drug works
- Drug effects on the breast fed infant

BREAST FEEDING AND MEDICATIONS

Taking medicines while breast feeding can also be cause for concern. Knowledge in this area has increased dramatically in recent years, but many questions still remain unanswered. For the most part, when a medicine passes into breast milk, the concentration of the drug has been diluted in comparison with the amount in the mother's bloodstream. So even though the medication may be measurable in breast milk, it may produce no effects or minimal negative effects on the baby. Many medicines, therefore, have a relatively safe track record when taken by nursing mothers.

On the other hand, some medications can produce extreme negative effects on the baby even in small amounts, so their use should be avoided during breast feeding, e.g., cancer chemotherapy agents. Still other medicines reach a high enough concentration in breast milk to be of serious concern. Lithium, for example, is known to reach levels in breast milk equivalent in the baby's bloodstream to about 40 percent of that in the mother's bloodstream, which can lead to the potential for serious harm to the baby. It is strongly recommended that women taking lithium not breast feed (American Society of Health System Pharmacists 2004).

The table on pages 220–21 presents a brief summary, by drug category, of some known information about medications and pregnancy and breast feeding. Also see information about specific medications in Part Two. If you have any concerns about a specific drug, discuss them thoroughly with your doctor.

THE ELDERLY

The aging process is associated with the appearance of multiple medical conditions, most of which will likely be treated with one or more medications. This can result in the risk of serious drug–drug interactions. To avoid such complications, it is essential that the doctor has a full medical history and a complete list of current medicines (including over-the-counter drugs).

In the past, certain mental health conditions were often not identified and treated in the elderly. That trend has changed. For example, it has become apparent that depression is not a normal part of aging and that the elderly do not have to suffer with untreated depression. Consequently, the aged population is more likely than ever to be receiving a psychiatric medication. When these are combined with medicines for physical illness, the chance of unintended drug interactions further increases.

Another problem associated with aging is the difficult time many people have in adhering to their prescribed medicines. Forgetfulness is sometimes the reason, especially for those who live alone. Many other causes have been identified, such as incomplete understanding of the medicine, impaired vision or hearing, or purposely taking less to avoid side effects. Limited or fixed incomes may mean that elderly people cannot pay for their medication regularly, causing intermittent compliance.

Furthermore, many biological systems change as a result of aging. Decreases in kidney and liver function are expected in the elderly. These changes increase the chance that medications can accumulate to seriously high levels in the body. Total body fat increases with age, which affects how some drugs are stored in the body (see Chapter 4 for a discussion of drug distribution within the body). Also, older people sometimes neglect their nutritional and fluid requirements. Being undernourished or dehydrated can create problems for people taking certain medications, such as lithium.

Neurotransmitter systems are also likely to change as a result of aging. This means that older people have different responses to a given drug than do younger people. Usually, the change is in the direction of increased sensitivity to the medicine, which can mean that the average adult dose is likely to be too much for an older person. Extreme sensitivity to side effects occurs in the elderly. The side effects listed below are of particular concern for older people who are taking psychiatric medications:

SIDE EFFECTS IN THE ELDERLY

- Changes in mental functioning: impaired memory, decreased alertness, confusion, lethargy, slowed reaction times.
- Changes in heart rate and blood pressure: a drop in blood pressure can lead to light-headedness and dizziness with an end result of falls and fractures. Other factors can combine to further increase the risk of fall, for

instance, arthritic conditions that impede mobility and balance, or nighttime awakening with disorientation.
- Drying effects: constipation, dry mouth, blurred vision, urinary retention.
- Movement disorders: pacing, rigid arms and legs, problems with walking.

Most medical practitioners are aware of the general steps that can be taken to minimize some of these difficulties. In addition, the following precautions should be observed:

- Nonmedication treatments should be considered and maximized (e.g., psychotherapy, exercise).
- Dosages generally should be reduced.
- Side effects should be recognized and treated promptly.
- If problems arise, they should be communicated immediately to a health care provider.

In recent years, many articles have been published about the aging population. Not only is the percentage of people sixty-five years and older increasing, but the number of the "old-old" (over eighty-five years old) is also increasing. The challenges associated with adequate medical and psychiatric treatment of this age group will be great. There is, however, good cause for optimism. Today, geriatric medicine and geriatric psychiatry are established specialty areas. Undoubtedly, increasing research and attention to this age group will result in more comprehensive and compassionate care.

CHAPTER 12

Natural Remedies

Many people suffering from psychological symptoms may choose not to be treated with psychiatric medications, even if they have a disorder that would be responsive to them. There are several reasons why this may be the case. Topping the list are concerns regarding the safety of psychotropic medications. Although many of these drugs, as mentioned in previous chapters, are safe, the fact remains that all medications do have some side effects, so this is an understandable concern.

A second reason is that some people are allergic to, or intolerant of various psychiatric medications and are unable to take them.

A third reason is cost. Many of the older-generation medications are currently available in generic form, and the cost is minimal. Some newer medications that are better tolerated and less toxic are also available in generic form. However, some of the newest drugs are available only in brand-name formulation (i.e., not generic), and can be very expensive. For example, some people being treated with the newer antipsychotics may have to pay between $5 and $15 per day. This can be a financial hardship for many people, particularly those who live on fixed incomes. Finally, of course, matter of personal choice comes into play, as some folks simply prefer to use nonmedical approaches to psychological problems (e.g., psychotherapy).

Many of the approaches addressed in this chapter can be used as adjuncts to medication treatment and/or psychotherapy. In fact, several of them are strongly recommended because of their track record of effectiveness in enhancing psychological wellness, especially physical exercise and techniques designed to improve sleep.

SLEEP: THE ROYAL ROAD TO MENTAL HEALTH

If one could identify the single most common stress symptom, seen in almost all types of psychiatric disorders, it would be sleep disturbance. Sleep is an incredibly important biological function. It is essential to restoring and maintaining both emotional and physical health. However, it is quite fragile and is prone to disruption by a host of factors. In the past three decades a significant amount of research has been accomplished in an attempt to understand more about sleep. Though much has been learned, much about the function of sleep is still mysterious.

What is clearly known is that sleep deprivation does a lot more than simply contribute to daytime drowsiness. With even a couple of nights of significantly disrupted sleep, most people will experience noticeable problems in thinking—in particular, an impaired ability to maintain attention and concentration. Most also will show signs of decreased emotional control. Sleep deprivation dramatically alters brain chemistry. Presumably, the ability of certain brain areas to regulate emotions becomes compromised; the result is increased emotional sensitivity, poor tolerance for frustration, and stronger emotional reactions (e.g., fearfulness or irritability). Thus, almost all psychiatric disorders are made a lot worse by a sleep disturbance. In addition, even a couple of nights of very poor sleep have been shown to have an adverse impact on the immune system and may be responsible for increased risk of infectious illnesses, such as colds or the flu. And, of course, there is daytime fatigue and drowsiness.

One of the most helpful things a person can do when experiencing any type of emotional distress is to improve the quality of sleep. When we suggest this to our clients, they often dismiss the advice. It seems like a trivial concern to them, especially when compared with the serious life events that are currently plaguing them. But we want to underscore how much disturbed sleep can contribute to emotional suffering and, conversely, how much enhanced sleep can be a direct way to improve emotional functioning. Guidelines to improve sleep are detailed in Chapter 9.

INFLUENCING SEROTONIN LEVELS IN THE BRAIN

In previous chapters we discussed the role of serotonin and its influence in various emotional disorders (e.g., depression, obsessive-compulsive disorder, and panic disorder). As you may have noticed, serotonin has also received a good deal of media attention. What's all the hype about serotonin?

Serotonin appears to be a sort of multipurpose stabilizing neurotransmitter. It functions in many parts of the brain to inhibit neuron firing, and it acts as a kind of braking mechanism, helping to regulate the internal chemical environment of the brain. In humans and other mammals, if serotonin levels are increased, aggression and irritability decrease. If serotonin is increased, it also decreases the likelihood of panic attacks. Furthermore, people suffering from major depression often recover when their serotonin levels are increased.

Certainly, one way to increase serotonin activity in the brain is to take antidepressants that have an impact on the serotonin system (i.e., the SSRIs, such as Prozac or Lexapro).

There may be nonpharmacologic ways of increasing serotonin, too. Some research supports the notion that the following activities may result in an increase in serotonin (Norden 1995):

- Exposure to bright light.
- Repetitive muscular movements. This may include such diverse activities as walking, knitting, chewing gum, or rocking in a rocking chair. Isn't it interesting how these activities are often experienced as relaxing or soothing? Have you ever wondered why rocking a crying baby can be so calming?
- Strenuous physical exercise.
- Eating a snack that contains complex carbohydrates (such as whole-grain bread or oatmeal). This may help to facilitate the absorption of amino acids into the brain, which is necessary for the production of neurotransmitters like serotonin.
- Crying *may* increase serotonin, although this is just speculation.
- Experiencing mastery.

Studies with monkeys have shown that if a new monkey is introduced into an established troop of monkeys, its initial serotonin levels will be either in the average range or somewhat below average. However, if this monkey establishes dominance and succeeds in becoming the dominant monkey, its serotonin levels increase.

Similarly, serotonin levels measured in college students have been found to be higher in those who were leaders or excelled in athletics. There is, of course, an interesting question here: What comes first—dominance and mastery or high serotonin levels? Current speculation holds that it can go either way: those with already high serotonin may be more likely to succeed. However, it may also be that as people—or monkeys for that matter—learn and practice how to be more assertive, powerful, or effective, these experiences may affect the brain by increasing serotonin levels.

"HEALTH FOODS" AND HERBS

For many years, vitamins, minerals, and other food supplements have been advocated as treatments for psychiatric symptoms. These recommendations were derived from the knowledge that many important brain chemicals (that is, neurotransmitters such as serotonin and norepinephrine) are produced in the brain and must use amino acids as their chemical building blocks.

Also, it has been discovered that some fairly rare psychiatric disorders can be caused by severe vitamin deficiencies (one example is Korsakoff's syndrome, which is most commonly seen in people with a history of severe alcoholism who suffer from malnutrition and vitamin B_1 deficiency). In the 1960s and 1970s, there was great hope that psychiatric disorders could be helped by treatment with megadoses of vitamins and improved diet. The results, however, have been disappointing. Such approaches aimed at treating schizophrenia and major depression have failed to produce the desired effects, and they have been successful only in the cases of Korsakoff's syndrome and other very rare diseases.

Although amino acids, such as tyrosine and tryptophan, and vitamins are important for the healthy functioning of the brain, it appears that almost everyone who eats a reasonably healthy diet receives ample supplies of these essential chemicals. Furthermore, even though a person might ingest large amounts of such supplements, these molecules have only a very limited capacity to enter the brain and thus have little if any impact on brain functioning. The one exception is 5-HTP, a precursor to serotonin. Some studies have shown 5-HTP to have antidepressant actions. It is important to be careful, because very high doses of vitamins have sometimes produced serious side effects and toxicity.

Typically, health food supplements are rarely subjected to carefully controlled research. In most instances, reports of "successful treatment" with vitamins and amino acids are only anecdotal and are not clearly substantiated by scientific research. Because most of these products are not regulated by the Food and Drug Administration, their strength and purity vary tremendously, and adequate studies that examine potential drug–drug interactions are rare. Thus, questions remain regarding the safety of these products. Still, despite the absence of solid research, health food supplements continue to be purchased by people seeking relief from emotional suffering.

Recent times, however, have seen the emergence of four products considered to be health food supplements that do appear to have some promise.

MELATONIN

Melatonin is a naturally produced hormone that is manufactured in the brain by the pineal gland. It is believed to play a role in regulating the circadian rhythm and sleep cycles in human beings and numerous other animals. It has received a good deal of media attention during the past few years, primarily as a treatment for sleep disorders.

Unlike many other so-called health foods, melatonin has been the subject of numerous research studies in the past twenty-five years. It does appear to have useful applications in the treatment of some sleep disorders, primarily jet lag and sleep problems caused by changing work-and-sleep schedules, as seen in shift workers. It must be stated, however, that the use of melatonin should still be considered experimental, and anyone considering taking this preparation should speak to his or her physician or pharmacist first. There have been indications that melatonin in high doses (e.g., 3 to 5 mg) *may* aggravate depression. Thus, at this time, high doses of melatonin are not advised to be taken by people who suffer from depression. Finally, there is a significant unknown; it is very unclear how melatonin interacts with other prescription medications. Until more research is done, this hormone should be taken with caution.

ST. JOHN'S WORT

Another preparation that has been subject to a lot of media attention is St. John's wort (the Latin name is *Hypericum perforatum*). This herbal treatment is derived from the flowers of the hypericum plant. It has been used in Germany during the past twenty years primarily to treat depression. The precise way that hypericum works is not known, but there is speculation that it increases the levels of serotonin, norepinephrine, and dopamine in the brain. St. John's wort, unlike most other herbal remedies, has been the subject of a fair amount of research. In two reviews of the literature, it has been shown to be effective in relieving symptoms of depression in those suffering from mild to moderate depression (Whiskey et al. 2001, Roder et al. 2004).

St. John's wort has few side effects and is generally well tolerated. Reports indicate that the time required for symptomatic improvement to become apparent may be longer than that for standard antidepressants (which sometimes require six weeks or more of treatment before the onset of positive effects). The drug, however, does not appear to be effective in treating severe depression, and, at the time of this writing, no long-term treatment studies are available.

St. John's wort may prove to be safe and useful for treating mild to moderate depression. However, it too must be considered an experimental treatment for the time being. Adverse drug-drug interactions can occur with St. John's wort; sometimes such interactions can be dangerous. Taken alone, St. John's wort is considered to be safe, but since it can interact in negative ways with some prescription drugs, anyone considering taking it should consult with their physician or pharmacist.

OMEGA-3 FATTY ACIDS

Omega-3 fatty acids were discussed in Chapter 6. This product, derived from fish oil, flax, or walnut oil, has been found to be an effective *adjunct* to standard psychiatric medications in the treatment of bipolar disorder. Some studies also show its efficacy in treating unipolar depression. At doses of 1–2 grams per day it is well tolerated and generally side-effect free.

SAM-e

SAM-e is the newest in over-the-counter products for the treatment of depression. This preparation is a naturally occurring chemical that facilitates several biochemical reactions in the body. It has been used in Europe for many years and does have some research support for the treatment of mild and moderately severe depression. Because of its very favorable side effect profile, SAM-e may be a viable alternative for the treatment of depression. However, it should be considered an experimental treatment until more research is conducted.

TWO CAUTIONARY NOTES

Since the FDA does not regulate the production of these over-the-counter preparations, consumers need to be careful when purchasing such remedies. According to several reports, some supplements contain contaminates. There are two regulatory agencies that evaluate herbal and other over-the-counter medications for purity. These organizations do not test for efficacy but do evaluate for the presence of contaminates, such as mercury, which has been found in some fish oil preparations. Look for one of these two seals on product labels to assure that they have undergone such testing: USP (United States Pharmacopeia) or NSF (National Sleep Foundation).

One final concern about health foods and supplements is that their availability as over-the-counter products can cause people to bypass the critical step of obtaining an accurate and thorough diagnosis from a trained professional. As indicated in several chapters of this book, many psychiatric disorders are best treated by a combination of medication and psychotherapy. The over-the-counter status of these products may lead some people to believe that depression, for instance, can be treated simply by a trip to the health food store. Potentially, psychotherapy could be ignored in favor of "natural" treatment with herbal remedies. The profoundly positive and often life-changing impact of psychotherapy would then be tragically absent from a person's attempts at a complete recovery.

PART TWO

A GUIDE TO PSYCHIATRIC DRUGS

NOTE

Most medications used to treat psychiatric disorders are FDA approved only for adults and older adolescents. However, many of these medications are used in the treatment of children and younger teenagers. This is referred to as "off label" use and is considered to be legal and ethical, despite the lack of FDA approval. There are exceptions: most notably, medications used to treat ADHD. The dosages for children depend on a number of factors, including the child's age and weight. Also it should be noted that prior to puberty, young bodies metabolize medications at a rate that is more rapid than adults. For this reason it is not uncommon for some children to be given doses that approach those used with adults. In most instances, there are not well established doses for children. Each child must be evaluated independently and generally started on a low dose of a medication, with the dose being raised if necessary and if tolerated. For these reasons childhood dosing guidelines are not listed here, unless the particular drug is FDA approved for use in children.

If you want information about a particular medication and you have only the brand name, see **Appendix 1** (pages 519–22) for a cross reference of brand names and generics.

ALPRAZOLAM (al-PRAZ-o-lam)

Drug Category: Antianxiety medicine

Requires prescription, controlled substance, moderate potential for abuse

COMMONLY USED BRAND-NAME PRODUCTS

Tablets
Xanax (and generic) 0.25mg, 0.5mg, 1mg, 2mg
Tablets, extended release
Xanax XR (and generic) 0.5mg, 1mg, 2mg, 3mg
Solution
(generic) 1mg/ml
Tablets, oral disintegrating
Niravam 0.25mg, 0.5mg, 1mg, 2mg

GENERAL INFORMATION

Used to treat anxiety and panic disorder. *This medicine is not intended to help with the stress of everyday life. Even when taken as prescribed, alprazolam may cause psychological and/or physical dependence.*

BEFORE TAKING THIS MEDICATION

Talk to your doctor about the benefits and risks associated with alprazolam. Make sure you understand how to take it safely and effectively. You and your family members should be very familiar with the side effects and signs of having too much in your system. Make sure your doctor has the following information in detail:

- Any allergic or bad reactions you have had to alprazolam or any other medication

- All prescription and over-the-counter medicines you are taking
- Your complete medical history, including mental health conditions
- If you are pregnant, could be pregnant, or are planning a pregnancy in the near future, alprazolam should not be taken
- If you are breast feeding, alprazolam can pass into breast milk and affect the baby

USUAL ADULT DOSAGE RANGE
Anxiety: 0.25–0.5 mg up to three times a day.
Panic disorder: 0.5–2mg up to four times a day. The extended release tablet form is given once daily.
Older adults are more susceptible to side effects and will generally require lower dosages.

DIRECTIONS FOR PROPER USE
- *Take exactly as prescribed. Do not take more or less than prescribed. Alprazolam levels that are too high can cause serious toxicity.*
- If you take alprazolam regularly for an extended period of time, do not stop taking it unless told to do so by your doctor. It may be necessary to gradually reduce the dose before stopping completely. If the medicine is stopped too quickly, your condition could become worse, or you could experience serious effects, such as seizures.
- May be taken with food to decrease stomach upset.
- If you miss a dose of the regular tablet form, take it as soon as possible. However, if the missed dose is within 4 hours of your next dose, skip the missed dose and resume with your next scheduled dose. Do not double the dose.
- If you are taking the long acting tablet form and you miss a dose, take it as soon as possible. However, if it is close to

the time of your next scheduled dose, skip the missed dose and resume with your next scheduled dose. Do not double the dose. Do not crush, chew, or break the tablets.

- If you are taking the liquid form, measure the dose in the dropper provided. Mix the medicine in water, soda, applesauce, or pudding immediately before taking your dose. Do not save any of the unused mixture for later.

- If you are taking the oral disintegrating form, place the tablet in your mouth, allow it to dissolve, and swallow. Water is not required. Keep the tablets in the original package until right before you take a tablet. Any rapidly dissolving tablets that have been exposed to air should be discarded.

PRECAUTIONS

- Alprazolam can cause drowsiness and slowed reaction times. Be cautious when driving, operating machinery, or doing jobs requiring alertness.

- Alcohol can cause extreme drowsiness when taken with alprazolam. *Alcohol should be avoided while taking alprazolam.*

SIDE EFFECTS

Not all side effects will occur. Many side effects will diminish with time. *However, some side effects may be warning signs of toxicity and will require attention from your doctor.* Check with your doctor immediately if you experience any of the following:

- Confusion, severe drowsiness, slurred speech, severe weakness, unusual thoughts, shortness of breath, excitement, hyperactivity, memory problems

Some side effects appear when you first start taking alprazolam and go away for most people. If the following side effects continue, contact your doctor:

- Dizziness, lightheadedness, drowsiness, blurred vision, stomach problems

DRUG INTERACTIONS

Alprazolam can adversely interact with the following frequently prescribed medications or foods:

- Cimetidine (Tagamet)—can cause high alprazolam levels
- Disulfiram (Antabuse)—can cause high alprazolam levels
- Birth control pills—can cause high alprazolam levels
- Levodopa—decreased effectiveness of levodopa
- Macrolide antibiotics (e.g., erythromycin)—can cause high alprazolam levels
- Oral antifungal agents—can cause high alprazolam levels
- HIV protease inhibitors—can cause high alprazolam levels
- Calcium channel blockers—can cause high alprazolam levels
- Serotonin-type antidepressants—can cause high alprazolam levels
- Digoxin—alprazolam can cause high digoxin levels
- Valproic acid—can cause high alprazolam levels
- Isoniazid—can cause high alprazolam levels
- Beta blockers—can cause high alprazolam levels
- Propoxyphene—can cause high alprazolam levels
- Carbamazepine—can lower alprazolam levels
- Grapefruit juice—can cause high alprazolam levels
- Drugs that depress certain functions of the nervous system, when combined with alprazolam, cause extreme drowsiness and slowed reaction times. Examples of these medicines are antihistamines, narcotics, muscle relaxants, and barbiturates.

MEDICAL CONSIDERATIONS

If you have any of the following medical conditions, make sure your doctor is aware of it.

- Liver disease or alcoholism—alprazolam levels may be higher than expected
- Kidney disease—alprazolam levels may be higher than expected
- Drug or alcohol dependence—dependence on alprazolam may occur
- Seizure disorder—stopping alprazolam abruptly may cause seizures
- Chronic lung disease—alprazolam can possibly make breathing more difficult
- Glaucoma—alprazolam may worsen your condition
- Sleep apnea—alprazolam may worsen your condition

AMITRIPTYLINE (am-ee-TRIP-tih-leen)
Drug Category: Antidepressant, tricyclic
Requires prescription

COMMONLY USED BRAND-NAME PRODUCTS
Tablets
Elavil (and generic) 10mg, 25mg, 50mg, 75mg, 100mg, 150mg

GENERAL INFORMATION
Used to treat major depression and the depressed phase of bipolar disorder. Because of its sedative effects, it is sometimes given in low doses to help with insomnia. It is also used to treat certain chronic pain disorders, such as migraine headache and diabetic neuropathy.

BEFORE TAKING THIS MEDICATION
Talk to your doctor about the benefits and risks associated with amitriptyline. Make sure you understand how to take it

safely and effectively. You and your family members should be very familiar with the side effects and signs of having too much in your system. Make sure your doctor has the following information in detail:

- Any allergic or bad reactions you have had to amitriptyline or any other medication
- All prescription and over-the-counter medicines you are taking
- Your complete medical history
- If you are pregnant, could be pregnant, or are planning a pregnancy in the near future, amitriptyline should not be taken
- If you are breast feeding, amitriptyline can pass into breast milk and affect the baby

USUAL ADULT DOSAGE RANGE

The starting dose of amitriptyline will be low and gradually be increased. Sometimes blood levels are tested to ensure that the dose you are taking is in the safe and effective range.

Depression: Starting dose 25–50mg at bedtime. Increased to 75–300 mg at bedtime over 2–3 weeks.

Insomnia: 10–50mg at bedtime

Chronic pain syndrome: 50–100mg daily.

Older adults are more susceptible to side effects and will generally require lower dosages.

DIRECTIONS FOR PROPER USE

- *Take exactly as prescribed. Do not take more or less than prescribed. Accidental or intended overdoses of amitriptyline are potentially fatal.*
- Do not abruptly stop taking amitriptyline unless instructed to do so by your doctor. Gradually reducing the dose can help prevent mood changes, headache, or diarrhea.

- If you miss a bedtime dose, do not take it the next morning, since it may make you drowsy. Do not double doses.
- It may take several weeks before you feel the full benefits.

PRECAUTIONS

- Amitriptyline can cause drowsiness and slowed reaction times. Be cautious when driving, operating machinery, or doing jobs requiring alertness.
- Alcohol can cause changes in mood and may interfere with amitriptyline's effectiveness. Alcohol can cause extreme drowsiness when taken with amitriptyline. *Alcohol should be avoided while taking amitriptyline.*
- Amitriptyline may cause your skin and eyes to be more sensitive to sunlight. Exposure to sunlight may cause a rash, skin discoloration, or sunburn. Limit direct exposure to sunlight, and use sunscreen when in direct sunlight. Avoid tanning booths and beds. Wear UV blocking sunglasses when outdoors.
- When taking amitriptyline, stand up slowly after sitting or lying down, since it may cause your blood pressure to drop and cause faintness or dizziness. Stand up slowly from a seated or lying position, especially when you first start taking amitriptyline.
- *Antidepressants may increase the risk of suicidal thinking and behavior in adolescents and children. When considering an antidepressant in a child or adolescent, the risk must be balanced with the need. Children and adolescents taking antidepressants should be closely monitored for worsening of symptoms, suicidality, or unusual changes in behavior.*
- Adolescents and children may be more susceptible to heart-related side effects of tricyclic antidepressants. Risk must be

balanced with need. Blood levels and heart function should be monitored in children and adolescents taking tricyclic antidepressants.

SIDE EFFECTS

Not all side effects will occur. Many side effects will diminish with time. *However, some side effects may require attention from your doctor.* Check with your doctor immediately if you experience any of the following:

- Seizure, changes in blood pressure, irregular heart rate, shortness of breath, problems with urination (difficult or painful urination, unable to urinate), confusion, extreme sedation, excitation or mania, increased skin sensitivity to sunlight, extreme constipation, yellow skin or eyes

Some side effects appear when you first start taking amitriptyline and go away for most people. If the following side effects continue, contact your doctor.

- Dizziness, blurred vision, dry mouth, mild to moderate constipation, increased appetite, weight gain, breast enlargement (men or women), discharge from the breast, sexual problems, tremor of the hands, persistent sore throat

DRUG INTERACTIONS

Amitriptyline can adversely interact with the following frequently prescribed medications:

- Cimetidine—can cause high amitriptyline levels
- SSRI antidepressants—can cause high amitriptyline levels
- MAOI antidepressants—severe reaction causing dangerously high blood pressure, high body temperature, seizures, or death
- Clonidine—if clonidine is being taken for high blood pressure, amitriptyline may cause clonidine to work less well
- Antipsychotics—may increase certain neurologic side effects

- Thyroid hormones—increased effects of both, especially excitation and changes in heart rate or rhythm
- Carbamazepine—can lower amitriptyline levels
- Bupropion—can increase amitriptyline levels
- Anticoagulants (blood thinners)—the effect of the anticoagulant can be increased
- Quinolones—increased risk of heart arrhythmias
- Amphetamines—increased blood pressure, irregular heart rate, or very high fever may result
- Drugs used during surgery—can cause increased blood pressure. Make sure your doctors are aware of upcoming planned surgeries.
- Drugs that depress certain functions of the nervous system, when combined with amitriptyline, cause extreme drowsiness and slowed reaction times: Examples of these medicines are antihistamines, narcotics, muscle relaxants, and barbiturates.

MEDICAL CONSIDERATIONS

If you have any of the following medical conditions, make sure your doctor is aware of it.

- Liver disease or alcoholism—amitriptyline levels may be higher than expected
- Kidney disease—amitriptyline levels may be higher than expected
- Glaucoma—amitriptyline can increase pressure inside the eye
- Heart problems—some heart problems can be made worse by amitriptyline; amitriptyline should not be taken by someone who has had a recent heart attack
- Urinary retention, prostate enlargement—urination may become more difficult
- Seizure disorder—amitriptyline can lower seizure threshold

- Diabetes mellitus (sugar diabetes)—blood sugar levels may be affected
- Thyroid disorders—amitriptyline may cause increased heart rate

AMOXAPINE (am-OX-uh-peen)
Drug Category: Antidepressant, tricyclic
Requires prescription

COMMONLY USED BRAND-NAME PRODUCTS
Tablets
Asendin (and generic) 25mg, 50mg, 100mg, 150mg

GENERAL INFORMATION
Used to treat major depression and the depressed phase of bipolar disorder.

BEFORE TAKING THIS MEDICATION
Talk to your doctor about the benefits and risks associated with amoxapine. Make sure you understand how to take it safely and effectively. You and your family members should be very familiar with the side effects and signs of having too much in your system. Make sure your doctor has the following information in detail:
- Any allergic or bad reactions you have had to amoxapine or any other medication
- All prescription and over-the-counter medicines you are taking
- Your complete medical history
- If you are pregnant, could be pregnant, or are planning a pregnancy in the near future, amoxapine should not be taken

- If you are breast feeding, amoxapine can pass into breast milk and affect the baby

USUAL ADULT DOSAGE RANGE

The starting dose of amoxapine will be low and will gradually be increased. Sometimes blood levels are tested to ensure that the dose you are taking is in the safe and effective range.

Adults: Starting dose is 50mg at bedtime, and is increased to 150–300mg at bedtime over 2–3 weeks.

Older adults are more susceptible to side effects and will generally require lower dosages.

DIRECTIONS FOR PROPER USE

- *Take exactly as prescribed. Do not take more or less than prescribed. Accidental or intended overdoses of amoxapine are potentially fatal.*
- Do not abruptly stop taking amoxapine unless instructed to do so by your doctor. Gradually reducing the dose can help prevent mood changes, headache, or diarrhea.
- If you miss a bedtime dose, do not take it the next morning, since it may make you drowsy. Do not double doses.
- It may take several weeks before you feel the full benefits.

PRECAUTIONS

- Amoxapine can cause drowsiness and slowed reaction times. Be cautious when driving, operating machinery, or doing jobs requiring alertness.
- Alcohol can cause changes in mood and may interfere with amoxapine's effectiveness. *Alcohol should be avoided when taking amoxapine.*
- Amoxapine may cause your skin and eyes to be more sensitive to sunlight. Exposure to sunlight may cause a rash, skin discoloration, or sunburn. Limit direct exposure to sunlight, and use sunscreen when in direct sunlight. Avoid

tanning booths and beds. Wear UV blocking sunglasses when outdoors.

- When taking amoxapine, stand up slowly after sitting or lying down, since it may cause your blood pressure to drop and cause faintness or dizziness. Stand up slowly from a seated or lying position, especially when you first start taking amoxapine.

- *Antidepressants may increase the risk of suicidal thinking and behavior in adolescents and children. When considering an antidepressant in a child or adolescent, the risk must be balanced with the need. Children and adolescents taking antidepressants should be closely monitored for worsening of symptoms, suicidality, or unusual changes in behavior.*

- Adolescents and children may be more susceptible to heart-related side effects of tricyclic antidepressants. Risk must be balanced with need. Blood levels and heart function should be monitored in children and adolescents taking tricyclic antidepressants.

SIDE EFFECTS

Not all side effects will occur. Many side effects will diminish with time. *However, some side effects may require attention from your doctor.* Check with your doctor immediately if you experience any of the following:

- Seizure, changes in blood pressure, irregular heart rate, shortness of breath, problems with urination (difficult or painful urination, unable to urinate), confusion, extreme sedation, excitation or mania, increased skin sensitivity to sunlight, extreme constipation, yellow skin or eyes
- Lip puckering; lip smacking; uncontrolled movements of the tongue; uncontrolled movements of the hands, arms, or legs; difficulty walking; rigid or stiff muscles; fever

Some side effects appear when you first start taking amoxapine and go away for most people. If the following side effects continue, contact your doctor.

- Dizziness, blurred vision, dry mouth, mild to moderate constipation, increased appetite, weight gain, breast enlargement (men or women), discharge from the breast, sexual problems, tremor of the hands, persistent sore throat

DRUG INTERACTIONS

Amoxapine can adversely interact with the following frequently prescribed medications:

- Cimetidine—can cause high amoxapine levels
- SSRI antidepressants—can cause high amoxapine levels
- MAOI antidepressants—severe reaction causing dangerously high blood pressure, high body temperature, seizures, or death
- Clonidine—if clonidine is being taken for high blood pressure, amoxapine may cause clonidine to work less well
- Antipsychotics—may increase certain neurologic side effects
- Thyroid hormones—increased effects of both, especially excitation and changes in heart rate or rhythm
- Carbamazepine—can lower amoxapine levels
- Bupropion—can increase amoxapine levels
- Anticoagulants (blood thinners)—the effect of the anticoagulant can be increased
- Quinolones—increased risk of heart arrhythmias
- Amphetamines—increased blood pressure, irregular heart rate, or very high fever may result
- Drugs used during surgery—can cause increased blood pressure. Make sure your doctors are aware of upcoming planned surgeries.

- Drugs that depress certain functions of the nervous system when combined with amoxapine, cause extreme drowsiness and slowed reaction times. Examples of these medicines are antihistamines, narcotics, muscle relaxants, and barbiturates.

MEDICAL CONSIDERATIONS

If you have any of the following medical conditions, make sure your doctor is aware of it.

- Liver disease, or alcoholism—amoxapine levels may be higher than expected
- Kidney disease—amoxapine levels may be higher than expected
- Glaucoma—amoxapine can increase pressure inside the eye
- Heart problems—some heart problems can be made worse by amoxapine; amoxapine should not be taken by someone who has had a recent heart attack
- Urinary retention, prostate enlargement—urination may become more difficult
- Seizure disorder—amoxapine can lower seizure threshold
- Diabetes mellitus (sugar diabetes)—blood sugar levels may be affected
- Thyroid disorders—amoxapine may cause increased heart rate

AMPHETAMINE (am-FET-a-meen)

Drug Category: Stimulant

Requires prescription, controlled substance, high potential for abuse, requires special prescription (triplicate, nonrefillable)

COMMONLY USED BRAND-NAME PRODUCTS

Amphetamine tablets
5mg, 10mg
Dextroamphetamine
Dexedrine (and generic) tablets 5mg, 10mg
Dexedrine long-acting capsules 5mg, 10mg, 15mg
Methamphetamine
Desoxyn tablets 5mg
Desoxyn long-acting tablets 5mg, 10mg, 15mg
Amphetamine mixture
Adderall (and generic) tablets 5mg, 7.5mg, 10mg, 12.5mg, 15mg, 20mg, 30mg
Adderall XR extended-release capsules 5mg, 10mg, 15mg, 20mg, 25mg, 30mg
Lisdexamfetamine
Vyvanse capsules 30mg, 50mg, 70mg

GENERAL INFORMATION

Used to treat attention deficit hyperactivity disorder, as part of a total program that includes psychological, educational, and social components. Amphetamines are sometimes used in the treatment of major depression in select patients when traditional antidepressants cannot be used.

BEFORE TAKING THIS MEDICATION

Talk to your doctor about the benefits and risks associated with amphetamines. Make sure you understand how to take it safely and effectively. You and your family members should be very familiar with the side effects and signs of having too much in your system. Make sure your doctor has the following information in detail:

- Any allergic or bad reactions you have had to amphetamines or any other medication

- All prescription and over-the-counter medicines you are taking
- Your complete medical history
- If you are pregnant, could be pregnant, or are planning a pregnancy in the near future, amphetamines should not be taken
- If you are breast feeding, amphetamines can pass into breast milk and affect the baby

DOSAGE

Adults and children over 6: Dosages are highly individualized, depending on response, age, and dosage form. For regular tablets, dosages can range from 5 to 20mg, at intervals of two to three times daily. For long-acting products, dosages can range from 10 to 70mg daily, at intervals of one to two times daily.

Older adults are more susceptible to side effects and will generally require lower dosages.

DIRECTIONS FOR PROPER USE

- *Take exactly as prescribed. Do not take more or less than prescribed. Accidental or intended overdoses of amphetamines are very serious.*
- If you take amphetamines regularly for an extended period of time, do not stop taking it unless told to do so by your doctor. It may be necessary to gradually reduce the dose before stopping completely.
- If you miss a dose of the regular tablets, take it as soon as possible, unless it is within 3 hours of your next scheduled dose; then skip the missed dose and resume with your next scheduled dose. If you miss a dose of the long-acting tablets, skip the dose and resume with your next scheduled dose.
- To prevent trouble sleeping, do not take the last dose later

than 6 pm for regular tablets and 3 pm for long-acting forms, unless otherwise directed by your doctor.

- If you are taking a long-acting form, swallow it whole; do not crush, chew or break. Some long-acting capsules can be sprinkled over food; make sure you are aware of how to take the particular medication prescribed for you.

- Treatment with these medications may last for months to years. Your doctor may discuss the option of "drug holidays." These are planned periods of time when you may not take the medicine—for example, during summer holidays from school.

PRECAUTIONS

- Amphetamines can mask some of the effects of alcohol. Routine alcohol use or alcohol withdrawal can increase the chance of seizures, as can amphetamines. *Alcohol should be avoided while taking amphetamines.*

- Amphetamines may cause your skin and eyes to be more sensitive to sunlight. Exposure to sunlight may cause a rash, skin discoloration, or sunburn. Limit direct exposure to sunlight, and use sunscreen when in direct sunlight. Avoid tanning booths and beds. Wear UV blocking sunglasses when outdoors.

SIDE EFFECTS

Not all side effects will occur. Many side effects will diminish with time. *However, some side effects may be warning signs of toxicity and will require attention from your doctor.* Check with your doctor immediately if you experience any of the following:

- Seizures; increased blood pressure; fast or irregular heartbeat; shortness of breath; confusion; agitation; excitement or mania; persistent throbbing headache; muscle twitches; tics or movement problems; unusual behavior; depressed mood; soreness of the mouth, gums, or throat; skin rash or itching; swelling of the face; any unusual bruising or bleeding; appearance of splotchy purplish darkening of the skin; vomiting; fatigue; weakness; fever, flulike symptoms; yellow tinge of the eyes or skin; dark-colored urine

Some side effects appear when you first start taking amphetamines and go away for most people. If the following side effects continue, contact your doctor.

- Dizziness, nervousness, blurred vision, difficulty sleeping, decreased appetite, weight loss, headache, nausea, dry mouth

DRUG INTERACTIONS

Amphetamines can adversely interact with the following frequently prescribed medications:

- MAOI antidepressants—severe reaction causing dangerously high blood pressure, high body temperature, seizures, or death
- Other stimulant medications such as decongestants, diet pills, some asthma medications, caffeine—can worsen side effects, especially nervousness, insomnia, high blood pressure
- Serotonin-type antidepressants—can worsen side effects, especially nervousness, insomnia, high blood pressure
- Thyroid medications—amphetamines can increase effects of thyroid drugs
- Tricyclic antidepressants—increased blood pressure, irregular heart rate, or very high fever may result
- Beta blockers—high blood pressure or decreased heart rate may result
- Meperidine—extremely low blood pressure, slowed breathing, or very high fever may results

- Digoxin—additive effects on the heart resulting in irregular heartbeat

MEDICAL CONSIDERATIONS

If you have any of the following medical conditions, make sure your doctor is aware of it.

- Liver disease or alcoholism—amphetamine levels may be higher than expected
- Kidney disease—amphetamine levels may be higher than expected
- Drug or alcohol dependence—dependence on amphetamines may occur
- Seizure disorder—stopping amphetamines abruptly may cause seizures
- Heart problems—some heart problems can be worsened by amphetamines
- High blood pressure—amphetamines may increase blood pressure
- Glaucoma—amphetamines may worsen your condition
- Tourette's syndrome—amphetamines may worsen tics
- Hyperthyroidism—thyroid hormone levels may increase

ANTICHOLINERGIC/ ANTIDYSKINETIC

Requires prescription

COMMONLY USED BRAND-NAME PRODUCTS

Benztropine (Cogentin and generic)
Trihexyphenidyl (Artane and generic)
Amantadine (Symmetrel and generic)

GENERAL INFORMATION

Anticholinergics are used to treat side effects caused by other medicines, such as hand tremor or severe restlessness. They are also used to treat Parkinson's disease.

BEFORE TAKING THIS MEDICATION

Talk to your doctor about the benefits and risks associated with an anticholinergic. Your doctor will need to know your complete medical history before prescribing an anticholinergic. Your doctor or pharmacist will need to be aware of all medicines you take to avoid drug interactions. Make sure you understand how to take an anticholinergic. Do not take more or less than prescribed. Do not suddenly stop taking an anticholinergic unless directed by your doctor.

PRECAUTIONS

- *Alcohol should be avoided while taking an anticholinergic.*

SIDE EFFECTS

Not all side effects will occur. Many side effects will diminish with time. *However, some side effects may require attention from your doctor.* Check with your doctor immediately if you experience any of the following:

- Confusion, extreme dizziness or light-headedness, fast heartbeat, eye pain, difficulty urinating, difficulty swallowing, rash or itching, unusual excitement, extreme restlessness

Some side effects appear when you first start taking anticholinergic and go away for most people. If the following side effects continue, contact your doctor.

- Blurred vision, severe fatigue, dry mouth, flushing of the skin, constipation

ANTIHISTAMINE

Requires prescription, some over-the-counter

COMMONLY USED BRAND-NAME PRODUCTS

Diphenhydramine (Benadryl and generic)

Hydroxyzine (Atarax, Vistaril, and generic)

GENERAL INFORMATION

Antihistamines may help some people treat anxiety symptoms or insomnia. They are also used to treat allergic conditions.

BEFORE TAKING THIS MEDICATION

Talk to your doctor about the benefits and risks associated with an antihistamine. Your doctor will need to know your complete medical history before prescribing an antihistamine. Your doctor or pharmacist will need to be aware of all medicines you take to avoid drug interactions. Make sure you understand how to take an antihistamine. Do not take more or less than prescribed. Do not suddenly stop taking an antihistamine unless directed by your doctor.

PRECAUTIONS

- *Alcohol should be avoided while taking an antihistamine.*

SIDE EFFECTS

Not all side effects will occur. Many side effects will diminish with time. *However, some side effects may require attention from your doctor.* Check with your doctor immediately if you experience any of the following:

- Confusion, extreme dizziness or light-headedness, fast heartbeat, difficulty urinating, rash or itching, unusual excitement, extreme restlessness

Some side effects appear when you first start taking antihistamine and go away for most people. If the following side effects continue, contact your doctor.

• Blurred vision, severe fatigue, dry mouth, flushing of the skin, constipation

ARIPIPRAZOLE (air-uh-PIP-ra-zole)

Drug Category: Neuroleptic; Antipsychotic
Requires prescription

COMMONLY USED BRAND-NAME PRODUCTS

Tablets
Abilify 2mg, 5mg, 10mg, 15mg, 20mg, 30mg
Tablets, oral disintegrating
Abilify Discmelt 10mg, 15mg
Solution
Abilify 1mg/ml

GENERAL INFORMATION

Used to treat psychotic symptoms, such as hallucinations and delusions. These symptoms occur in schizophrenia, schizoaffective disorder, bipolar disorder, or major depression with psychotic features. Because of its mood-stabilizing properties, aripiprazole may be used in the treatment of bipolar disorder, especially acute manic episodes. For difficult-to-treat depression, it may be used in combination with an antidepressant. Aripiprazole can be used for short-term management of aggressive, out-of-control behaviors or feelings of anger and rage.

BEFORE TAKING THIS MEDICATION

Talk to your doctor about the benefits and risks associated with aripiprazole. Make sure you understand how to take it safely and effectively. You and your family members should be very familiar with its side effects. *Your doctor may periodically monitor your weight, blood pressure, blood sugar, and blood lipid levels while you are taking aripiprazole.* Make sure your doctor has the following information in detail:

- Any allergic or bad reactions you have had to aripiprazole or any other medication
- All prescription and over-the-counter medicines you are taking
- Your complete medical history
- If you are pregnant, could be pregnant, or are planning a pregnancy in the near future, aripiprazole has not been shown to be absolutely safe
- If you are breast feeding, aripiprazole can pass into breast milk and affect the baby

USUAL ADULT DOSAGE RANGE
Adults and adolescents: 5–30mg daily.
Older adults are *extremely* susceptible to side effects and will generally require lower dosages. *Should not be used in elderly patients to treat dementia-related psychosis or behavioral disturbances.*

DIRECTIONS FOR PROPER USE
- *Take exactly as prescribed. Do not take more or less than prescribed. Aripiprazole levels that are too high can cause serious toxicity.*
- If you miss a dose, take it as soon as possible. However, if the missed dose is within 4 hours of your next dose, skip the missed dose and resume with your next scheduled dose. Do not double the dose.
- If you are taking the oral disintegrating form, place the tablet in your mouth, allow it to dissolve, and swallow. Water is not required. Keep the tablets in the original package

until right before you take a tablet. Any rapidly dissolving tablets that have been exposed to air should be discarded.

- It may be several weeks before you feel the full benefits.

PRECAUTIONS

- Aripiprazole can cause drowsiness and slowed reaction times. Be cautious when driving, operating machinery, or doing jobs requiring alertness.
- Alcohol can cause extreme drowsiness when taken with aripiprazole. *Alcohol should be avoided while taking aripiprazole.*
- Aripiprazole may cause your body temperature to increase and could result in heat stroke. Be extra careful in hot weather, when exercising, or when taking hot baths or saunas not to become overheated.
- When taking aripiprazole, stand up slowly after sitting or lying down, since it may cause your blood pressure to drop and cause faintness or dizziness. Stand up slowly from a seated or lying position, especially when you first start taking aripiprazole.

SIDE EFFECTS

Not all side effects will occur. Many side effects will diminish with time. *However, some side effects may be warning signs of toxicity and will require attention from your doctor.* Check with your doctor immediately if you experience any of the following:

- Seizure; high fever; fast or irregular heartbeat; very low blood pressure; faintness; any abnormal movements of the mouth, tongue, neck, arms, or legs; difficulty speaking or swallowing; imbalance or difficulty walking normally; severe muscle stiffness; discoloration of the skin or eyes; confusion; significant drowsiness; restlessness; difficulty urinating; sexual problems; vomiting; diarrhea; unusual bruising or bleeding; serious skin reaction to sunlight (burning or blistering); severe constipation; breast pain or enlargement

Some side effects appear when you first start taking aripiprazole and go away for most people. If the following side effects continue, contact your doctor.

- Dry mouth, mild to moderate constipation, dizziness, hand tremor, stuffy nose, weight gain

DRUG INTERACTIONS

Aripiprazole can adversely interact with the following frequently prescribed medications or foods:

- Lithium—increased neurologic side effects
- Levodopa—decreased effectiveness of levodopa
- Amphetamines—increased psychotic symptoms are possible
- Anticonvulsants—decreased aripiprazole levels
- Tricyclic antidepressants—increased tricyclic antidepressant levels
- Macrolide antibiotics (e.g., erythromycin)—can cause high aripiprazole levels
- Oral antifungal agents—can cause high aripiprazole levels
- HIV protease inhibitors—can cause high aripiprazole levels
- Cimetidine—can cause high aripiprazole levels
- Serotonin-type antidepressants—can cause high aripiprazole levels
- Caffeine—can cause high aripiprazole levels
- Drugs that depress certain functions of the nervous system, when combined with aripiprazole, cause extreme drowsiness and slowed reaction times. Examples of these medicines are antihistamines, narcotics, muscle relaxants, and barbiturates.

MEDICAL CONSIDERATIONS

If you have any of the following medical conditions, make sure your doctor is aware of it:

- Kidney disease—aripiprazole levels may be higher than expected
- Liver disease—aripiprazole levels may be higher than expected
- Heart problems—some heart problems can be made worse by aripiprazole
- Seizure disorder—aripiprazole can lower seizure threshold
- Urinary retention, prostate enlargement—urination may be more difficult
- Glaucoma—aripiprazole can increase pressure inside the eye
- Parkinson's disease—some Parkinson's symptoms may be worsened
- Breast cancer—may increase risk of cancer progression
- Overweight/obesity—aripiprazole can cause weight gain
- Diabetes—aripiprazole can make this condition worse
- Elevated lipid (cholesterol and triglycerides) levels—aripiprazole can make this condition worse
- High blood pressure—aripiprazole can make this condition worse

ATOMOXETINE (a-tow-MOX-a-teen)

Drug Category: NRI (norepinephrine reuptake inhibitor)

Requires prescription

COMMONLY USED BRAND-NAME PRODUCTS

Capsules

Strattera 10mg, 18mg, 25mg, 40mg, 60mg, 80mg

GENERAL INFORMATION

Used to treat attention deficit hyperactivity disorder, as part of a total program that includes psychological, educational, and social components.

BEFORE TAKING THIS MEDICATION

Talk to your doctor about the benefits and risks associated with atomoxetine. Make sure you understand how to take it safely and effectively. You and your family members should be very familiar with the side effects and signs of having too much in your system. Make sure your doctor has the following information in detail:

- Any allergic or bad reactions you have had to atomoxetine or any other medication
- All prescription and over-the-counter medicines you are taking
- Your complete medical history
- If you are pregnant, could be pregnant, or are planning a pregnancy in the near future, atomoxetine should not be taken
- If you are breast feeding, atomoxetine can pass into breast milk and affect the baby

DOSAGE

Adults and children over 150 lbs: 40–80mg, one to two times daily. Dosages are highly individualized, depending on response.

Older adults are more susceptible to side effects and will generally require lower dosages.

DIRECTIONS FOR PROPER USE

- *Take exactly as prescribed. Do not take more or less than prescribed. Accidental or intended overdoses of atomoxetine are very serious.*

- If you take atomoxetine regularly for an extended period of time, do not stop taking it unless told to do so by your doctor. It may be necessary to gradually reduce the dose before stopping completely.
- If you miss a dose of the regular tablets, take it as soon as possible, unless it is within 3 hours of your next scheduled dose. Then, skip the missed dose and resume with your next scheduled dose. Do not double the dose.
- Treatment with these medications may last for months to years. Your doctor may discuss the option of "drug holidays." These are planned periods of time when you may not take the medicine—for example, during summer holidays from school.

PRECAUTIONS

- Atomoxetine can cause drowsiness and slowed reaction times. Be cautious when driving, operating machinery, or doing jobs requiring alertness.
- Alcohol can cause changes in mood and may interfere with atomoxetine's effectiveness. Alcohol can cause extreme drowsiness when taken with atomoxetine. *Alcohol should be avoided while taking atomoxetine.*
- *Atomoxetine may increase the risk of suicidal thinking and behavior in adolescents and children. When considering an antidepressant in a child or adolescent, the risk must be balanced with the need. Children and adolescents taking antidepressants should be closely monitored for worsening of symptoms, suicidality, or unusual changes in behavior.*

SIDE EFFECTS

Not all side effects will occur. Many side effects will diminish with time. *However, some side effects may be warning signs of toxicity and will require attention from your doctor.* Check with your doctor immediately if you experience any of the following:

- Seizures; increased blood pressure; fast or irregular heartbeat; shortness of breath; confusion; agitation; excitement or mania; persistent throbbing headache; muscle twitches; tics or movement problems; unusual behavior; depressed mood; soreness of the mouth, gums, or throat; skin rash or itching; swelling of the face; any unusual bruising or bleeding; appearance of splotchy purplish darkening of the skin; vomiting; fatigue; weakness; fever; flulike symptoms; yellow tinge of the eyes or skin; dark-colored urine

Some side effects appear when you first start taking atomoxetine and go away for most people. If the following side effects continue, contact your doctor.

- Dizziness, nervousness, blurred vision, difficulty sleeping, decreased appetite, weight loss, headache, nausea, dry mouth

DRUG INTERACTIONS
Atomoxetine can adversely interact with the following frequently prescribed medications:

- MAOI antidepressants—severe reaction causing dangerously high blood pressure, high body temperature, seizures, or death
- Serotonin-type antidepressants—can worsen side effects, especially nervousness, insomnia, high blood pressure
- Tricyclic antidepressants—increased blood pressure, irregular heart rate, or very high fever may result
- Albuterol—increased excitatory side effects (heart rate, tremor)
- Antiarrhythmics or other drugs that can affect the heartbeat—when taken with atomoxetine can cause serious disturbances of heart rhythm

- Drugs that depress certain functions of the nervous system, when combined with atomoxetine, cause extreme drowsiness and slowed reaction times. Examples of these medicines are antihistamines, narcotics, muscle relaxants, and barbiturates.

MEDICAL CONSIDERATIONS

If you have any of the following medical conditions, make sure your doctor is aware of it.

- Liver disease or alcoholism—atomoxetine levels may be higher than expected
- Kidney disease—atomoxetine levels may be higher than expected
- Seizure disorder—stopping atomoxetine abruptly may cause seizures
- Heart problems—some heart problems can be worsened by atomoxetine
- High blood pressure—atomoxetine may increase blood pressure
- Glaucoma—atomoxetine may worsen your condition

BETA BLOCKER

Requires prescription

COMMONLY USED BRAND-NAME PRODUCTS

Atenolol (Tenormin and generic)
Metoprolol (Lopressor and generic)
Nadolol (Corgard and generic)
Pindolol (Visken)
Propranolol (Inderal and generic)

GENERAL INFORMATION

Beta blockers are used to help relieve certain symptoms of panic disorder, such as increased heart rate. They also can be used to treat side effects resulting from other medicines, such as hand tremor and severe restlessness, and they sometimes are used to relieve severe anxiety symptoms associated with stressful situations like public speaking. Beta blockers are primarily used to treat a variety of conditions such as high blood pressure, irregular heart rate, and heart disease.

BEFORE TAKING THIS MEDICATION

Talk to your doctor about the benefits and risks associated with a beta blocker. Your doctor will need to know your complete medical history before prescribing a beta blocker. Your doctor or pharmacist will need to be aware of all medicines that you take to avoid drug interactions. Make sure you understand how to take a beta blocker. Do not take more or less than prescribed. Do not suddenly stop taking a beta blocker unless directed by your doctor.

PRECAUTIONS

Alcohol should be avoided while taking a beta blocker.

SIDE EFFECTS

Not all side effects will occur. Many side effects will diminish with time. *However, some side effects may require attention from your doctor.* Check with your doctor immediately if you experience any of the following:

- Difficulty breathing, depressed mood, slow heart rate, irregular heart rate, chest pain, dizziness, light-headedness, swelling of the feet or ankles, confusion, extreme fatigue, sweating

Some side effects appear when you first start taking a beta

blocker and go away for most people. If the following side effects continue, contact your doctor.

- Mild fatigue, dizziness, sexual problems

BUPROPION (bewe-PRO-pi-on)

Drug Category: Antidepressant, cyclic
Requires prescription

COMMONLY USED BRAND-NAME PRODUCTS

Tablets
Wellbutrin (and generic) 75mg, 100mg
Tablets, sustained release
Wellbutrin SR (and generic) 100mg, 150mg, 200mg
Tablets, extended release
Wellbutrin XL (and generic) 150mg, 300mg

GENERAL INFORMATION

Used to treat major depression and the depressed phase of bipolar disorder. Also used to aid in smoking cessation as part of an overall program.

BEFORE TAKING THIS MEDICATION

Talk to your doctor about the benefits and risks associated with bupropion. Make sure you understand how to take it safely and effectively. You and your family members should be very familiar with the side effects and the signs of having too much in your system. Make sure your doctor has the following information in detail:

- Any allergic or bad reactions you have had to bupropion or any other medication
- All prescription and over-the-counter medicines you are taking

- Your complete medical history
- If you are pregnant, could be pregnant, or are planning a pregnancy in the near future, bupropion should not be taken
- If you are breast feeding, bupropion can pass into breast milk and affect the baby

USUAL ADULT DOSAGE RANGE

The starting dose of bupropion will be low and gradually be increased.

75–150mg two times daily. Doses of immediate-release tablets should be at least 4 hours apart; sustained-release tablets at least 8 hours apart; extended-release tablets 24 hours apart.

Older adults are more susceptible to side effects and will generally require lower dosages.

DIRECTIONS FOR PROPER USE

- *Take exactly as prescribed. Do not take more or less than prescribed. Accidental or intended overdoses of bupropion can be potentially fatal.*
- *Bupropion is associated with a higher occurrence of seizures than other antidepressants. Taking bupropion exactly as directed can reduce the risk of seizures.*
- *Make sure your doctor is aware if you are taking a bupropion-containing product for smoking cessation so that the total dose of bupropion is not too high.*
- Do not abruptly stop taking bupropion unless instructed to do so by your doctor. Gradually reducing the dose can help prevent mood changes, headache, diarrhea.
- If you miss a dose, take it as soon as possible, unless it is within 6 hours of your next scheduled dose, then skip the missed dose and resume with your next scheduled dose. Do not double doses.
- If you are taking a long-acting tablet form and you miss a

dose, take it as soon as possible within 1 to 2 hours of the missed dose. However, if it is more than 2 hours after the missed dose, skip the missed dose and resume with your next scheduled dose. Swallow tablets whole; do not crush, chew, or break.

- It may take several weeks before you feel the full benefits of bupropion.

PRECAUTIONS
- Bupropion can cause drowsiness and slowed reaction times. Be cautious when driving, operating machinery, or doing jobs requiring alertness.
- Alcohol can cause changes in mood and may interfere with bupropion's effectiveness. Alcohol can cause extreme drowsiness when taken with bupropion. *Alcohol should be avoided while taking bupropion.*
- *Antidepressants may increase the risk of suicidal thinking and behavior in adolescents and children. When considering an antidepressant in a child or adolescent, the risk must be balanced with the need. Children and adolescents taking antidepressants should be closely monitored for worsening of symptoms, suicidality, or unusual changes in behavior.*

SIDE EFFECTS
Not all side effects will occur. Many side effects will diminish with time. *However, some side effects may require attention from your doctor.* Check with your doctor immediately if you experience any of the following:
- Seizure, changes in blood pressure, irregular heart rate, shortness of breath, problems with urination (difficult or painful urination, unable to urinate), confusion, extreme

sedation, excitement or mania, extreme constipation, yellow skin or eyes, significant weight loss, severe headache

Some side effects appear when you first start taking bupropion and go away for most people. If the following side effects continue, contact your doctor.

- Dizziness, blurred vision, dry mouth, mild to moderate constipation, increased appetite, weight gain, sexual problems, tremor of the hands

DRUG INTERACTIONS

Bupropion can adversely interact with the following frequently prescribed medications or foods:

- MAOI antidepressants—severe reaction causing dangerously high blood pressure, high body temperature, seizures, or death
- TCA antidepressants—dosage adjustment of one or both drugs may be necessary
- SSRI antidepressants—dosage adjustment of one or both drugs may be necessary
- Some nonsedating antihistamines—cardiac (heart) toxicity
- Clonidine—if clonidine is being taken for high blood pressure, bupropion may cause clonidine to work less well
- Antipsychotics—may increase certain neurologic side effects
- Drugs used during surgery—can cause increased blood pressure; make sure your doctors are aware of upcoming planned surgeries
- Caffeine in large amounts or other stimulants—can increase the risk of seizure
- Drugs that depress certain functions of the nervous system, when combined with bupropion, cause extreme drowsiness and slowed reaction times. Examples of these medicines are

antihistamines, narcotics, muscle relaxants, and barbiturates.

MEDICAL CONSIDERATIONS

If you have any of the following medical conditions, make sure your doctor is aware of it.

- Liver disease or alcoholism—bupropion levels may be higher than expected
- Seizure disorder—bupropion may increase the chance of seizures
- Kidney disease—bupropion levels may be higher than expected
- Heart problems—some heart problems can be made worse by bupropion; bupropion should not be taken by someone who has had a recent heart attack
- Urinary retention, prostate enlargement—urination may become more difficult
- Bulimia or anorexia—there is an increased risk of seizure

BUSPIRONE (byou-SPI-rone)
Drug Category: Antianxiety medicine
Requires prescription

COMMONLY USED BRAND-NAME PRODUCTS
Tablets
BuSpar (and generic) 5mg, 7.5mg, 10mg
Dividose Tablets
BuSpar 7.5mg, 15mg, 30 mg

GENERAL INFORMATION
Used to treat anxiety. *This medicine is not intended to help with the stress of everyday life. Even when taken as prescribed, buspirone may cause psychological and/or physical dependence.*

BEFORE TAKING THIS MEDICATION

Talk to your doctor about the benefits and risks associated with buspirone. Make sure you understand how to take it safely and effectively. You and your family members should be very familiar with the side effects and signs of having too much in your system. Make sure your doctor has the following information in detail:

- Any allergic or bad reactions you have had to buspirone or any other medication
- All prescription and over-the-counter medicines you are taking
- Your complete medical history, including mental health conditions
- If you are pregnant, could be pregnant, or are planning a pregnancy in the near future, buspirone should not be taken
- If you are breast feeding, buspirone can pass into breast milk and affect the baby

USUAL ADULT DOSAGE RANGE

5–10mg two to three times a day.

Older adults are more susceptible to side effects and will generally require lower dosages.

DIRECTIONS FOR PROPER USE

- *Take exactly as prescribed. Do not take more or less than prescribed. Buspirone levels that are too high can cause serious toxicity.*
- If you take buspirone regularly for an extended period of time, do not stop taking it unless told to do so by your doctor. It may be necessary to gradually reduce the dose before stopping completely.
- Always take buspirone the same way, either always with food or always without food.

- If you miss a dose, take it as soon as possible. However, if the missed dose is within 4 hours of your next dose, skip the missed dose and resume with your next scheduled dose. Do not double the dose.
- Several weeks may elapse before you begin to feel the full benefit of buspirone.

PRECAUTIONS
- Buspirone can cause drowsiness and slowed reaction times. Be cautious when driving, operating machinery, or doing jobs requiring alertness.
- Alcohol can cause extreme drowsiness when taken with buspirone. *Alcohol should be avoided while taking buspirone.*

SIDE EFFECTS
Not all side effects will occur. Many side effects will diminish with time. *However, some side effects may be warning signs of toxicity and will require attention from your doctor.* Check with your doctor immediately if you experience any of the following:
- Confusion, depressed mood, severe drowsiness, slurred speech, severe weakness, unusual thoughts, shortness of breath, excitement, extreme muscle pain or stiffness, severe nausea, vomiting

Some side effects appear when you first start taking buspirone and go away for most people. If the following side effects continue, contact your doctor.
- Dizziness, lightheadedness, drowsiness, blurred vision, stomach problems, sexual problems

DRUG INTERACTIONS
Buspirone can adversely interact with the following frequently prescribed medications or foods:

- Monoamine oxidase inhibitors—a severe reaction, causing dangerously high blood pressure, high body temperature, seizures, or death, is possible
- Cimetidine—can cause high buspirone levels
- Macrolide antibiotics (e.g., erythromycin)—can cause high buspirone levels
- Oral antifungal agents—can cause high buspirone levels
- HIV protease inhibitors—can cause high buspirone levels
- Carbamazepine—can lower buspirone levels
- Phenytoin—can lower buspirone levels
- Grapefruit juice—can cause high buspirone levels
- Drugs that depress certain functions of the nervous system, when combined with buspirone, cause extreme drowsiness and slowed reaction times. Examples of these medicines are antihistamines, narcotics, muscle relaxants, and barbiturates.

MEDICAL CONSIDERATIONS

If you have any of the following medical conditions, make sure your doctor is aware of it.

- Liver disease or alcoholism—buspirone levels may be higher than expected
- Kidney disease—buspirone levels may be higher than expected
- Parkinson's disease—buspirone may make this condition worse

CARBAMAZEPINE (car-bum-AZE-e-peen)

Drug Category: Mood stabilizer
Requires prescription

COMMONLY USED BRAND-NAME PRODUCTS

Tablets

Tegretol chewable tablets (also as generic) 100mg

Tegretol, Epitol tablets (also as generic) 200mg

Tablets, extended release

Tegretol XR 100mg, 200mg, 400mg

Suspension

Tegretol 100mg/5ml

Capsules, extended release

Equetro 100mg, 200mg, 300mg

GENERAL INFORMATION

Used to treat bipolar disorder, especially hard-to-treat cases, such as rapid cycling. Also reduces the number and severity of subsequent episodes of both mania and depression. Can be used alone or in combination with other mood stabilizers. It is also used to treat schizoaffective disorder, usually in combination with other medications called antipsychotics. There is some evidence that it can help people who have significant problems with impulse control, by reducing anger or temper outbursts and aggressive behaviors.

BEFORE TAKING THIS MEDICATION

Talk to your doctor about the benefits and risks associated with carbamazepine. Make sure you understand how to take it safely and effectively. You and your family members should be very familiar with the side effects and signs of having too much in your system. Make sure your doctor has the following information in detail:

- Any allergic or bad reactions you have had to carbamazepine or any other medication
- All prescription and over-the-counter medicines you are taking
- Your complete medical history

- If you are pregnant, could be pregnant, or are planning a pregnancy in the near future, carbamazepine should not be taken
- If you are breast feeding, carbamazepine can pass into breast milk and affect the baby

USUAL ADULT DOSAGE RANGE

The starting dose of carbamazepine will be adjusted on the basis of your response and blood levels. You may require more carbamazepine during and immediately following an acute manic episode than when your symptoms have stabilized.

Acute mania: 600–1600 mg per day, divided in two to four doses daily.

Older adults are more susceptible to side effects and will generally require lower dosages.

DIRECTIONS FOR PROPER USE

- *Take exactly as prescribed. Do not take more or less than prescribed. Carbamazepine levels that are too high can cause serious toxicity.*
- If you take carbamazepine regularly for an extended period of time, do not stop taking it unless told to do so by your doctor. It may be necessary to gradually reduce the dose before stopping completely.
- Take carbamazepine with meals or a snack. This will help relieve stomach upset or diarrhea.
- If you are taking the liquid form, it should be shaken well to evenly disperse all the medication. Do not mix it with other liquid medications or beverages.
- If you miss a dose of the regular tablet or liquid form, take it as soon as possible. However, if you discover the missed dose and it is very close to the time for the next dose, skip the missed dose, and resume with your next scheduled dose. Do not double doses.

If you are taking a long-acting form:

- Swallow the tablet or capsule whole. Do not crush, split, or chew it.
- If you miss a dose, take it as soon as possible. However, if the missed dose is within 6 hours of your next dose, skip the missed dose and resume with your next scheduled dose.
- Long-acting forms are not interchangeable with regular carbamazepine tablets or liquid forms.
- It may take several weeks before you feel the full benefits of carbamazepine.
- Laboratory tests are necessary to determine if the amount of carbamazepine in your bloodstream is in the correct range.

PRECAUTIONS

- Carbamazepine can cause drowsiness and slowed reaction times. Be cautious when driving, operating machinery, or doing jobs requiring alertness.
- Alcohol can cause changes in mood and may interfere with carbamazepine's effectiveness. Alcohol can cause extreme drowsiness when taken with carbamazepine. *Alcohol should be avoided while taking carbamazepine.*
- **Carbamazepine may cause suicidal thoughts. Notify your doctor immediately if you notice changes in your mood, behavior, or actions or have thoughts of harming yourself.**

SIDE EFFECTS

Not all side effects will occur. Many side effects will diminish with time. *However, some side effects may be warning signs of toxicity and will require attention from your doctor.* Check with your doctor immediately if you experience any of the following:

- Unusual bleeding or bruising, black stools, blood in the urine, difficulty urinating, confusion, significant drowsiness, irregular heartbeat, difficulty breathing, swelling of the feet or hands, yellow eyes or skin

Check with your doctor as soon as possible if you experience any of the following side effects:

- Back-and-forth movement of the eyes, blurred or double vision, skin rash or hives, severe diarrhea

Some side effects appear when you first start taking carbamazepine and go away for most people. If the following side effects continue, contact your doctor.

- Mild hand tremor, mild nausea, mild dizziness, diarrhea or constipation, increased sensitivity of the skin to sunlight, dry mouth

DRUG INTERACTIONS

Carbamazepine can adversely interact with the following frequently prescribed medications or foods:

- Anticoagulants (blood thinners)—the effect of the anticoagulant can be decreased
- Certain medications for high blood pressure
- Calcium channel blockers—can cause increased carbamazepine levels
- Cimetidine (Tagamet)—carbamazepine levels can be increased
- Erythromycin and similar antibiotics—can cause increased carbamazepine levels
- Propoxyphene (Darvon)—carbamazepine levels can be increased
- Birth control pills—carbamazepine may cause birth control pills to work less well
- Tricyclic antidepressants—increased sedation, change in blood levels of carbamazepine or the antidepressant

- Buspirone—carbamazepine can lower buspirone levels
- Grapefruit juice—can increase carbamazepine levels
- Anticonvulsants—decreased levels of other anticonvulsants
- Isoniazid—can cause liver toxicity
- Monoamine oxidase-inhibitors—severe reaction causing dangerously high blood pressure, high body temperature, seizures or death
- Oral antifungal agents—can cause high carbamazepine levels
- HIV protease inhibitors—carbamazepine can increase levels of protease inhibitors
- Drugs that depress certain functions of the nervous system, when combined with carbamazepine, cause extreme drowsiness and slowed reaction times. Examples of these medicines are antihistamines, narcotics, muscle relaxants, and barbiturates.

MEDICAL CONSIDERATIONS

If you have any of the following medical conditions, make sure your doctor is aware of it.

- Liver disease or alcoholism—carbamazepine levels may be higher than expected
- Kidney disease—carbamazepine levels may be higher than expected
- Anemia or other blood problems—these conditions can be made worse by carbamazepine
- Heart problems—some heart problems can be made worse by carbamazepine, usually in the elderly
- Problem with urination—carbamazepine may worsen this condition
- Glaucoma—carbamazepine may worsen this condition
- Diabetes mellitus (sugar diabetes)—urine sugar levels can be increased

- Hyponatremia (low sodium)—carbamazepine may worsen this condition

CHLORDIAZEPOXIDE (klor-dye-az-ep-OX-ide)

Drug Category: Antianxiety medicine
Requires prescription, controlled substance, modest potential for abuse

COMMONLY USED BRAND-NAME PRODUCTS

Capsules
Librium (and generic) 5mg, 10mg, 25mg

GENERAL INFORMATION

Used to treat anxiety and symptoms of alcohol withdrawal. *This medicine is not intended to help with the stress of everyday life. Even when taken as prescribed, chlordiazepoxide may cause psychological and/or physical dependence.*

BEFORE TAKING THIS MEDICATION

Talk to your doctor about the benefits and risks associated with chlordiazepoxide. Make sure you understand how to take it safely and effectively. You and your family members should be very familiar with the side effects and signs of having too much in your system. Make sure your doctor has the following information in detail:

- Any allergic or bad reactions you have had to chlordiazepoxide or any other medication
- All prescription and over-the-counter medicines you are taking
- Your complete medical history, including mental health conditions

- If you are pregnant, could be pregnant, or are planning a pregnancy in the near future, chlordiazepoxide should not be taken
- If you are breast feeding, chlordiazepoxide can pass into breast milk and affect the baby

USUAL ADULT DOSAGE RANGE
5–25 mg two to four times a day.
Older adults are more susceptible to side effects and will generally require lower dosages.

DIRECTIONS FOR PROPER USE
- *Take exactly as prescribed. Do not take more or less than prescribed. Chlordiazepoxide levels that are too high can cause serious toxicity.*
- If you will be taking chlordiazepoxide regularly for an extended period of time, do not stop taking it unless told to do so by your doctor. It may be necessary to gradually reduce the dose of chlordiazepoxide before stopping completely. If the medicine is stopped too quickly, your condition could become worse, or you could experience serious effects, such as seizures.
- May be taken with food to decrease stomach upset.
- If you miss a dose, take it as soon as possible. However, if the missed dose is within 6 hours of your next dose, skip the missed dose and resume with your next scheduled dose. Do not double the dose.

PRECAUTIONS
- Chlordiazepoxide can cause drowsiness and slowed reaction times. Be cautious when driving, operating machinery, or doing jobs requiring alertness.
- Alcohol can cause extreme drowsiness when taken with

chlordiazepoxide. *Alcohol should be avoided while taking chlordiazepoxide.*

SIDE EFFECTS

Not all side effects will occur. Many side effects will diminish with time. *However, some side effects may be warning signs of toxicity and will require attention from your doctor.* Check with your doctor immediately if you experience any of the following:

- Confusion, severe drowsiness, slurred speech, severe weakness, unusual thoughts, shortness of breath, excitement, hyperactivity, memory problems

Some side effects appear when you first start taking chlordiazepoxide and go away for most people. If the following side effects continue, contact your doctor.

- Dizziness, lightheadedness, drowsiness, blurred vision, stomach problems

DRUG INTERACTIONS

Chlordiazepoxide can adversely interact with the following frequently prescribed medications or foods:

- Cimetidine (Tagamet)—can cause high chlordiazepoxide levels
- Disulfiram (Antabuse)—can cause high chlordiazepoxide levels
- Birth control pills—can cause high chlordiazepoxide levels
- Levodopa—decreased effectiveness of levodopa
- Macrolide antibiotics (e.g., erythromycin)—can cause high chlordiazepoxide levels
- Oral antifungal agents—can cause high chlordiazepoxide levels
- HIV protease inhibitors—can cause high chlordiazepoxide levels

- Calcium channel blockers—can cause high chlordiazepoxide levels
- Serotonin-type antidepressants—can cause high chlordiazepoxide levels
- Digoxin—chlordiazepoxide can cause high digoxin levels
- Valproic acid—can cause high chlordiazepoxide levels
- Isoniazid—can cause high chlordiazepoxide levels
- Beta blockers—can cause high chlordiazepoxide levels
- Propoxyphene—can cause high chlordiazepoxide levels
- Carbamazepine—can lower chlordiazepoxide levels
- Grapefruit juice—can cause high chlordiazepoxide levels
- Drugs that depress certain functions of the nervous system, when combined with chlordiazepoxide, cause extreme drowsiness and slowed reaction times. Examples of these medicines are antihistamines, narcotics, muscle relaxants and barbiturates.

MEDICAL CONSIDERATIONS

If you have any of the following medical diagnoses, chlordiazepoxide may affect your condition.

- Liver disease or alcoholism—chlordiazepoxide levels may be higher than expected
- Kidney disease—chlordiazepoxide levels may be higher than expected
- Drug dependence or alcohol dependence—dependence on chlordiazepoxide may occur
- Seizure disorder—stopping chlordiazepoxide abruptly may cause seizures
- Chronic lung disease—chlordiazepoxide can possibly make breathing more difficult
- Glaucoma—chlordiazepoxide may worsen your condition
- Sleep apnea—chlordiazepoxide may worsen your condition

CHLORPROMAZINE (Thorazine)
Drug Category: Neuroleptic; Antipsychotic
Requires prescription

COMMONLY USED BRAND-NAME PRODUCTS
Tablets
Thorazine (and generic), 10mg, 25mg, 50mg, 100mg, 200mg
Liquids
Thorazine (and generic) Syrup, 10mg/5ml
Concentrate, 30mg/ml, 100mg/ml

GENERAL INFORMATION
Used to treat psychotic symptoms, such as hallucinations and delusions. These symptoms occur in schizophrenia, schizo-affective disorder, bipolar disorder, or major depression with psychotic features. Chlorpromazine can be used for short-term management of aggressive, out-of-control behaviors or feelings of anger and rage.

BEFORE TAKING THIS MEDICATION
Talk to your doctor about the benefits and risks associated with chlorpromazine. Make sure you understand how to take it safely and effectively. You and your family members should be very familiar with its side effects. Make sure your doctor has the following information in detail:
- Any allergic or bad reactions you have had to chlorpromazine or any other medication
- All prescription and over-the-counter medicines you are taking
- Your complete medical history
- If you are pregnant, could be pregnant, or are planning a pregnancy in the near future, chlorpromazine has not been shown to be absolutely safe

- If you are breast feeding, chlorpromazine can pass into breast milk and affect the baby

USUAL ADULT DOSAGE RANGE

100–1600mg daily. There is a wide effective dosage range. *Older adults* are *extremely* susceptible to side effects and will generally require lower dosages.

DIRECTIONS FOR PROPER USE

- *Take exactly as prescribed. Do not take more or less than prescribed. Chlorpromazine levels that are too high can cause serious toxicity.*
- If you miss a dose, take it as soon as possible. However, if the missed dose is within 4 hours of your next dose, skip the missed dose and resume with your next scheduled dose. Do not double the dose.
- If you are taking a liquid form, avoid contacting the skin with the medicine. Irritation can result if the medicine comes in contact with skin. Do not use the liquid form if the medicine becomes very discolored (dark yellow) or has a sediment at the bottom of the bottle.
- It may be several weeks before you feel the full benefits.

PRECAUTIONS

- Chlorpromazine can cause drowsiness and slowed reaction times. Be cautious when driving, operating machinery, or doing jobs requiring alertness.
- Alcohol can cause extreme drowsiness when taken with chlorpromazine. *Alcohol should be avoided while taking chlorpromazine.*
- Chlorpromazine may cause your body temperature to increase and could result in heat stroke. Be extra careful in hot weather, when exercising, or when taking hot baths or saunas not to become overheated.

- Chlorpromazine may cause your skin and eyes to be more sensitive to sunlight. Exposure to sunlight may cause a rash, skin discoloration, or sunburn. Limit direct exposure to sunlight, and use sunscreen when in direct sunlight. Avoid tanning booths and beds. Wear UV-blocking sunglasses when outdoors.
- When taking chlorpromazine, stand up slowly after sitting or lying down, since it may cause your blood pressure to drop and cause faintness or dizziness. Stand up slowly from a seated or lying position, especially when you first start taking chlorpromazine.

SIDE EFFECTS

Not all side effects will occur. Many side effects will diminish with time. *However, some side effects may be warning signs of toxicity and will require attention from your doctor.* Check with your doctor immediately if you experience any of the following:

- Seizure; high fever; fast or irregular heartbeat; very low blood pressure; faintness; any abnormal movements of the mouth, tongue, neck, arms, or legs; difficulty speaking or swallowing; imbalance or difficulty walking normally; severe muscle stiffness; discoloration of the skin or eyes; confusion; significant drowsiness; restlessness; difficulty urinating; sexual problems; vomiting; diarrhea; unusual bruising or bleeding; serious skin reaction to sunlight (burning or blistering); severe constipation; breast pain or enlargement

Some side effects appear when you first start taking chlorpromazine and go away for most people. If the following side effects continue, contact your doctor.

- Dry mouth, mild to moderate constipation, dizziness, hand tremor, stuffy nose, weight gain

DRUG INTERACTIONS

Chlorpromazine can adversely interact with the following frequently prescribed medications:

- Lithium—increased neurologic side effects
- Levodopa—decreased effectiveness of levodopa
- Amphetamines—increased psychotic symptoms are possible
- Anticonvulsants—decreased chlorpromazine levels
- Tricyclic antidepressants—increased TCA levels
- Serotonin-type antidepressants—can cause high chlorpromazine levels
- Beta blockers—can cause high chlorpromazine levels
- HIV protease inhibitors—can cause high chlorpromazine levels
- Drugs that depress certain functions of the nervous system, when combined with chlorpromazine, cause extreme drowsiness and slowed reaction times. Examples of these medicines are antihistamines, narcotics, muscle relaxants, and barbiturates.

MEDICAL CONSIDERATIONS

If you have any of the following medical conditions, make sure your doctor is aware of it.

- Kidney disease—chlorpromazine levels may be higher than expected
- Liver disease—chlorpromazine levels may be higher than expected
- Heart problems—some heart problems can be made worse by chlorpromazine
- Seizure disorder—chlorpromazine can lower seizure threshold
- Urinary retention, prostate enlargement—urination may be more difficult

- Glaucoma—chlorpromazine can increase pressure inside the eye
- Parkinson's disease—some Parkinson's symptoms may be worsened
- Breast cancer—may increase risk of cancer progression

CITALOPRAM (sit-AL-oh-pram)

Drug Category: Antidepressant, SSRI (serotonin specific reuptake inhibitor)

Requires prescription

COMMONLY USED BRAND-NAME PRODUCTS

Tablets

Celexa (and generic) 10mg, 20mg, 40mg

Solution

10mg/5ml

GENERAL INFORMATION

Used to treat major depression, the depressed phase of bipolar disorder, and obsessive compulsive disorder (OCD). Also used to treat panic disorder.

BEFORE TAKING THIS MEDICATION

Talk to your doctor about the benefits and risks associated with citalopram. Make sure you understand how to take it safely and effectively. You and your family members should be very familiar with the side effects and signs of having too much in your system. Make sure your doctor has the following information in detail:

- Any allergic or bad reactions you have had to citalopram or any other medication

- All prescription and over-the-counter medicines you are taking
- Your complete medical history
- If you are pregnant, could be pregnant, or are planning a pregnancy in the near future, citalopram should not be taken
- If you are breast feeding, citalopram can pass into breast milk and affect the baby

USUAL ADULT DOSAGE RANGE

20–60mg daily. Dosage increases should occur no more often than weekly.

Older adults are more susceptible to side effects and will generally require lower dosages.

DIRECTIONS FOR PROPER USE

- ***Take exactly as prescribed. Do not take more or less than prescribed.***
- Do not abruptly stop taking citalopram unless instructed to do so by your doctor.
- May be taken with food or meals to lessen stomach upset.
- If you miss a dose, do not try to make it up. Wait and take your next scheduled dose. Do not double doses.
- It may take several weeks before you feel the full benefits.

PRECAUTIONS

- Citalopram can cause drowsiness and slowed reaction times. Be cautious when driving, operating machinery, or doing jobs requiring alertness.
- Alcohol can cause changes in mood and may interfere with citalopram's effectiveness. Alcohol can cause extreme drowsiness when taken with citalopram. ***Alcohol should be avoided while taking citalopram.***
- Citalopram may cause your skin and eyes to be more sensi-

tive to sunlight. Exposure to sunlight may cause a rash, skin discoloration, or sunburn. Limit direct exposure to sunlight, and use sunscreen when in direct sunlight. Avoid tanning booths and beds. Wear UV-blocking sunglasses when outdoors.

- *Antidepressants may increase the risk of suicidal thinking and behavior in adolescents and children. When considering an antidepressant in a child or adolescent, the risk must be balanced with the need. Children and adolescents taking antidepressants should be closely monitored for worsening of symptoms, suicidality, or unusual changes in behavior.*

SIDE EFFECTS

Not all side effects will occur. Many side effects will diminish with time. *However, some side effects may require attention from your doctor.* Check with your doctor immediately if you experience any of the following:

- Skin rash or hives, shortness of breath, chills or fever, swelling of the hands or feet, seizures, bleeding or bruising

Some side effects appear when you first start taking citalopram and go away for most people. If the following side effects continue, contact your doctor.

- Agitation, anxiety, insomnia, dizziness, sexual problems, sweating, blurred vision, dry mouth, mild to moderate constipation, change in appetite, change in weight, tremor of the hands

DRUG INTERACTIONS

Citalopram can adversely interact with the following frequently prescribed medications or foods:

- Anticoagulants (blood thinners)—the effect of the anticoagulant can be increased
- Some nonsedating antihistamines—cardiac (heart) toxicity

- Diet pills—severe reaction causing dangerously high blood pressure, high body temperature, seizures, or death
- Products containing L-tryptophan—severe reaction causing dangerously high blood pressure, high body temperature, seizures, or death
- Cimetidine—can cause high citalopram levels
- Bupropion—dosage adjustment of one or both drugs may be necessary
- Amphetamines—increased blood pressure, irregular heart rate, or very high fever may result
- Tricyclic antidepressants—can cause high TCA levels
- Monoamine oxidase inhibitors—severe reaction causing dangerously high blood pressure, high body temperature, seizures, or death
- Antipsychotics—may increase certain neurologic side effects
- Lithium—increased lithium levels causing possible confusion, dizziness, tremor
- Anticonvulsants—increased anticonvulsant levels or decreased citalopram levels
- Antiarrhythmic drugs—may require dosage adjustment of antiarrhythmics and/or closer heart monitoring
- Benzodiazepines—citalopram can increase benzodiazepine levels
- Beta blockers—citalopram can increase beta blocker levels
- Aspirin, NSAIDs–increased chance of bleeding
- HIV protease inhibitors—citalopram can increase levels of protease inhibitors
- Drugs that depress certain functions of the nervous system, when combined with citalopram, cause extreme drowsiness and slowed reaction times. Examples of these medicines are antihistamines, narcotics, muscle relaxants, and barbiturates.

MEDICAL CONSIDERATIONS

If you have any of the following medical conditions, make sure your doctor is aware of it.

- Liver disease or alcoholism—citalopram levels may be higher than expected
- Kidney disease—citalopram levels may be higher than expected
- Seizure disorder—citalopram can lower seizure threshold
- Diabetes mellitus (sugar diabetes)—blood sugar levels may be affected
- Low sodium—citalopram may worsen this condition
- Bleeding disorder—citalopram may worsen this condition

CLOMIPRAMINE (cloe-MIP-ra-meen)

Drug Category: Antidepressant, tricyclic
Requires prescription

COMMONLY USED BRAND-NAME PRODUCTS

Capsules
Anafranil (and generic) 25mg, 50mg, 75mg

GENERAL INFORMATION

Used to treat obsessive compulsive disorder (OCD). May be used to treat major depression, the depressed phase of bipolar disorder, and panic disorder.

BEFORE TAKING THIS MEDICATION

Talk to your doctor about the benefits and risks associated with clomipramine. Make sure you understand how to take it safely and effectively. You and your family members should be very familiar with the side effects and signs of having too much

in your system. Make sure your doctor has the following information in detail:

- Any allergic or bad reactions you have had to clomipramine or any other medication
- All prescription and over-the-counter medicines you are taking
- Your complete medical history
- If you are pregnant, could be pregnant, or are planning a pregnancy in the near future, clomipramine should not be taken
- If you are breast feeding, clomipramine can pass into breast milk and affect the baby

USUAL ADULT DOSAGE RANGE

The starting dose of clomipramine will be low and will gradually be increased. Sometimes blood levels are tested to ensure that the dose you are taking is in the safe and effective range.

OCD, depression: Starting dose 25 mg at bedtime. Increased to 100–250 mg at bedtime over 2 to 3 weeks.

Panic disorder: 25–200mg daily.

Older adults are more susceptible to side effects and will generally require lower dosages.

DIRECTIONS FOR PROPER USE

- *Take exactly as prescribed. Do not take more or less than prescribed. Accidental or intended overdoses of clomipramine are potentially fatal.*
- Do not abruptly stop taking clomipramine unless instructed to do so by your doctor. Gradually reducing the dose can help prevent mood changes, headache, or diarrhea.
- Take with food or milk to reduce stomach upset.

- If you miss a bedtime dose, do not take it the next morning, since it may make you drowsy. Do not double doses.
- It may take several weeks before you feel the full benefits.

PRECAUTIONS

- Clomipramine can cause drowsiness and slowed reaction times. Be cautious when driving, operating machinery, or doing jobs requiring alertness.
- Alcohol can cause changes in mood and may interfere with clomipramine's effectiveness. Alcohol can cause extreme drowsiness when taken with clomipramine. *Alcohol should be avoided while taking clomipramine.*
- Clomipramine may cause your skin and eyes to be more sensitive to sunlight. Exposure to sunlight may cause a rash, skin discoloration, or sunburn. Limit direct exposure to sunlight, and use sunscreen when in direct sunlight. Avoid tanning booths and beds. Wear UV-blocking sunglasses when outdoors.
- When taking clomipramine, stand up slowly after sitting or lying down, since it may cause your blood pressure to drop and cause faintness or dizziness. Stand up slowly from a seated or lying position, especially when you first start taking clomipramine.
- *Antidepressants may increase the risk of suicidal thinking and behavior in adolescents and children. When considering an antidepressant in a child or adolescent, the risk must be balanced with the need. Children and adolescents taking antidepressants should be closely monitored for worsening of symptoms, suicidality, or unusual changes in behavior.*
- Adolescents and children may be more susceptible to the heart-related side effects of tricyclic antidepressants. Risk

must be balanced with need. Blood levels and heart function should be monitored in children and adolescents taking tricyclic antidepressants.

SIDE EFFECTS

Not all side effects will occur. Many side effects will diminish with time. *However, some side effects may require attention from your doctor.* Check with your doctor immediately if you experience any of the following:

- Seizure, changes in blood pressure, irregular heart rate, shortness of breath, problems with urination (difficult or painful urination, unable to urinate), confusion, extreme sedation, excitation or mania, increased skin sensitivity to the sunlight, extreme constipation, yellow skin or eyes

Some side effects appear when you first start taking clomipramine and go away for most people. If the following side effects continue, contact your doctor.

- Dizziness, blurred vision, dry mouth, mild to moderate constipation, increased appetite, weight gain, breast enlargement (men or women), discharge from the breast, sexual problems, tremor of the hands, persistent sore throat

DRUG INTERACTIONS

Clomipramine can adversely interact with the following frequently prescribed medications:

- Cimetidine—can cause high clomipramine levels
- SSRI antidepressants—can cause high clomipramine levels
- MAOI antidepressants—severe reaction causing dangerously high blood pressure, high body temperature, seizures, or death
- Clonidine—if clonidine is being taken for high blood pressure, clomipramine may cause clonidine to work less well

- Antipsychotics—may increase certain neurologic side effects
- Thyroid hormones—increased effects of both, especially excitation and changes in heart rate or rhythm
- Carbamazepine—can lower clomipramine levels
- Bupropion—can increase clomipramine levels
- Anticoagulants (blood thinners)—the effect of the anticoagulant can be increased
- Quinolones—increased risk of heart arrhythmias
- Amphetamines—increased blood pressure, irregular heart rate, or very high fever may result
- Drugs used during surgery—can cause increased blood pressure. Make sure your doctors are aware of upcoming planned surgeries.
- Drugs that depress certain functions of the nervous system, when combined with clomipramine, cause extreme drowsiness and slowed reaction times. Examples of these medicines are antihistamines, narcotics, muscle relaxants, and barbiturates.

MEDICAL CONSIDERATIONS

If you have any of the following medical conditions, make sure your doctor is aware of it.

- Liver disease or alcoholism—clomipramine levels may be higher than expected
- Kidney disease—clomipramine levels may be higher than expected
- Glaucoma—clomipramine can increase pressure inside the eye
- Heart problems—some heart problems can be made worse by clomipramine; clomipramine should not be taken by someone who has had a recent heart attack

- Urinary retention, prostate enlargement—urination may become more difficult
- Seizure disorder—clomipramine can lower seizure threshold
- Diabetes mellitus (sugar diabetes)—blood sugar levels may be affected
- Thyroid disorders—clomipramine may cause increased heart rate

CLONAZEPAM (klon-AZ-e-pam)

Drug Category: Antianxiety medicine
Requires prescription, controlled substance, moderate potential for abuse

COMMONLY USED BRAND-NAME PRODUCTS

Tablets
Klonopin (and generic) 0.5mg, 1mg, 2mg
Tablets, oral disintegrating
Klonopin (and generic) 0.25mg, 0.5mg, 1mg, 2mg

GENERAL INFORMATION

Used to treat anxiety and panic disorder. *This medicine is not intended to help with the stress of everyday life. Even when taken as prescribed, clonazepam may cause psychological and/or physical dependence.*

BEFORE TAKING THIS MEDICATION

Talk to your doctor about the benefits and risks associated with clonazepam. Make sure you understand how to take it safely and effectively. You and your family members should be very familiar with the side effects and signs of having too much

in your system. Make sure your doctor has the following information in detail:

- Any allergic or bad reactions you have had to clonazepam or any other medication
- All prescription and over-the-counter medicines you are taking
- Your complete medical history, including mental health conditions
- If you are pregnant, could be pregnant, or are planning a pregnancy in the near future, clonazepam should not be taken
- If you are breast.feeding, clonazepam can pass into breast milk and affect the baby

USUAL ADULT DOSAGE RANGE

1–4 mg daily, in divided doses.
Older adults are more susceptible to side effects and will generally require lower dosages.

DIRECTIONS FOR PROPER USE

- *Take exactly as prescribed. Do not take more or less than prescribed. Clonazepam levels that are too high can cause serious toxicity.*
- If you take clonazepam regularly for an extended period of time, do not stop taking it unless told to do so by your doctor. It may be necessary to gradually reduce the dose before stopping completely. If the medicine is stopped too quickly, your condition could become worse, or you could experience serious effects, such as seizures.
- May be taken with food to decrease stomach upset.
- If you miss a dose, take it as soon as possible. However, if the missed dose is within 6 hours of your next dose, skip the missed dose and resume with your next scheduled dose. Do not double the dose.

- If you are taking the oral disintegrating form, place the tablet in your mouth, allow it to dissolve, and swallow. Water is not required. Keep the tablets in the original package until right before you take a tablet. Any rapidly dissolving tablets that have been exposed to air should be discarded.

PRECAUTIONS
- Clonazepam can cause drowsiness and slowed reaction times. Be cautious when driving, operating machinery, or doing jobs requiring alertness.
- Alcohol can cause extreme drowsiness when taken with clonazepam. *Alcohol should be avoided while taking clonazepam.*

SIDE EFFECTS
Not all side effects will occur. Many side effects will diminish with time. *However, some side effects may be warning signs of toxicity and will require attention from your doctor.* Check with your doctor immediately if you experience any of the following:
- Confusion, severe drowsiness, slurred speech, severe weakness, unusual thoughts, shortness of breath, excitement, hyperactivity, memory problems

Some side effects appear when you first start taking clonazepam and go away for most people. If the following side effects continue, contact your doctor.
- Dizziness, lightheadedness, drowsiness, blurred vision, stomach problems

DRUG INTERACTIONS
Clonazepam can adversely interact with the following frequently prescribed medications or foods:
- Cimetidine (Tagamet)—can cause high clonazepam levels
- Disulfiram (Antabuse)—can cause high clonazepam levels

- Birth control pills—can cause high clonazepam levels
- Levodopa—decreased effectiveness of levodopa
- Macrolide antibiotics (e.g., erythromycin)—can cause high clonazepam levels
- Oral antifungal agents—can cause high clonazepam levels
- HIV protease inhibitors—can cause high clonazepam levels
- Calcium channel blockers—can cause high clonazepam levels
- Serotonin-type antidepressants—can cause high clonazepam levels
- Digoxin—clonazepam can cause high digoxin levels
- Valproic acid—can cause high clonazepam levels
- Isoniazid—can cause high clonazepam levels
- Beta blockers—can cause high clonazepam levels
- Propoxyphene—can cause high clonazepam levels
- Carbamazepine—can lower clonazepam levels
- Grapefruit juice—can cause high clonazepam levels
- Drugs that depress certain functions of the nervous system, when combined with clonazepam, cause extreme drowsiness and slowed reaction times. Examples of these medicines are antihistamines, narcotics, muscle relaxants, and barbiturates.

MEDICAL CONSIDERATIONS

If you have any of the following medical conditions, make sure your doctor is aware of it.

- Liver disease or alcoholism—clonazepam levels may be higher than expected
- Kidney disease—clonazepam levels may be higher than expected
- Drug or alcohol dependence—dependence on clonazepam may occur

- Seizure disorder—stopping clonazepam abruptly may cause seizures
- Glaucoma—clonazepam may worsen your condition
- Sleep apnea—clonazepam may worsen your condition

CLONIDINE (Klon-UH-deen)

Requires prescription

COMMONLY USED BRAND-NAME PRODUCTS

Catapres (and generic) tablets, skin patch

GENERAL INFORMATION

Typically used to treat high blood pressure. Sometimes used to treat aggression, hostility, or violent behaviors associated with a psychiatric or neurological disorder, and attention deficit hyperactivity disorder.

BEFORE TAKING THIS MEDICATION

Talk to your doctor about the benefits and risks associated with clonidine. Your doctor will need to know your complete medical history before prescribing clonidine. Your doctor or pharmacist will need to be aware of all medicines that you take to avoid drug interactions. Make sure you understand how to take clonidine. Do not take more or less than prescribed. Do not suddenly stop taking clonidine unless directed by your doctor.

PRECAUTIONS

- Clonidine can cause drowsiness and slowed reaction times. Be cautious when driving, operating machinery, or doing jobs requiring alertness.
- Alcohol can cause extreme drowsiness when taken with clonidine. *Alcohol should be avoided while taking clonidine.*

SIDE EFFECTS

Not all side effects will occur. Many side effects will diminish with time. *However, some side effects may require attention from your doctor.* Check with your doctor immediately if you experience any of the following:

- Difficulty breathing, slow or irregular heart rate, dizziness, light-headedness, swelling of the feet or ankles, confusion, extreme fatigue, red or itchy skin

Some side effects appear when you first start taking clonidine and go away for most people. If the following side effects continue, contact your doctor.

- Mild fatigue, dizziness, dry mouth, constipation

CLORAZEPATE (klor-AZE-uh-pate)

Drug Category: Antianxiety medicine
Requires prescription, controlled substance, moderate potential for abuse

COMMONLY USED BRAND-NAME PRODUCTS

Tablets
Tranxene (and generic) 3.75mg, 7.5mg, 15mg
Tablets, long acting
Tranxene SD 11.25mg, 22.5mg

GENERAL INFORMATION

Used to treat anxiety and symptoms of alcohol withdrawal. *This medicine is not intended to help with the stress of everyday life. Even when taken as prescribed, clorazepate may cause psychological and/or physical dependence.*

BEFORE TAKING THIS MEDICATION

Talk to your doctor about the benefits and risks associated with clorazepate. Make sure you understand how to take it

safely and effectively. You and your family members should be very familiar with the side effects and signs of having too much in your system. Make sure your doctor has the following information in detail:

- Any allergic or bad reactions you have had to clorazepate or any other medication
- All prescription and over-the-counter medicines you are taking
- Your complete medical history, including mental health conditions
- If you are pregnant, could be pregnant, or are planning a pregnancy in the near future, clorazepate should not be taken
- If you are breast feeding, clorazepate can pass into breast milk and affect the baby

USUAL ADULT DOSAGE RANGE

7.5–60 mg daily, in divided doses. The long-acting tablet form may be given once daily.

Older adults are more susceptible to side effects and will generally require lower dosages.

DIRECTIONS FOR PROPER USE

- *Take exactly as prescribed. Do not take more or less than prescribed. Clorazepate levels that are too high can cause serious toxicity.*
- If you take clorazepate regularly for an extended period of time, do not stop taking it unless told to do so by your doctor. It may be necessary to gradually reduce the dose before stopping completely. If the medicine is stopped too quickly, your condition could become worse, or you could experience serious effects, such as seizures.
- May be taken with food to decrease stomach upset.

- If you miss a dose, take it as soon as possible. However, if the missed dose is within 6 hours of your next dose, skip the missed dose and resume with your next scheduled dose. Do not double the dose.
- If you are taking the long-acting tablet form and you miss a dose, take it as soon as possible within 1 to 2 hours of the missed dose. However, if it is more than 2 hours after the missed dose, skip the missed dose and resume with your next scheduled dose. Swallow the tablets whole; do not crush, chew, or break them.

PRECAUTIONS
- Clorazepate can cause drowsiness and slowed reaction times. Be cautious when driving, operating machinery, or doing jobs requiring alertness.
- Alcohol can cause extreme drowsiness when taken with clorazepate. *Alcohol should be avoided while taking clorazepate.*

SIDE EFFECTS
Not all side effects will occur. Many side effects will diminish with time. *However, some side effects may be warning signs of toxicity and will require attention from your doctor.* Check with your doctor immediately if you experience any of the following:
- Confusion, severe drowsiness, slurred speech, severe weakness, unusual thoughts, shortness of breath, excitement, hyperactivity, memory problems

Some side effects appear when you first start taking clorazepate and go away for most people. If the following side effects continue, contact your doctor.
- Dizziness, lightheadedness, drowsiness, blurred vision, stomach problems

DRUG INTERACTIONS

Clorazepate can adversely interact with the following frequently prescribed medications or foods:

- Cimetidine (Tagamet)—can cause high clorazepate levels
- Disulfiram (Antabuse)—can cause high clorazepate levels
- Birth control pills—can cause high clorazepate levels
- Levodopa—decreased effectiveness of levodopa
- Macrolide antibiotics (e.g., erythromycin)—can cause high clorazepate levels
- Oral antifungal agents—can cause high clorazepate levels
- HIV protease inhibitors—can cause high clorazepate levels
- Calcium channel blockers—can cause high clorazepate levels
- Serotonin-type antidepressants—can cause high clorazepate levels
- Digoxin—clorazepate can cause high digoxin levels
- Valproic acid—can cause high clorazepate levels
- Isoniazid—can cause high clorazepate levels
- Beta blockers—can cause high clorazepate levels
- Propoxyphene—can cause high clorazepate levels
- Carbamazepine—can lower clorazepate levels
- Grapefruit juice—can cause high clorazepate levels
- Drugs that depress certain functions of the nervous system, when combined with clorazepate, cause extreme drowsiness and slowed reaction times. Examples of these medicines are antihistamines, narcotics, muscle relaxants, and barbiturates.

MEDICAL CONSIDERATIONS

If you have any of the following medical conditions, make sure your doctor is aware of it.

- Liver disease or alcoholism—clorazepate levels may be higher than expected
- Kidney disease—clorazepate levels may be higher than expected
- Drug or alcohol dependence—dependence on clorazepate may occur
- Seizure disorder—stopping clorazepate abruptly may cause seizures
- Chronic lung disease—clorazepate may make breathing more difficult
- Glaucoma—clorazepate may worsen your condition
- Sleep apnea—clorazepate may worsen your condition

CLOZAPINE (KLO-zuh-peen)
Drug Category: Neuroleptic; Antipsychotic
Requires prescription

COMMONLY USED BRAND-NAME PRODUCTS
Tablets, rapidly dissolving
Clozaril (and generic) 12.5mg, 25mg, 100mg, 200mg

GENERAL INFORMATION
Used to treat schizophrenia, reducing psychotic symptoms such as hallucinations and delusions. Also especially helpful with symptoms such as lack of motivation, emotional blunting, and withdrawing from others.

BEFORE TAKING THIS MEDICATION
Talk to your doctor about the benefits and risks associated with clozapine. Make sure you understand how to take it safely and effectively. You and your family members should be

very familiar with its side effects. *Your doctor may periodically monitor your weight, blood pressure, blood sugar, and blood lipid levels while you are taking clozapine.*

You and your family must be able to follow the special laboratory monitoring requirements necessary for safe use. For the first 6 months you are taking clozapine, you will be able to receive only a 7-day supply at a time and only if your weekly blood tests show it is safe to continue taking. After the first 6 months, your doctor will assess whether you can receive a 2-week supply, and only if your blood tests every 2 weeks show it is safe. After 1 year, your doctor will assess whether you can receive a 4-week supply, and only if your monthly blood tests show it is safe. The distribution of clozapine is restricted, and each manufacturer has its own system. You and your family will need to work closely with your doctor, laboratory, and pharmacy to make sure you understand the steps involved in obtaining your medication.

Make sure your doctor has the following information in detail:

- Any allergic or bad reactions you have had to clozapine or any other medication
- All prescription and over-the-counter medicines you are taking
- Your complete medical history
- If you are pregnant, could be pregnant, or are planning a pregnancy in the near future, clozapine has not been shown to be absolutely safe
- If you are breast feeding, clozapine can pass into breast milk and affect the baby

USUAL ADULT DOSAGE RANGE
300–900mg daily.

Older adults are *extremely* susceptible to side effects and will generally require lower dosages. ***Should not be used in elderly patients to treat dementia-related psychosis or behavioral disturbances.***

DIRECTIONS FOR PROPER USE

- ***Take exactly as prescribed. Do not take more or less than prescribed. Clozapine levels that are too high can cause serious toxicity.***
- ***Get laboratory tests done as directed by your doctor to check your white blood cell count. If you do not get these tests done, or if your white blood cell count drops too much, clozapine will have to be stopped.***
- ***Get all other tests done as directed by your doctor.***
- If you miss a dose, take it as soon as possible. However, if the missed dose is within 4 hours of your next dose, skip the missed dose and resume with your next scheduled dose. Do not double the dose.

If you are taking the rapidly dissolving form:

- Place the tablet in your mouth, allow it to dissolve, and swallow. Water is not required, but you can take it with water if you like. Keep the tablets in the original package until right before you take a tablet. Any rapidly dissolving tablets that have been exposed to air should be discarded.
- If you miss a dose, take it as soon as possible. However, if the missed dose is within 6 hours of your next dose, skip the missed dose and resume with your next scheduled dose.
- It may be several weeks before you feel the full benefits.

PRECAUTIONS

- Clozapine can cause drowsiness and slowed reaction times. Be cautious when driving, operating machinery, or doing jobs requiring alertness.

- Alcohol can cause extreme drowsiness when taken with clozapine. *Alcohol should be avoided while taking clozapine.*
- Clozapine may cause your body temperature to increase and could result in heat stroke. Be extra careful in hot weather, when exercising, or when taking hot baths or saunas not to become overheated.
- When taking clozapine, stand up slowly after sitting or lying down, since it may cause your blood pressure to drop and cause faintness or dizziness. Stand up slowly from a seated or lying position, especially when you first start taking clozapine.

SIDE EFFECTS

Not all side effects will occur. Many side effects will diminish with time. *However, some side effects may be warning signs of toxicity and will require attention from your doctor.* Check with your doctor immediately if you experience any of the following:

- Seizure; high fever; fast or irregular heartbeat; very low blood pressure; faintness; any abnormal movements of the mouth, tongue, neck, arms, or legs; difficulty speaking or swallowing; imbalance or difficulty walking normally; severe muscle stiffness; discoloration of the skin or eyes; confusion; significant drowsiness; restlessness; difficulty urinating; sexual problems; vomiting; diarrhea; unusual bruising or bleeding; serious skin reaction to sunlight (burning or blistering); severe constipation; breast pain or enlargement

Some side effects appear when you first start taking clozapine and go away for most people. If the following side effects continue, contact your doctor.

- Dry mouth, mild to moderate constipation, dizziness, hand tremor, stuffy nose, weight gain

DRUG INTERACTIONS

Clozapine can adversely interact with the following frequently prescribed medications or foods:

- Lithium—increased neurologic side effects
- Levodopa—decreased effectiveness of levodopa
- Amphetamines—increased psychotic symptoms are possible
- Anticonvulsants—decreased clozapine levels
- Tricyclic antidepressants—increased TCA levels
- Macrolide antibiotics (e.g., erythromycin)—can cause high clozapine levels
- Oral antifungal agents—can cause high clozapine levels
- HIV protease inhibitors—can cause high clozapine levels
- Cimetidine—can cause high clozapine levels
- Serotonin-type antidepressants—can cause high clozapine levels
- Cancer chemotherapy drugs—clozapine can interact to lower the white blood cell count
- Caffeine—can cause high clozapine levels
- Drugs that depress certain functions of the nervous system, when combined with clozapine, cause extreme drowsiness and slowed reaction times. Examples of these medicines are antihistamines, narcotics, muscle relaxants, and barbiturates.

MEDICAL CONSIDERATIONSS

If you have the following medical conditions, make sure your doctor is aware of it.

- Kidney disease—clozapine levels may be higher than expected

- Liver disease—clozapine levels may be higher than expected
- Heart problems—some heart problems can be made worse by clozapine
- Seizure disorder—clozapine can lower seizure threshold
- Urinary retention, prostate enlargement—urination may be more difficult
- Glaucoma—clozapine can increase pressure inside the eye
- Parkinson's disease—Some Parkinson's symptoms may be worsened
- Breast cancer—may increase risk of cancer progression
- Overweight/obesity—clozapine can cause weight gain
- Diabetes—clozapine can make this condition worse
- Elevated lipid (cholesterol and triglycerides) levels—clozapine can make this condition worse
- High blood pressure—clozapine can make this condition worse

DESIPRAMINE (dess-IP-ruh-meen)

Drug Category: Antidepressant, tricyclic
Requires prescription

COMMONLY USED BRAND-NAME PRODUCTS

Tablets
Norpramin (and generic) 10mg, 25mg, 50mg, 75mg, 100mg, 150mg

GENERAL INFORMATION

Used to treat major depression and the depressed phase of bipolar disorder. Also used to treat certain chronic pain disorders, such as migraine headache and diabetic neuropathy. Sometimes used to treat bulimia.

BEFORE TAKING THIS MEDICATION

Talk to your doctor about the benefits and risks associated with desipramine. Make sure you understand how to take it safely and effectively. You and your family members should be very familiar with the side effects and signs of having too much in your system. Make sure your doctor has the following information in detail:

- Any allergic or bad reactions you have had to desipramine or any other medication
- All prescription and over-the-counter medicines you are taking
- Your complete medical history
- If you are pregnant, could be pregnant, or are planning a pregnancy in the near future, desipramine should not be taken
- If you are breast feeding, desipramine can pass into breast milk and affect the baby

USUAL ADULT DOSAGE RANGE

The starting dose of desipramine will be low and will gradually be increased. Sometimes blood levels are tested to ensure that the dose you are taking is in the safe and effective range.

Depression: 75–300mg at bedtime over 2 to 3 weeks.

Chronic pain syndrome: 25–100mg daily.

Older adults are more susceptible to side effects and will generally require lower dosages.

DIRECTIONS FOR PROPER USE

- *Take exactly as prescribed. Do not take more or less than prescribed. Accidental or intended overdoses of desipramine are potentially fatal.*
- Do not abruptly stop taking desipramine unless instructed

to do so by your doctor. Gradually reducing the dose can help prevent mood changes, headache, or diarrhea.
- If you miss a bedtime dose, do not take it the next morning, since it may make you drowsy. Do not double doses.
- It may take several weeks before you feel the full benefits.

PRECAUTIONS
- Desipramine can cause drowsiness and slowed reaction times. Be cautious when driving, operating machinery, or doing jobs requiring alertness.
- Alcohol can cause changes in mood and may interfere with desipramine's effectiveness. Alcohol can cause extreme drowsiness when taken with desipramine. *Alcohol should be avoided while taking desipramine.*
- Desipramine may cause your skin and eyes to be more sensitive to sunlight. Exposure to sunlight may cause a rash, skin discoloration, or sunburn. Limit direct exposure to sunlight, and use sunscreen when in direct sunlight. Avoid tanning booths and beds. Wear UV-blocking sunglasses when outdoors.
- When taking desipramine, stand up slowly after sitting or lying down, since it may cause your blood pressure to drop and cause faintness or dizziness. Stand up slowly from a seated or lying position, especially when you first start taking desipramine.
- *Antidepressants may increase the risk of suicidal thinking and behavior in adolescents and children. When considering an antidepressant in a child or adolescent, the risk must be balanced with the need. Children and adolescents taking antidepressants should be closely monitored for worsening of symptoms, suicidality, or unusual changes in behavior.*
- Adolescents and children may be more susceptible to heart-

related side effects of tricyclic antidepressants. Risk must be balanced with need. Blood levels and heart function should be monitored in children and adolescents taking tricyclic antidepressants.

SIDE EFFECTS

Not all side effects will occur. Many side effects will diminish with time. *However, some side effects may require attention from your doctor.* Check with your doctor immediately if you experience any of the following:

- Seizure, changes in blood pressure, irregular heart rate, shortness of breath, problems with urination (difficult or painful urination; unable to urinate), confusion, extreme sedation, excitement or mania, increased skin sensitivity to the sunlight, extreme constipation, yellow skin or eyes

Some side effects appear when you first start taking desipramine and go away for most people. If the following side effects continue, contact your doctor.

- Dizziness, blurred vision, dry mouth, mild to moderate constipation, increased appetite, weight gain, breast enlargement (men or women), discharge from the breast, sexual problems, tremor of the hands, persistent sore throat

DRUG INTERACTIONS

Desipramine can adversely interact with the following frequently prescribed medications:

- Cimetidine—can cause high desipramine levels
- SSRI antidepressants—can cause high desipramine levels
- MAOI antidepressants—severe reaction causing dangerously high blood pressure, high body temperature, seizures, or death
- Clonidine—if clonidine is being taken for high blood pressure, desipramine may cause clonidine to work less well

- Antipsychotics—may increase certain neurologic side effects
- Thyroid hormones—increased effects of both, especially excitation and changes in heart rate or rhythm
- Carbamazepine—can lower desipramine levels
- Bupropion—can increase desipramine levels
- Anticoagulants (blood thinners)—the effect of the anticoagulant can be increased
- Quinolones—increased risk of heart arrhythmias
- Amphetamines—increased blood pressure, irregular heart rate, or very high fever may result
- Drugs used during surgery—can cause increased blood pressure. Make sure your doctors are aware of upcoming planned surgeries.
- Drugs that depress certain functions of the nervous system, when combined with desipramine, cause extreme drowsiness and slowed reaction times. Examples of these medicines are antihistamines, narcotics, muscle relaxants, and barbiturates.

MEDICAL CONSIDERATIONS

If you have any of the following medical conditions, make sure your doctor is aware of it.

- Liver disease or alcoholism—desipramine levels may be higher than expected
- Kidney disease—desipramine levels may be higher than expected
- Glaucoma—desipramine can increase pressure inside the eye
- Heart problems—some heart problems can be made worse by desipramine; desipramine should not be taken by someone who has had a recent heart attack

- Urinary retention, prostate enlargement—urination may become more difficult
- Seizure disorder—desipramine can lower seizure threshold
- Diabetes mellitus (sugar diabetes)—blood sugar levels may be affected
- Thyroid disorders—desipramine may cause increased heart rate

DESVENLAFAXINE (des-ven-la-FAX-een)

Drug Category: Antidepressant, SNRI (serotonin, norepinephrine reuptake inhibitor)

Requires prescription

COMMONLY USED BRAND-NAME PRODUCTS

Tablets, extended release

Pristiq 50mg, 100mg

GENERAL INFORMATION

Used to treat major depression.

BEFORE TAKING THIS MEDICATION

Talk to your doctor about the benefits and risks associated with desvenlafaxine. Make sure you understand how to take it safely and effectively. You and your family members should be very familiar with the side effects and signs of having too much in your system. Make sure your doctor has the following information in detail:

- Any allergic or bad reactions you have had to desvenlafaxine or any other medication

- All prescription and over-the-counter medicines you are taking
- Your complete medical history
- If you are pregnant, could be pregnant, or are planning a pregnancy in the near future, desvenlafaxine should not be taken
- If you are breast feeding, desvenlafaxine can pass into breast milk and affect the baby

DOSAGE

Adults: 50–400mg daily. When you first start taking desvenlafaxine, your initial dose will be lower and will be gradually increased depending on how you are doing and the side effects you might be experiencing.

Older adults are more susceptible to side effects and will generally require lower dosages.

DIRECTIONS FOR PROPER USE

- *Take exactly as prescribed. Do not take more or less than prescribed.*
- Do not abruptly stop taking desvenlafaxine unless instructed to do so by your doctor.
- If you miss a dose, take it as soon as possible within 1 to 2 hours of the missed dose. However, if it is more than 2 hours after the missed dose, skip the missed dose and resume with your next scheduled dose. Do not double doses.
- Swallow capsules whole with liquid; do not crush, chew, or break.
- It may take several weeks before you feel the full benefits of desvenlafaxine.

PRECAUTIONS

- Desvenlafaxine can cause drowsiness and slowed reaction times. Be cautious when driving, operating machinery, or doing jobs requiring alertness.
- Alcohol can cause changes in mood and may interfere with desvenlafaxine's effectiveness. Alcohol can cause extreme drowsiness when taken with desvenlafaxine. *Alcohol should be avoided while taking desvenlafaxine.*
- *Antidepressants may increase the risk of suicidal thinking and behavior in adolescents and children. When considering an antidepressant in a child or adolescent, the risk must be balanced with the need. Children and adolescents taking antidepressants should be closely monitored for worsening of symptoms, suicidality, or unusual changes in behavior.*

SIDE EFFECTS

Not all side effects will occur. Many side effects will diminish with time. *However, some side effects may require attention from your doctor.* Check with your doctor immediately if you experience any of the following:

- Increased blood pressure, increased heart rate, skin rash or hives, shortness of breath, chills or fever, swelling of the hands or feet, seizures

Some side effects appear when you first start taking desvenlafaxine and go away for most people. If the following side effects continue, contact your doctor.

- Agitation, anxiety, insomnia, dizziness, sexual problems, sweating, blurred vision, dry mouth, mild to moderate constipation, change in appetite, change in weight, tremor of the hands

DRUG INTERACTIONS

Desvenlafaxine can adversely interact with the following frequently prescribed medications or foods:

- Anticoagulants (blood thinners)—the effect of the anticoagulant can be increased
- Some nonsedating antihistamines—cardiac (heart) toxicity
- Diet pills—severe reaction causing dangerously high blood pressure, high body temperature, seizures, or death
- Products containing L-tryptophan or with serotonin activity—severe reaction causing dangerously high blood pressure, high body temperature, seizures, or death
- Cimetidine—can cause high desvenlafaxine levels
- TCA antidepressants—can cause high TCA levels
- MAOI antidepressants—severe reaction causing dangerously high blood pressure, high body temperature, seizures, or death
- Antipsychotics—may increase certain neurologic side effects
- Lithium—increased lithium levels causing possible confusion, dizziness, tremor
- Anticonvulsants—increased anticonvulsant levels or decreased desvenlafaxine levels
- Drugs that depress certain functions of the nervous system, when combined with desvenlafaxine, cause extreme drowsiness and slowed reaction times. Examples of these medicines are antihistamines, narcotics, muscle relaxants, and barbiturates.

MEDICAL CONSIDERATIONS

If you have any of the following medical conditions, make sure your doctor is aware of it.

- Liver disease or alcoholism—desvenlafaxine levels may be higher than expected

- Kidney disease—desvenlafaxine levels may be higher than expected
- Seizure disorder—desvenlafaxine can lower seizure threshold
- Diabetes mellitus (sugar diabetes)—blood sugar levels may be affected

DEXMETHYLPHENIDATE (dex-meth-ill-PHEN-i-date)

Drug Category: Stimulant

Requires prescription, controlled substance, high potential for abuse, requires special prescription (triplicate, nonrefillable)

COMMONLY USED BRAND-NAME PRODUCTS

Tablets
Focalin 2.5mg, 5mg, 10mg
Capsules, extended release
Focalin XR 5mg, 10mg, 15mg, 20mg

GENERAL INFORMATION

Used to treat Attention Deficit Hyperactivity Disorder, as part of a total program that includes psychological, educational, and social components.

BEFORE TAKING THIS MEDICATION

Talk to your doctor about the benefits and risks associated with dexmethylphenidate. Make sure you understand how to take it safely and effectively. You and your family members should be very familiar with the side effects and signs of having too much in your system. Make sure your doctor has the following information in detail:

- Any allergic or bad reactions you have had to dexmethylphenidate or any other medication

- All prescription and over-the-counter medicines you are taking
- Your complete medical history
- If you are pregnant, could be pregnant, or are planning a pregnancy in the near future, dexmethylphenidate should not be taken
- If you are breast feeding, dexmethylphenidate can pass into breast milk and affect the baby

DOSAGE

Adults and children over 6: Dosages are highly individualized, depending on response, age, and dosage form. For regular tablets, dosages can range from 5 to 20mg, usually two times daily. For long-acting capsules, dosages can range from 5 to 20mg daily.

Older adults are more susceptible to side effects and will generally require lower dosages.

DIRECTIONS FOR PROPER USE

- ***Take exactly as prescribed. Do not take more or less than prescribed. Accidental or intended overdoses of dexmethylphenidate are very serious.***
- If you take dexmethylphenidate regularly for an extended period of time, do not stop taking it unless told to do so by your doctor. It may be necessary to gradually reduce the dose before stopping completely.
- If you miss a dose of the regular tablets, take it as soon as possible, unless it is within 3 hours of your next scheduled dose; then skip the missed dose and resume with your next scheduled dose. Do not double the dose.
- If you miss a dose of the long-acting tablets, skip the dose and resume with your next scheduled dose. To prevent trouble sleeping, do not take the last dose later than 6 pm

for regular tablets and 3 pm for long-acting forms, unless otherwise directed by your doctor.

- If you are taking a long-acting form, swallow it whole. Do not crush, chew, or break. The long-acting capsules can be sprinkled over applesauce; make sure you are aware of how to take it.
- Treatment with these medications may last for months to years. Your doctor may discuss the option of "drug holidays." These are planned periods of time when you may not take the medicine—for example, during summer holidays from school.

PRECAUTIONS

Dexmethylphenidate can mask some of the effects of alcohol. Routine alcohol use, or alcohol withdrawal, can increase the chance of seizures, as can dexmethylphenidate. *Alcohol should be avoided while taking dexmethylphenidate.*

SIDE EFFECTS

Not all side effects will occur. Many side effects will diminish with time. *However, some side effects may be warning signs of toxicity and will require attention from your doctor.* Check with your doctor immediately if you experience any of the following:

- Seizures; increased blood pressure; fast or irregular heart-beat; shortness of breath; confusion; agitation; excitement or mania; persistent throbbing headache; muscle twitches; tics or movement problems; unusual behavior; depressed mood; soreness of the mouth, gums, or throat; skin rash or itching; swelling of the face; any unusual bruising or bleeding; appearance of splotchy purplish darkening of the skin; vomiting; fatigue; weakness; fever or flu-like symptoms; yellow tinge of the eyes or skin; dark-colored urine

Some side effects appear when you first start taking dexmethylphenidate and go away for most people. If the following side effects continue, contact your doctor.

- Dizziness, nervousness, blurred vision, difficulty sleeping, decreased appetite, weight loss, headache, nausea, dry mouth

DRUG INTERACTIONS

Dexmethylphenidate can adversely interact with the following frequently prescribed medications:

- Anticoagulants (blood thinners)—the effect of the anticoagulant can be increased
- MAOI antidepressants—severe reaction causing dangerously high blood pressure, high body temperature, seizures, or death
- Other stimulant medications such as decongestants, diet pills, some asthma medications, caffeine—can worsen side effects, especially nervousness, insomnia, high blood pressure
- Serotonin-type antidepressants—can worsen side effects, especially nervousness, insomnia, high blood pressure
- Tricyclic antidepressants—dexmethylphenidate can increase tricyclic levels
- Digoxin—additive effects on the heart resulting in irregular heartbeat
- Anticonvulsants—dexmethylphenidate can increase anticonvulsant levels
- Pimozide—dexmethylphenidate may worsen tics
- Clonidine and other medications used to treat high blood pressure—dexmethylphenidate may make these drugs less effective

MEDICAL CONSIDERATIONS

If you have any of the following medical conditions, make sure your doctor is aware of it.

- Liver disease or alcoholism—dexmethylphenidate levels may be higher than expected
- Kidney disease—dexmethylphenidate levels may be higher than expected
- Drug or alcohol dependence—dependence on dexmethylphenidate may occur
- Seizure disorder—stopping dexmethylphenidate abruptly may cause seizures
- Heart problems—some heart problems can be worsened by dexmethylphenidate
- High blood pressure—dexmethylphenidate may increase blood pressure
- Glaucoma—dexmethylphenidate may worsen the condition
- Tourette's syndrome—dexmethylphenidate may worsen tics
- Hyperthyroidism—thyroid hormone levels may increase

DIAZEPAM (dye-A-ze-pam)

Drug Category: Antianxiety medicine

Requires prescription, controlled substance, moderate potential for abuse

COMMONLY USED BRAND-NAME PRODUCTS

Tablets

Valium (and generic) 2mg, 5mg, 10mg

Liquid

Valium (and generic) 5mg/ml (concentrate), 5mg/5ml

GENERAL INFORMATION

Used to treat anxiety and symptoms of alcohol withdrawal. *This medicine is not intended to help with the stress of everyday life. Even when taken as prescribed, diazepam may cause psychological and/or physical dependence.*

BEFORE TAKING THIS MEDICATION

Talk to your doctor about the benefits and risks associated with diazepam. Make sure you understand how to take it safely and effectively. You and your family members should be very familiar with the side effects and signs of having too much in your system. Make sure your doctor has the following information in detail:

- Any allergic or bad reactions you have had to diazepam or any other medication
- All prescription and over-the-counter medicines you are taking
- Your complete medical history, including mental health conditions
- If you are pregnant, could be pregnant, or are planning a pregnancy in the near future, diazepam should not be taken
- If you are breast feeding, diazepam can pass into breast milk and affect the baby

USUAL ADULT DOSAGE RANGE

5–40 mg daily, in divided doses.
Older adults are more susceptible to side effects and will generally require lower dosages.

DIRECTIONS FOR PROPER USE

- *Take exactly as prescribed. Do not take more or less than prescribed. Diazepam levels that are too high can cause serious toxicity.*
- If you take diazepam regularly for an extended period of

time, do not stop taking it unless told to do so by your doctor. It may be necessary to gradually reduce the dose before stopping completely. If the medicine is stopped too quickly, your condition could become worse, or you could experience serious effects, such as seizures.

- May be taken with food to decrease stomach upset.
- If you miss a dose, take it as soon as possible. However, if the missed dose is within 4 hours of your next dose, skip the missed dose and resume with your next scheduled dose. Do not double the dose.
- If you are taking the concentrated liquid form, mix your dose in water, fruit juice (but not grapefruit juice), applesauce, or pudding before taking. Measure the dose carefully. Take immediately; do not save for later use.

PRECAUTIONS

- Diazepam can cause drowsiness and slowed reaction times. Be cautious when driving, operating machinery, or doing jobs requiring alertness.
- Alcohol can cause extreme drowsiness when taken with diazepam. *Alcohol should be avoided while taking diazepam.*

SIDE EFFECTS

Not all side effects will occur. Many side effects will diminish with time. *However, some side effects may be warning signs of toxicity and will require attention from your doctor.* Check with your doctor immediately if you experience any of the following:

- Confusion, severe drowsiness, slurred speech, severe weakness, unusual thoughts, shortness of breath, excitement, hyperactivity, memory problems

Some side effects appear when you first start taking diazepam and go away for most people. If the following side effects continue, contact your doctor.

- Dizziness, lightheadedness, drowsiness, blurred vision, stomach problems

DRUG INTERACTIONS

Diazepam can adversely interact with the following frequently prescribed medications or foods:

- Cimetidine (Tagamet)—can cause high diazepam levels
- Disulfiram (Antabuse)—can cause high diazepam levels
- Birth control pills—can cause high diazepam levels
- Levodopa—decreased effectiveness of levodopa
- Macrolide antibiotics (e.g., erythromycin)—can cause high diazepam levels
- Oral antifungal agents—can cause high diazepam levels
- HIV protease inhibitors—can cause high diazepam levels
- Calcium channel blockers—can cause high diazepam levels
- Serotonin-type antidepressants—can cause high diazepam levels
- Digoxin—diazepam can cause high digoxin levels
- Valproic acid—can cause high diazepam levels
- Isoniazid—can cause high diazepam levels
- Beta blockers—can cause high diazepam levels
- Propoxyphene—can cause high diazepam levels
- Carbamazepine—can lower diazepam levels
- Grapefruit juice—can cause high diazepam levels
- Drugs that depress certain functions of the nervous system, when combined with diazepam, cause extreme drowsiness and slowed reaction times. Examples of these medicines are antihistamines, narcotics, muscle relaxants, and barbiturates.

MEDICAL CONSIDERATIONS

If you have any of the following medical conditions, make sure your doctor is aware of it.

- Liver disease or alcoholism—diazepam levels may be higher than expected
- Kidney disease—diazepam levels may be higher than expected
- Drug or alcohol dependence—dependence on diazepam may occur
- Seizure disorder—stopping diazepam abruptly may cause seizures
- Chronic lung disease—diazepam may make breathing more difficult
- Glaucoma—diazepam may worsen the condition
- Sleep apnea—diazepam may worsen the condition

DOXEPIN (dox-e-pin)
Drug Category: Antidepressant, tricyclic
Requires prescription

COMMONLY USED BRAND-NAME PRODUCTS
Capsules
Sinequan, Adapin (and generic) 10mg, 25mg, 50mg, 75mg, 100mg, 150mg
Solution
Doxepin, 10mg/ml

GENERAL INFORMATION
Used to treat major depression and the depressed phase of bipolar disorder. Because of its sedative effects, it is sometimes given in low doses to help with insomnia. Also used to treat certain chronic pain disorders, such as migraine headache and diabetic neuropathy.

BEFORE TAKING THIS MEDICATION

Talk to your doctor about the benefits and risks associated with doxepin. Make sure you understand how to take it safely and effectively. You and your family members should be very familiar with the side effects and signs of having too much in your system. Make sure your doctor has the following information in detail:

- Any allergic or bad reactions you have had to doxepin or any other medication
- All prescription and over-the-counter medicines you are taking
- Your complete medical history
- If you are pregnant, could be pregnant, or are planning a pregnancy in the near future, doxepin should not be taken
- If you are breast feeding, doxepin can pass into breast milk and affect the baby

USUAL ADULT DOSAGE RANGE

The starting dose of doxepin will be low and gradually be increased. Sometimes blood levels are tested to ensure that the dose you are taking is in the safe and effective range.

Depression: Starting dose 25–50mg at bedtime. Increased to 75–300mg at bedtime over 2 to 3 weeks.

Insomnia: 10–50mg at bedtime.

Chronic pain syndrome: 50–100mg daily.

Older adults are more susceptible to side effects and will generally require lower dosages.

DIRECTIONS FOR PROPER USE

- *Take exactly as prescribed. Do not take more or less than prescribed. Accidental or intended overdoses of doxepin are potentially fatal.*
- Do not abruptly stop taking doxepin unless instructed to

do so by your doctor. Gradually reducing the dose can help prevent mood changes, headache, or diarrhea.

- If you miss a bedtime dose, do not take it the next morning, since it may make you drowsy. Do not double doses.
- If you are taking the liquid form of doxepin, it must be mixed in liquid before taking. Use the dropper that comes with the original bottle. Doxepin must be mixed in 4 ounces of water, milk, citrus juice, or tomato or prune juice before taking. Do not mix in grape or carbonated beverages. Take immediately after mixing. Do not store for later use.
- It may take several weeks before you feel the full benefits.

PRECAUTIONS
- Doxepin can cause drowsiness and slowed reaction times. Be cautious when driving, operating machinery, or doing jobs requiring alertness.
- Alcohol can cause changes in mood and may interfere with doxepin's effectiveness. Alcohol can cause extreme drowsiness when taken with doxepin. ***Alcohol should be avoided while taking doxepin.***
- Doxepin may cause your skin and eyes to be more sensitive to sunlight. Exposure to sunlight may cause a rash, skin discoloration, or sunburn. Limit direct exposure to sunlight, and use sunscreen when in direct sunlight. Avoid tanning booths and beds. Wear UV-blocking sunglasses when outdoors.
- When taking doxepin, stand up slowly after sitting or lying down, since it may cause your blood pressure to drop and cause faintness or dizziness. Stand up slowly from a seated or lying position, especially when you first start taking doxepin.

- *Antidepressants may increase the risk of suicidal thinking and behavior in adolescents and children. When considering an antidepressant in a child or adolescent, the risk must be balanced with the need. Children and adolescents taking antidepressants should be closely monitored for worsening of symptoms, suicidality, or unusual changes in behavior.*

- Adolescents and children may be more susceptible to heart-related side effects of tricyclic antidepressants. Risk must be balanced with need. Blood levels and heart function should be monitored in children and adolescents taking tricyclic antidepressants.

SIDE EFFECTS

Not all side effects will occur. Many side effects will diminish with time. *However, some side effects may require attention from your doctor.* Check with your doctor immediately if you experience any of the following:

- Seizure, changes in blood pressure, irregular heart rate, shortness of breath, problems with urination (difficult or painful urination, unable to urinate), confusion, extreme sedation, excitation or mania, increased skin sensitivity to the sunlight, extreme constipation, yellow skin or eyes

Some side effects appear when you first start taking doxepin and go away for most people. If the following side effects continue, contact your doctor.

- Dizziness, blurred vision, dry mouth, mild to moderate constipation, increased appetite, weight gain, breast enlargement (men or women), discharge from the breast, sexual problems, tremor of the hands, persistent sore throat

DRUG INTERACTIONS

Doxepin can adversely interact with the following frequently prescribed medications:

- Cimetidine—can cause high doxepin levels
- SSRI antidepressants—can cause high doxepin levels
- MAOI antidepressants—severe reaction causing dangerously high blood pressure, high body temperature, seizures, or death
- Clonidine—if clonidine is being taken for high blood pressure, doxepin may cause clonidine to work less well
- Antipsychotics—may increase certain neurologic side effects
- Thyroid hormones—increased effects of both, especially excitation and changes in heart rate or rhythm
- Carbamazepine—can lower doxepin levels
- Bupropion—can increase doxepin levels
- Anticoagulants (blood thinners)—the effect of the anticoagulant can be increased
- Quinolones—increased risk of heart arrhythmias
- Amphetamines—increased blood pressure, irregular heart rate, or very high fever may result
- Drugs used during surgery—can cause increased blood pressure; make sure your doctors are aware of upcoming planned surgeries
- Drugs that depress certain functions of the nervous system, when combined with doxepin, cause extreme drowsiness and slowed reaction times. Examples of these medicines are antihistamines, narcotics, muscle relaxants, and barbiturates.

MEDICAL CONSIDERATIONS

If you have any of the following medical conditions, make sure your doctor is aware of it.

- Liver disease or alcoholism—doxepin levels may be higher than expected
- Kidney disease—doxepin levels may be higher than expected
- Glaucoma—doxepin can increase pressure inside the eye
- Heart problems—some heart problems can be made worse by doxepin; doxepin should not be taken by someone who has had a recent heart attack
- Urinary retention, prostate enlargement—urination may become more difficult
- Seizure disorder—doxepin can lower seizure threshold
- Diabetes mellitus (sugar diabetes)—blood sugar levels may be affected
- Thyroid disorders—doxepin may cause increased heart rate

DULOXETINE (due-LOX-uh-teen)

Drug Category: Antidepressant, SNRI (serotonin, norepinephrine reuptake inhibitor)

Requires prescription

COMMONLY USED BRAND-NAME PRODUCTS

Capsules, delayed release

Cymbalta 20mg, 30mg, 60mg

GENERAL INFORMATION

Used to treat major depression and the depressed phase of bipolar disorder. Also used to treat generalized anxiety disorder. Used to treat nerve pain in diabetic patients.

BEFORE TAKING THIS MEDICATION

Talk to your doctor about the benefits and risks associated with duloxetine. Make sure you understand how to take it safely and effectively. You and your family members should be very familiar with the side effects and signs of having too much in your system. Make sure your doctor has the following information in detail:

- Any allergic or bad reactions you have had to duloxetine or any other medication
- All prescription and over-the-counter medicines you are taking
- Your complete medical history
- If you are pregnant, could be pregnant, or are planning a pregnancy in the near future, duloxetine should not be taken
- If you are breast feeding, duloxetine can pass into breast milk and affect the baby

USUAL ADULT DOSAGE RANGE

20–30mg twice daily or 40–60mg once daily.
Older adults are more susceptible to side effects and will generally require lower dosages.

DIRECTIONS FOR PROPER USE

- *Take exactly as prescribed. Do not take more or less than prescribed.*
- Do not abruptly stop taking duloxetine unless instructed to do so by your doctor. Gradually reducing the dose can help prevent mood changes, headache, or diarrhea.
- If you miss a dose, take it as soon as possible within 1 to 2 hours of the missed dose. However, if it is more than 2 hours after the missed dose, skip the missed dose and resume with your next scheduled dose. Do not double doses. Swallow capsules whole. Do not crush, chew, or break.

- It may take several weeks before you feel the full benefits of duloxetine.

PRECAUTIONS

- Duloxetine can cause drowsiness and slowed reaction times. Be cautious when driving, operating machinery, or doing jobs requiring alertness.
- Alcohol can cause changes in mood and may interfere with duloxetine's effectiveness. Alcohol can cause extreme drowsiness when taken with duloxetine. *Alcohol should be avoided while taking duloxetine.*
- When taking duloxetine, stand up slowly after sitting or lying down, since it may cause your blood pressure to drop and cause faintness or dizziness. Stand up slowly from a seated or lying position, especially when you first start taking duloxetine.
- *Antidepressants may increase the risk of suicidal thinking and behavior in adolescents and children. When considering an antidepressant in a child or adolescent, the risk must be balanced with the need. Children and adolescents taking antidepressants should be closely monitored for worsening of symptoms, suicidality, or unusual changes in behavior.*

SIDE EFFECTS

Not all side effects will occur. Many side effects will diminish with time. *However, some side effects may require attention from your doctor.* Check with your doctor immediately if you experience any of the following:

- Increased blood pressure, increased heart rate, skin rash or hives, shortness of breath, chills or fever, swelling of the hands or feet, seizures, bruising/bleeding, dark urine or stools

Some side effects appear when you first start taking duloxetine and go away for most people. If the following side effects continue, contact your doctor.

- Agitation, anxiety, insomnia, dizziness, sexual problems, sweating, blurred vision, dry mouth, mild to moderate constipation, change in appetite, change in weight, tremor of the hands

DRUG INTERACTIONS

Duloxetine can adversely interact with the following frequently prescribed medications:

- Anticoagulants (blood thinners)—the effect of the anticoagulant can be increased
- Diet pills—severe reaction causing dangerously high blood pressure, high body temperature, seizures, or death
- Products containing L-tryptophan or with serotonin activity—severe reaction causing dangerously high blood pressure, high body temperature, seizures, or death
- Cimetidine—can cause high duloxetine levels
- TCA antidepressants—can cause high TCA levels
- MAOI antidepressants—severe reaction causing dangerously high blood pressure, high body temperature, seizures, or death
- Antipsychotics—may increase certain neurologic side effects
- Lithium—increased lithium levels causing possible confusion, dizziness, tremor
- Quinolones—can cause high duloxetine levels
- Antiarryhthmics—increased risk of heart arrhythmias
- Anticonvulsants—increased anticonvulsant levels or decreased duloxetine levels
- Drugs that depress certain functions of the nervous system,

when combined with duloxetine, cause extreme drowsiness and slowed reaction times. Examples of these medicines are antihistamines, narcotics, muscle relaxants, and barbiturates.

MEDICAL CONSIDERATIONS

If you have any of the following medical conditions, make sure your doctor is aware of it.

- Liver disease or alcoholism—duloxetine levels may be higher than expected
- Kidney disease—duloxetine levels may be higher than expected
- Glaucoma—duloxetine can increase pressure inside the eye
- Seizure disorder—duloxetine can lower seizure threshold
- Diabetes mellitus (sugar diabetes)—blood sugar levels may be affected

ESCITALOPRAM (es-SIT-al-oh-pram)

Drug Category: Antidepressant, SSRI (serotonin specific reuptake inhibitor)

Requires prescription

COMMONLY USED BRAND-NAME PRODUCTS

Tablets

Lexapro 5mg, 10mg, 20mg

Solution

5mg/5ml

GENERAL INFORMATION

Used to treat major depression and the depressed phase of bipolar disorder. Also used to treat generalized anxiety disorder.

BEFORE TAKING THIS MEDICATION

Talk to your doctor about the benefits and risks associated with escitalopram. Make sure you understand how to take it safely and effectively. You and your family members should be very familiar with the side effects and signs of having too much in your system. Make sure your doctor has the following information in detail:

- Any allergic or bad reactions you have had to escitalopram or any other medication
- All prescription and over-the-counter medicines you are taking
- Your complete medical history
- If you are pregnant, could be pregnant, or are planning a pregnancy in the near future, escitalopram should not be taken
- If you are breast feeding, escitalopram can pass into breast milk and affect the baby

USUAL ADULT DOSAGE RANGE

10–20mg daily. Dosage increases should occur no more often than weekly.

Older adults are more susceptible to side effects and will generally require lower dosages.

DIRECTIONS FOR PROPER USE

- ***Take exactly as prescribed. Do not take more or less than prescribed.***
- Do not abruptly stop taking escitalopram unless instructed to do so by your doctor.
- May be taken with food or meals to lessen stomach upset.
- If you miss a dose, do not try to make it up. Wait and take your next scheduled dose. Do not double doses.
- It may take several weeks before you feel the full benefits.

PRECAUTIONS

- Escitalopram can cause drowsiness and slowed reaction times. Be cautious when driving, operating machinery, or doing jobs requiring alertness.
- Alcohol can cause changes in mood and may interfere with escitalopram's effectiveness. Alcohol can cause extreme drowsiness when taken with escitalopram. *Alcohol should be avoided while taking escitalopram.*
- Escitalopram may cause your skin and eyes to be more sensitive to sunlight. Exposure to sunlight may cause a rash, skin discoloration, or sunburn. Limit direct exposure to sunlight, and use sunscreen when in direct sunlight. Avoid tanning booths and beds. Wear UV-blocking sunglasses when outdoors.
- *Antidepressants may increase the risk of suicidal thinking and behavior in adolescents and children. When considering an antidepressant in a child or adolescent, the risk must be balanced with the need. Children and adolescents taking antidepressants should be closely monitored for worsening of symptoms, suicidality, or unusual changes in behavior.*

SIDE EFFECTS

Not all side effects will occur. Many side effects will diminish with time. *However, some side effects may require attention from your doctor.* Check with your doctor immediately if you experience any of the following:

- Skin rash or hives, shortness of breath, chills or fever; swelling of the hands or feet, seizures, bleeding or bruising

Some side effects appear when you first start taking escitalopram and go away for most people. If the following side effects continue, contact your doctor.

- Agitation, anxiety, insomnia, dizziness, sexual problems,

sweating, blurred vision, dry mouth, mild to moderate constipation, change in appetite, change in weight, tremor of the hands

DRUG INTERACTIONS

Escitalopram can adversely interact with the following frequently prescribed medications or foods:

- Anticoagulants (blood thinners)—the effect of the anticoagulant can be increased
- Some nonsedating antihistamines—cardiac (heart) toxicity
- Diet pills—severe reaction causing dangerously high blood pressure, high body temperature, seizures, or death
- Products containing L-tryptophan—severe reaction causing dangerously high blood pressure, high body temperature, seizures, or death
- Cimetidine—can cause high escitalopram levels
- Bupropion—dosage adjustment of one or both drugs may be necessary
- Amphetamines—increased blood pressure, irregular heart rate, or very high fever may result
- TCA antidepressants—can cause high TCA levels
- MAOI antidepressants—severe reaction causing dangerously high blood pressure, high body temperature, seizures, or death
- Antipsychotics—may increase certain neurologic side effects
- Lithium—increased lithium levels causing possible confusion, dizziness, tremor
- Anticonvulsants—increased anticonvulsant levels or decreased escitalopram levels
- Antiarrhythmic drugs—increased risk of arrhythmias
- Benzodiazepines—escitalopram can increase benzodiazepine levels

- Beta blockers—escitalopram can increase beta blocker levels
- Aspirin, NSAIDs—increased chance of bleeding
- HIV protease inhibitors—escitalopram can increase levels of protease inhibitors
- Drugs that depress certain functions of the nervous system, when combined with escitalopram, cause extreme drowsiness and slowed reaction times. Examples of these medicines are antihistamines, narcotics, muscle relaxants, and barbiturates.

MEDICAL CONSIDERATIONS

If you have any of the following medical conditions, make sure your doctor is aware of it.

- Liver disease or alcoholism—escitalopram levels may be higher than expected
- Kidney disease—escitalopram levels may be higher than expected
- Seizure disorder—escitalopram can lower seizure threshold
- Diabetes mellitus (sugar diabetes)—blood sugar levels may be affected
- Low sodium—escitalopram may worsen this condition
- Bleeding disorder—escitalopram may worsen this condition

ESTAZOLAM (es-TAZ-o-lam)

Drug Category: Insomnia medicine

Requires prescription, controlled substance, moderate potential for abuse

COMMONLY USED BRAND-NAME PRODUCTS

Tablets

ProSom (and generic) 1mg, 2mg

GENERAL INFORMATION

Used to treat insomnia. *Even when taken as prescribed, estazolam may cause psychological and/or physical dependence. Not intended for long-term use.*

BEFORE TAKING THIS MEDICATION

Talk to your doctor about the benefits and risks associated with estazolam. Make sure you understand how to take it safely and effectively. You and your family members should be very familiar with the side effects and signs of having too much in your system. Make sure your doctor has the following information in detail:

- Any allergic or bad reactions you have had to estazolam or any other medication
- All prescription and over-the-counter medicines you are taking
- Your complete medical history, including mental health conditions
- If you are pregnant, could be pregnant, or are planning a pregnancy in the near future, estazolam should not be taken
- If you are breast feeding, estazolam can pass into breast milk and affect the baby

USUAL ADULT DOSAGE RANGE

1–2mg at bedtime

Older adults are more susceptible to side effects and will generally require lower dosages.

DIRECTIONS FOR PROPER USE

- *Take exactly as prescribed. Do not take more or less than prescribed. Estazolam levels that are too high can cause serious toxicity.*
- If you take estazolam regularly for an extended period of

time, do not stop taking it unless told to do so by your doctor. It may be necessary to gradually reduce the dose before stopping completely.

- If you miss a dose, take it as soon as possible if it is within 1 hour of the scheduled time. However, estazolam should be taken only if you are sure you will get a full night's sleep of at least 7 to 8 hours.

PRECAUTIONS

- Estazolam can cause drowsiness and slowed reaction times. Be cautious when driving, operating machinery, or doing jobs requiring alertness.
- Alcohol can cause extreme drowsiness when taken with estazolam. *Alcohol should be avoided while taking estazolam.*
- Estazolam may cause a severe allergic reaction and/or severe facial swelling, which can occur as early as the first dose.
- Estazolam can cause complex sleep-related behaviors, which may include sleep-driving, making phone calls, and preparing and eating food (while asleep).

SIDE EFFECTS

Not all side effects will occur. Many side effects will diminish with time. *However, some side effects may be warning signs of toxicity and will require attention from your doctor.* Check with your doctor immediately if you experience any of the following:

- Confusion, severe drowsiness, slurred speech, severe weakness, unusual thoughts, shortness of breath, excitement, hyperactivity, memory problems

Some side effects appear when you first start taking estazolam and go away for most people. If the following side effects continue, contact your doctor.

- Dizziness, lightheadedness, daytime drowsiness, blurred vision

DRUG INTERACTIONS

Estazolam can adversely interact with the following frequently prescribed medications or foods:

- Cimetidine (Tagamet)—can cause high estazolam levels
- Disulfiram (Antabuse)—can cause high estazolam levels
- Birth control pills—can cause high estazolam levels
- Levodopa—decreased effectiveness of levodopa
- Macrolide antibiotics (e.g., erythromycin)—can cause high estazolam levels
- Oral antifungal agents—can cause high estazolam levels
- HIV protease inhibitors—can cause high estazolam levels
- Calcium channel blockers—can cause high estazolam levels
- Serotonin-type antidepressants—can cause high estazolam levels
- Digoxin—estazolam can cause high digoxin levels
- Valproic acid—can cause high estazolam levels
- Isoniazid—can cause high estazolam levels
- Beta blockers—can cause high estazolam levels
- Propoxyphene—can cause high estazolam levels
- Carbamazepine—can lower estazolam levels
- Grapefruit juice—can cause high estazolam levels
- Drugs that depress certain functions of the nervous system, when combined with estazolam, cause extreme drowsiness and slowed reaction times. Examples of these medicines are antihistamines, narcotics, muscle relaxants, and barbiturates.

MEDICAL CONSIDERATIONS

If you have any of the following medical conditions, make sure your doctor is aware of it.

- Liver disease or alcoholism—estazolam levels may be higher than expected
- Kidney disease—estazolam levels may be higher than expected
- Drug or alcohol dependence—dependence on estazolam may occur
- Seizure disorder—stopping estazolam abruptly may cause seizures
- Chronic lung disease—estazolam may make breathing more difficult
- Glaucoma—estazolam may worsen the condition
- Sleep apnea—estazolam may worsen the condition

ESZOPICLONE (es-ZOE-pi-clone)

Drug Category: Insomnia medicine
Requires prescription, controlled substance, moderate potential for abuse

COMMONLY USED BRAND-NAME PRODUCTS
Tablets
Lunesta 1mg, 2mg, 3mg

GENERAL INFORMATION
Used to treat insomnia. *Even when taken as prescribed, eszopiclone may cause psychological and/or physical dependence. Not intended for long-term use.*

BEFORE TAKING THIS MEDICATION
Talk to your doctor about the benefits and risks associated with eszopiclone. Make sure you understand how to take it safely and effectively. You and your family members should be very familiar with the side effects and signs of having too much

in your system. Make sure your doctor has the following information in detail:

- Any allergic or bad reactions you have had to eszopiclone or any other medication
- All prescription and over-the-counter medicines you are taking
- Your complete medical history, including mental health conditions
- If you are pregnant, could be pregnant, or are planning a pregnancy in the near future, eszopiclone should not be taken
- If you are breast feeding, eszopiclone can pass into breast milk and affect the baby

USUAL ADULT DOSAGE RANGE
1–3mg at bedtime.
Older adults are more susceptible to side effects and will generally require lower dosages.

DIRECTIONS FOR PROPER USE
- ***Take exactly as prescribed. Do not take more or less than prescribed. Eszopiclone levels that are too high can cause serious toxicity.***
- If you take eszopiclone regularly for an extended period of time, do not stop taking it unless told to do so by your doctor. It may be necessary to gradually reduce the dose before stopping completely.
- Do not take with or immediately after a high-fat meal.
- Take immediately before bedtime and only if you are sure you will get a full night's sleep of at least 8 hours.
- Swallow the tablet whole; do not crush, break, or chew.

PRECAUTIONS

- Eszopiclone can cause drowsiness and slowed reaction times. Be cautious when driving, operating machinery, or doing jobs requiring alertness.
- Alcohol can cause extreme drowsiness when taken with eszopiclone. *Alcohol should be avoided while taking eszopiclone.*
- Eszopiclone may cause a severe allergic reaction and/or severe facial swelling, which can occur as early as the first dose.
- Eszopiclone can cause complex sleep-related behaviors, which may include sleep-driving, making phone calls, and preparing and eating food (while asleep).

SIDE EFFECTS

Not all side effects will occur. Many side effects will diminish with time. *However, some side effects may be warning signs of toxicity and will require attention from your doctor.* Check with your doctor immediately if you experience any of the following:

- Confusion, severe drowsiness, slurred speech, severe weakness, unusual thoughts, shortness of breath, excitement, hyperactivity, memory problems, abnormal addictive behaviors

Some side effects appear when you first start taking eszopiclone and go away for most people. If the following side effects continue, contact your doctor.

- Dizziness, lightheadedness, daytime drowsiness, blurred vision

DRUG INTERACTIONS

Eszopiclone can adversely interact with the following frequently prescribed medications:

- Macrolide antibiotics (e.g., erythromycin)—can cause high eszopiclone levels
- Oral antifungal agents—can cause high eszopiclone levels
- HIV protease inhibitors—can cause high eszopiclone levels
- Anticonvulsants—can cause lower eszopiclone levels
- Drugs that depress certain functions of the nervous system, when combined with eszopiclone, cause extreme drowsiness and slowed reaction times. Examples of these medicines are antihistamines, narcotics, muscle relaxants, and barbiturates.

MEDICAL CONSIDERATIONS

If you have any of the following medical conditions, make sure your doctor is aware of it.

- Liver disease or alcoholism—eszopiclone levels may be higher than expected
- Kidney disease—eszopiclone levels may be higher than expected
- Drug or alcohol dependence—dependence on eszopiclone may occur
- Chronic lung disease—eszopiclone may make breathing more difficult

FLUOXETINE (flew-OX-un-teen)

Drug Category: Antidepressant, SSRI (serotonin specific reuptake inhibitor)

Requires prescription

COMMONLY USED BRAND-NAME PRODUCTS

Capsules and Tablets

Prozac (and generic) 10mg, 20mg, 40mg

Capsules, delayed release 90mg
Prozac Weekly.
Solution
Prozac 20mg/5ml

GENERAL INFORMATION
Used to treat major depression, the depressed phase of bipolar disorder, and obsessive compulsive disorder (OCD). Effective in treating panic disorder. May be useful in treating bulimia and premenstrual dysphoric disorder (PMDD).

BEFORE TAKING THIS MEDICATION
Talk to your doctor about the benefits and risks associated with fluoxetine. Make sure you understand how to take it safely and effectively. You and your family members should be very familiar with the side effects and signs of having too much in your system. Make sure your doctor has the following information in detail:

- Any allergic or bad reactions you have had to fluoxetine or any other medication
- All prescription and over-the-counter medicines you are taking
- Your complete medical history
- If you are pregnant, could be pregnant, or are planning a pregnancy in the near future, fluoxetine should not be taken
- If you are breast feeding, fluoxetine can pass into breast milk and affect the baby

USUAL ADULT DOSAGE RANGE
Depression, panic disorder, bulimia, PMDD: 10–40mg daily. Sometimes higher doses are required. Dosage increases should not be more often than every 4 weeks.

OCD: 20–80mg daily.
Bulimia: 60mg daily.
Older adults are more susceptible to side effects and will generally require lower dosages.

DIRECTIONS FOR PROPER USE

- *Take exactly as prescribed. Do not take more or less than prescribed.*
- Do not abruptly stop taking fluoxetine unless instructed to do so by your doctor.
- May be taken with food or meals to lessen stomach upset.
- If you miss a dose, do not try to make it up. Wait and take your next scheduled dose. Do not double doses.
- If you are taking the weekly dosage form, swallow the capsule whole; do not crush, chew, or break.
- It may take several weeks before you feel the full benefits.

PRECAUTIONS

- Fluoxetine can cause drowsiness and slowed reaction times. Be cautious when driving, operating machinery, or doing jobs requiring alertness.
- Alcohol can cause changes in mood and may interfere with fluoxetine's effectiveness. Alcohol can cause extreme drowsiness when taken with fluoxetine. *Alcohol should be avoided while taking fluoxetine.*
- Fluoxetine may cause your skin and eyes to be more sensitive to sunlight. Exposure to sunlight may cause a rash, skin discoloration, or sunburn. Limit direct exposure to sunlight, and use sunscreen when in direct sunlight. Avoid tanning booths and beds. Wear UV-blocking sunglasses when outdoors.
- *Antidepressants may increase the risk of suicidal thinking and behavior in adolescents and children. When considering an antidepressant in a child or adolescent, the risk*

must be balanced with the need. Children and adolescents taking antidepressants should be closely monitored for worsening of symptoms, suicidality, or unusual changes in behavior.

SIDE EFFECTS

Not all side effects will occur. Many side effects will diminish with time. *However, some side effects may require attention from your doctor.* Check with your doctor immediately if you experience any of the following:

- Skin rash or hives, shortness of breath, chills or fever, swelling of the hands or feet, seizures, bleeding or bruising

Some side effects appear when you first start taking fluoxetine and go away for most people. If the following side effects continue, contact your doctor.

- Agitation, anxiety, insomnia, dizziness, sexual problems, sweating, blurred vision, dry mouth, mild to moderate constipation, change in appetite, change in weight, tremor of the hands

DRUG INTERACTIONS

Fluoxetine can adversely interact with the following frequently prescribed medications or foods:

- Anticoagulants (blood thinners)—the effect of the anticoagulant can be increased
- Some nonsedating antihistamines—cardiac (heart) toxicity
- Diet pills—severe reaction causing dangerously high blood pressure, high body temperature, seizures, or death
- Products containing L-tryptophan—severe reaction causing dangerously high blood pressure, high body temperature, seizures, or death
- Cimetidine—can cause high fluoxetine levels
- Bupropion—dosage adjustment of one or both drugs may be necessary

- Amphetamines—increased blood pressure, irregular heart rate, or very high fever may result
- TCA antidepressants—can cause high TCA levels
- MAOI antidepressants—severe reaction causing dangerously high blood pressure, high body temperature, seizures, or death
- Antipsychotics—may increase certain neurologic side effects
- Lithium—increased lithium levels causing possible confusion, dizziness, tremor
- Anticonvulsants—increased anticonvulsant levels or decreased fluoxetine levels
- Antiarrhythmic drugs—increased risk of arrhythmias
- Benzodiazepines—fluoxetine can increase benzodiazepine levels
- Beta blockers—fluoxetine can increase beta blocker levels
- Aspirin, NSAIDs—increased chance of bleeding
- HIV protease inhibitors—fluoxetine can increase levels of protease inhibitors
- Drugs that depress certain functions of the nervous system when combined with fluoxetine cause extreme drowsiness and slowed reaction times. Examples of these medicines are antihistamines, narcotics, muscle relaxants, and barbiturates.

MEDICAL CONSIDERATIONS

If you have any of the following medical conditions, make sure your doctor is aware of it.

- Liver disease, or alcoholism—fluoxetine levels may be higher than expected
- Kidney disease—fluoxetine levels may be higher than expected
- Seizure disorder—fluoxetine can lower seizure threshold

- Diabetes mellitus (sugar diabetes)—blood sugar levels may be affected
- Low sodium—fluoxetine may worsen this condition
- Bleeding disorder—fluoxetine may worsen this condition

FLUPHENAZINE (flew-FEN-uh-zeen)

Drug Category: Neuroleptic; Antipsychotic
Requires prescription

COMMONLY USED BRAND-NAME PRODUCTS

Tablets
Prolixin (and generic), 1mg, 2.5mg, 5mg, 10mg
Liquid
Prolixin (and generic) solution 2.5mg/5ml (contains alcohol), 5mg/ml

GENERAL INFORMATION

Used to treat psychotic symptoms, such as hallucinations and delusions. These symptoms occur in schizophrenia, schizoaffective disorder, bipolar disorder, or major depression with psychotic features. Fluphenazine can be used for short-term management of aggressive, out-of-control behaviors or feelings of anger and rage.

BEFORE TAKING THIS MEDICATION

Talk to your doctor about the benefits and risks associated with fluphenazine. Make sure you understand how to take it safely and effectively. You and your family members should be very familiar with its side effects. Make sure your doctor has the following information in detail:

- Any allergic or bad reactions you have had to fluphenazine or any other medication

- All prescription and over-the-counter medicines you are taking
- Your complete medical history
- If you are pregnant, could be pregnant, or are planning a pregnancy in the near future, fluphenazine has not been shown to be absolutely safe
- If you are breast feeding, fluphenazine can pass into breast milk and affect the baby

USUAL ADULT DOSAGE RANGE

5–80mg daily. There is a wide effective dosage range.

Older adults are *extremely* susceptible to side effects and will generally require lower dosages.

DIRECTIONS FOR PROPER USE

- ***Take exactly as prescribed. Do not take more or less than prescribed. Fluphenazine levels that are too high can cause serious toxicity.***
- If you miss a dose, take it as soon as possible. However, if the missed dose is within 4 hours of your next dose, skip the missed dose and resume with your next scheduled dose. Do not double the dose.
- If you are taking a liquid form, avoid contacting the skin with the medicine. Irritation can result by the medicine coming in contact with skin. Do not use the liquid form if the medicine becomes very discolored (dark yellow) or has a sediment at the bottom of the bottle.
- The long-acting shot form of fluphenazine can have an effect for up to 4 weeks after the shot is given.
- It may be several weeks before you feel the full benefits.

PRECAUTIONS

- Fluphenazine can cause drowsiness and slowed reaction times. Be cautious when driving, operating machinery, or doing jobs requiring alertness.
- Alcohol can cause extreme drowsiness when taken with fluphenazine. *Alcohol should be avoided while taking fluphenazine.*
- Fluphenazine may cause your body temperature to increase and could result in heat stroke. Be extra careful in hot weather, when exercising, or when taking hot baths or saunas not to become overheated.
- Fluphenazine may cause your skin and eyes to be more sensitive to sunlight. Exposure to sunlight may cause a rash, skin discoloration, or sunburn. Limit direct exposure to sunlight and use sunscreen when in direct sunlight. Avoid tanning booths and beds. Wear UV-blocking sunglasses when outdoors.
- When taking fluphenazine, stand up slowly after sitting or lying down, since it may cause your blood pressure to drop and cause faintness or dizziness. Stand up slowly from a seated or lying position, especially when you first start taking fluphenazine.

SIDE EFFECTS

Not all side effects will occur. Many side effects will diminish with time. *However, some side effects may be warning signs of toxicity and will require attention from your doctor.* Check with your doctor immediately if you experience any of the following:

- Seizure; high fever; fast or irregular heartbeat; very low blood pressure; faintness; any abnormal movements of the mouth, tongue, neck, arms, or legs; difficulty speaking or swallowing; imbalance or difficulty walking normally; severe muscle stiffness; discoloration of the skin or eyes; confusion; significant drowsiness; restlessness, difficulty urinating; sexual problems; vomiting; diarrhea; unusual bruising or bleeding; serious skin reaction to sunlight (burning or blistering); severe constipation; breast pain or enlargement

Some side effects appear when you first start taking fluphenazine and go away for most people. If the following side effects continue, contact your doctor.

- Dry mouth, mild to moderate constipation, dizziness, hand tremor, stuffy nose, weight gain

DRUG INTERACTIONS

Fluphenazine can adversely interact with the following frequently prescribed medications:

- Lithium—increased neurologic side effects
- Levodopa—decreased effectiveness of levodopa
- Amphetamines—increased psychotic symptoms are possible
- Anticonvulsants—decreased fluphenazine levels
- Tricyclic antidepressants—increased TCA levels
- Serotonin-type antidepressants—can cause high fluphenazine levels
- Beta blockers—can cause high fluphenazine levels
- HIV protease inhibitors—can cause high fluphenazine levels
- Drugs that depress certain functions of the nervous system, when combined with fluphenazine, cause extreme drowsiness and slowed reaction times. Examples of these medicines are antihistamines, narcotics, muscle relaxants, and barbiturates.

MEDICAL CONSIDERATIONS

If you have any of the following medical conditions, make sure your doctor is aware of it.

- Kidney disease—fluphenazine levels may be higher than expected
- Liver disease—fluphenazine levels may be higher than expected
- Heart problems—some heart problems can be made worse by fluphenazine
- Seizure disorder—fluphenazine can lower seizure threshold
- Urinary retention, prostate enlargement—urination may be more difficult
- Glaucoma—fluphenazine can increase pressure inside the eye
- Parkinson's disease—some Parkinson's symptoms may be worsened
- Breast cancer—may increase risk of cancer progression

FLURAZEPAM (flur-AZ-e-pam)

Drug Category: Insomnia medicine
Requires prescription, controlled substance, moderate potential for abuse

COMMONLY USED BRAND-NAME PRODUCTS

Capsules
Dalmane (and generic), 15mg, 30mg

GENERAL INFORMATION

Used to treat insomnia. *Even when taken as prescribed, flurazepam may cause psychological and/or physical dependence. Not intended for long-term use.*

BEFORE TAKING THIS MEDICATION

Talk to your doctor about the benefits and risks associated with flurazepam. Make sure you understand how to take it

safely and effectively. You and your family members should be very familiar with the side effects and signs of having too much in your system. Make sure your doctor has the following information in detail:

- Any allergic or bad reactions you have had to flurazepam or any other medication
- All prescription and over-the-counter medicines you are taking
- Your complete medical history, including mental health conditions
- If you are pregnant, could be pregnant, or are planning a pregnancy in the near future, flurazepam should not be taken
- If you are breast feeding, flurazepam can pass into breast milk and affect the baby

USUAL ADULT DOSAGE RANGE
15–30 mg at bedtime.
Older adults are more susceptible to side effects and will generally require lower dosages.

DIRECTIONS FOR PROPER USE
- *Take exactly as prescribed. Do not take more or less than prescribed. Flurazepam levels that are too high can cause serious toxicity.*
- If you take flurazepam regularly for an extended period of time, do not stop taking it unless told to do so by your doctor. It may be necessary to gradually reduce the dose before stopping completely.
- If you miss a dose, take it as soon as possible if it is within 1 hour of the scheduled time. However, flurazepam should be taken only if you are sure you will get a full night's sleep of at least 7 to 8 hours.

PRECAUTIONS

- Flurazepam can cause drowsiness and slowed reaction times. Be cautious when driving, operating machinery, or doing jobs requiring alertness.
- Alcohol can cause extreme drowsiness when taken with flurazepam. *Alcohol should be avoided while taking flurazepam.*
- Flurazepam may cause a severe allergic reaction and/or severe facial swelling, which can occur as early as the first dose.
- Flurazepam can cause complex sleep-related behaviors, which may include sleep-driving, making phone calls, and preparing and eating food (while asleep).

SIDE EFFECTS

Not all side effects will occur. Many side effects will diminish with time. *However, some side effects may be warning signs of toxicity and will require attention from your doctor.* Check with your doctor immediately if you experience any of the following:

- Confusion, severe drowsiness, slurred speech, severe weakness, unusual thoughts, shortness of breath, excitement, hyperactivity, memory problems

Some side effects appear when you first start taking flurazepam and go away for most people. If the following side effects continue, contact your doctor.

- Dizziness, lightheadedness, daytime drowsiness, blurred vision

DRUG INTERACTIONS

Flurazepam can adversely interact with the following frequently prescribed medications or foods:

- Cimetidine (Tagamet)—can cause high flurazepam levels
- Disulfiram (Antabuse)—can cause high flurazepam levels

- Birth control pills—can cause high flurazepam levels
- Levodopa—decreased effectiveness of levodopa
- Macrolide antibiotics (e.g., erythromycin)—can cause high flurazepam levels
- Oral antifungal agents—can cause high flurazepam levels
- HIV protease inhibitors—can cause high flurazepam levels
- Calcium channel blockers—can cause high flurazepam levels
- Serotonin-type antidepressants—can cause high flurazepam levels
- Digoxin—flurazepam can cause high digoxin levels
- Valproic acid—can cause high flurazepam levels
- Isoniazid—can cause high flurazepam levels
- Beta blockers—can cause high flurazepam levels
- Propoxyphene—can cause high flurazepam levels
- Carbamazepine—can lower flurazepam levels
- Grapefruit juice—can cause high flurazepam levels
- Drugs that depress certain functions of the nervous system, when combined with flurazepam, cause extreme drowsiness and slowed reaction times. Examples of these medicines are antihistamines, narcotics, muscle relaxants, and barbiturates.

MEDICAL CONSIDERATIONS

If you have any of the following medical conditions, make sure your doctor is aware of it.

- Liver disease or alcoholism—flurazepam levels may be higher than expected
- Kidney disease—flurazepam levels may be higher than expected
- Drug or alcohol dependence—dependence on flurazepam may occur

- Seizure disorder—stopping flurazepam abruptly may cause seizures
- Chronic lung disease—flurazepam may make breathing more difficult
- Glaucoma—flurazepam may worsen your condition
- Sleep apnea—flurazepam may worsen your condition

FLUVOXAMINE (flu-VOX-a-meen)

Drug Category: Antidepressant, SSRI (serotonin specific reuptake inhibitor)

Requires prescription

COMMONLY USED BRAND-NAME PRODUCTS

Tablets

Luvox (and generic) 25mg, 50mg, 100mg

GENERAL INFORMATION

Used to treat obsessive compulsive disorder (OCD). Also used to treat major depression.

BEFORE TAKING THIS MEDICATION

Talk to your doctor about the benefits and risks associated with fluvoxamine. Make sure you understand how to take it safely and effectively. You and your family members should be very familiar with the side effects and signs of having too much in your system. Make sure your doctor has the following information in detail:

- Any allergic or bad reactions you have had to fluvoxamine or any other medication
- All prescription and over-the-counter medicines you are taking
- Your complete medical history

- If you are pregnant, could be pregnant, or are planning a pregnancy in the near future, fluvoxamine should not be taken
- If you are breast feeding, fluvoxamine can pass into breast milk and affect the baby

USUAL ADULT DOSAGE RANGE

50–300mg daily. The starting dose will be low and will gradually be increased depending on the response and side effects. *Older adults* are more susceptible to side effects and will generally require lower dosages.

DIRECTIONS FOR PROPER USE

- *Take exactly as prescribed. Do not take more or less than prescribed.*
- Do not abruptly stop taking fluvoxamine unless instructed to do so by your doctor.
- May be taken with food or meals to lessen stomach upset.
- If you miss a dose, do not try to make it up. Wait and take your next scheduled dose. Do not double doses.
- It may take several weeks before you feel the full benefits.

PRECAUTIONS

- Fluvoxamine can cause drowsiness and slowed reaction times. Be cautious when driving, operating machinery, or doing jobs requiring alertness.
- Alcohol can cause changes in mood and may interfere with fluvoxamine's effectiveness. Alcohol can cause extreme drowsiness when taken with fluvoxamine. *Alcohol should be avoided while taking fluvoxamine*
- Fluvoxamine may cause your skin and eyes to be more sensitive to sunlight. Exposure to sunlight may cause a rash, skin discoloration, or sunburn. Limit direct exposure to sunlight, and use sunscreen when in direct sunlight. Avoid

tanning booths and beds. Wear UV-blocking sunglasses when outdoors.

- *Antidepressants may increase the risk of suicidal thinking and behavior in adolescents and children. When considering an antidepressant in a child or adolescent, the risk must be balanced with the need. Children and adolescents taking antidepressants should be closely monitored for worsening of symptoms, suicidality, or unusual changes in behavior.*

SIDE EFFECTS

Not all side effects will occur. Many side effects will diminish with time. *However, some side effects may require attention from your doctor.* Check with your doctor immediately if you experience any of the following:

- Skin rash or hives, shortness of breath, chills or fever, swelling of the hands or feet, seizures, bleeding or bruising

Some side effects appear when you first start taking fluvoxamine and go away for most people. If the following side effects continue, contact your doctor.

- Agitation, anxiety, insomnia, dizziness, sexual problems, sweating, blurred vision, dry mouth, mild to moderate constipation, change in appetite, change in weight, tremor of the hands

DRUG INTERACTIONS

Fluvoxamine can adversely interact with the following frequently prescribed medications or foods:

- Anticoagulants (blood thinners)—the effect of the anticoagulant can be increased
- Some nonsedating antihistamines—cardiac (heart) toxicity
- Diet pills—severe reaction causing dangerously high blood pressure, high body temperature, seizures, or death
- Products containing L-tryptophan—severe reaction caus-

ing dangerously high blood pressure, high body temperature, seizures, or death

- Cimetidine—can cause high fluvoxamine levels
- Bupropion—dosage adjustment of one or both drugs may be necessary
- Amphetamines—increased blood pressure, irregular heart rate, or very high fever may result
- TCA antidepressants—can cause high TCA levels
- MAOI antidepressants—severe reaction causing dangerously high blood pressure, high body temperature, seizures, or death
- Antipsychotics—may increase certain neurologic side effects
- Lithium—increased lithium levels causing possible confusion, dizziness, tremor
- Anticonvulsants—increased anticonvulsant levels or decreased fluvoxamine levels
- Antiarrhythmic drugs—increased risk of arrhythmias
- Benzodiazepines—fluvoxamine can increase benzodiazepine levels
- Beta blockers—fluvoxamine can increase levels of beta blockers
- Aspirin, NSAIDs—increased chance of bleeding
- HIV protease inhibitors—fluvoxamine can increase levels of protease inhibitors
- Drugs that depress certain functions of the nervous system, when combined with fluvoxamine, cause extreme drowsiness and slowed reaction times. Examples of these medicines are antihistamines, narcotics, muscle relaxants, and barbiturates.

MEDICAL CONSIDERATIONS

If you have any of the following medical conditions, make sure your doctor is aware of it.

- Liver disease or alcoholism—fluvoxamine levels may be higher than expected
- Kidney disease—fluvoxamine levels may be higher than expected
- Seizure disorder—fluvoxamine can lower seizure threshold
- Diabetes mellitus (sugar diabetes)—blood sugar levels may be affected
- Low sodium—fluvoxamine may worsen this condition
- Bleeding disorder—fluvoxamine may worsen this condition

HALOPERIDOL (hal-o-PAIR-ih-dahl)

Drug Category: Neuroleptic; Antipsychotic
Requires prescription

COMMONLY USED BRAND-NAME PRODUCTS

Tablets
Haldol (and generic), 0.5mg, 1mg, 2.5mg, 5mg, 10mg, 20mg
Liquid
Haldol (and generic) solution 2mg/ml
Injection, long acting
50mg/ml, 100mg/ml

GENERAL INFORMATION

Used to treat psychotic symptoms, such as hallucinations and delusions. These symptoms occur in schizophrenia, schizoaffective disorder, bipolar disorder, or major depression with psychotic features. Also effective in treating Tourette's syndrome, to help reduce motor tics and vocalization. Haloperidol can be used for short-term management of aggressive, out-of-control behaviors or feelings of anger and rage.

BEFORE TAKING THIS MEDICATION

Talk to your doctor about the benefits and risks associated with haloperidol. Make sure you understand how to take it safely and effectively. You and your family members should be very familiar with its side effects. Make sure your doctor has the following information in detail:

- Any allergic or bad reactions you have had to haloperidol or any other medication
- All prescription and over-the-counter medicines you are taking
- Your complete medical history
- If you are pregnant, could be pregnant, or are planning a pregnancy in the near future, haloperidol has not been shown to be absolutely safe
- If you are breast feeding, haloperidol can pass into breast milk and affect the baby

USUAL ADULT DOSAGE RANGE

5–80mg daily. There is a wide effective dosage range.
Older adults are *extremely* susceptible to side effects and will generally require lower dosages.

DIRECTIONS FOR PROPER USE

- ***Take exactly as prescribed. Do not take more or less than prescribed. Haloperidol levels that are too high can cause serious toxicity.***
- If you miss a dose, take it as soon as possible. However, if the missed dose is within 4 hours of your next dose, skip the missed dose and resume with your next scheduled dose. Do not double the dose.
- If you are taking a liquid form, avoid contacting the skin

with the medicine. Irritation can result by the medicine coming in contact with skin. Do not use the liquid form if the medicine becomes very discolored (dark yellow) or has a sediment at the bottom of the bottle.

- The long-acting shot form of haloperidol may have an effect for up to 6 weeks.
- It may be several weeks before you feel the full benefits.

PRECAUTIONS

- Haloperidol can cause drowsiness and slowed reaction times. Be cautious when driving, operating machinery, or doing jobs requiring alertness.
- Alcohol can cause extreme drowsiness when taken with haloperidol. *Alcohol should be avoided while taking haloperidol.*
- Haloperidol may cause your body temperature to increase and could result in heat stroke. Be extra careful in hot weather, when exercising, or when taking hot baths or saunas not to become overheated.
- Haloperidol may cause your skin and eyes to be more sensitive to sunlight. Exposure to sunlight may cause a rash, skin discoloration, or sunburn. Limit direct exposure to sunlight, and use sunscreen when in direct sunlight. Avoid tanning booths and beds. Wear UV-blocking sunglasses when outdoors.
- When taking haloperidol, stand up slowly after sitting or lying down, since it may cause your blood pressure to drop and cause faintness or dizziness. Stand up slowly from a seated or lying position, especially when you first start taking haloperidol.

SIDE EFFECTS

Not all side effects will occur. Many side effects will diminish with time. *However, some side effects may be warning signs of toxicity and will require attention from your doctor.* Check with your doctor immediately if you experience any of the following:

- Seizure; high fever; fast or irregular heartbeat; very low blood pressure; faintness; any abnormal movements of the mouth, tongue, neck, arms, or legs; difficulty speaking or swallowing; imbalance or difficulty walking normally; severe muscle stiffness; discoloration of the skin or eyes; confusion; significant drowsiness; restlessness; difficulty urinating; sexual problems; vomiting; diarrhea; unusual bruising or bleeding; serious skin reaction to sunlight (burning or blistering); severe constipation; breast pain or enlargement

Some side effects appear when you first start taking haloperidol and go away for most people. If the following side effects continue, contact your doctor.

- Dry mouth, mild to moderate constipation, dizziness, hand tremor, stuffy nose, weight gain

DRUG INTERACTIONS

Haloperidol can adversely interact with the following frequently prescribed medications:

- Lithium—increased neurologic side effects
- Levodopa—decreased effectiveness of levodopa
- Amphetamines—increased psychotic symptoms are possible
- Anticonvulsants—decreased haloperidol levels
- Tricyclic antidepressants—increased TCA levels
- Serotonin-type antidepressants—can cause high haloperidol levels
- Beta blockers—can cause high haloperidol levels
- HIV protease inhibitors—can cause high haloperidol levels
- Drugs that depress certain functions of the nervous system, when combined with haloperidol, cause extreme drowsi-

ness and slowed reaction times. Examples of these medicines are antihistamines, narcotics, muscle relaxants, and barbiturates.

MEDICAL CONSIDERATIONS

If you have any of the following medical conditions, make sure your doctor is aware of it.

- Kidney disease—haloperidol levels may be higher than expected
- Liver disease—haloperidol levels may be higher than expected
- Heart problems—some heart problems can be made worse by haloperidol
- Seizure disorder—haloperidol can lower seizure threshold
- Urinary retention, prostate enlargement—urination may be more difficult
- Glaucoma—haloperidol can increase pressure inside the eye
- Parkinson's disease—Some Parkinson's symptoms may be worsened
- Breast cancer—may increase risk of cancer progression

IMIPRAMINE (im-IP-rah-meen)

Drug Category: Antidepressant, tricyclic
Requires prescription

COMMONLY USED BRAND-NAME PRODUCTS

Tablets
Tofranil (and generic) 10mg, 25mg, 50mg
Capsules, as pamoate
Tofranil PM 75mg, 100mg, 125mg, 150mg

GENERAL INFORMATION

Used to treat major depression and the depressed phase of bipolar disorder. Also used to treat certain chronic pain disorders, such as migraine headache and diabetic neuropathy.

BEFORE TAKING THIS MEDICATION

Talk to your doctor about the benefits and risks associated with imipramine. Make sure you understand how to take it safely and effectively. You and your family members should be very familiar with the side effects and signs of having too much in your system. Make sure your doctor has the following information in detail:

- Any allergic or bad reactions you have had to imipramine or any other medication
- All prescription and over-the-counter medicines you are taking
- Your complete medical history
- If you are pregnant, could be pregnant, or are planning a pregnancy in the near future, imipramine should not be taken
- If you are breast feeding, imipramine can pass into breast milk and affect the baby

USUAL ADULT DOSAGE RANGE

The starting dose of imipramine will be low and will gradually be increased. Sometimes blood levels are tested to ensure that the dose you are taking is in the safe and effective range.

Depression: Starting dose 25–50mg at bedtime. Increased to 75–300 mg at bedtime over 2 to 3 weeks.

Chronic pain syndrome: 50–100mg daily.

Older adults are more susceptible to side effects and will generally require lower dosages.

DIRECTIONS FOR PROPER USE

- *Take exactly as prescribed. Do not take more or less than prescribed. Accidental or intended overdoses of imipramine are potentially fatal.*
- Do not abruptly stop taking imipramine unless instructed to do so by your doctor. Gradually reducing the dose can help prevent mood changes, headache, or diarrhea.
- If you miss a bedtime dose, do not take it the next morning, since it may make you drowsy. Do not double doses.
- It may take several weeks before you feel the full benefits.

PRECAUTIONS

- Imipramine can cause drowsiness and slowed reaction times. Be cautious when driving, operating machinery, or doing jobs requiring alertness.
- Alcohol can cause changes in mood and may interfere with imipramine's effectiveness. Alcohol can cause extreme drowsiness when taken with imipramine. *Alcohol should be avoided while taking imipramine.*
- Imipramine may cause your skin and eyes to be more sensitive to sunlight. Exposure to sunlight may cause a rash, skin discoloration, or sunburn. Limit direct exposure to sunlight, and use sunscreen when in direct sunlight. Avoid tanning booths and beds. Wear UV-blocking sunglasses when outdoors.
- When taking imipramine, stand up slowly after sitting or lying down, since it may cause your blood pressure to drop and cause faintness or dizziness. Stand up slowly from a seated or lying position, especially when you first start taking imipramine.
- *Antidepressants may increase the risk of suicidal thinking and behavior in adolescents and children. When considering an antidepressant in a child or adolescent, the risk*

must be balanced with the need. Children and adolescents taking antidepressants should be closely monitored for worsening of symptoms, suicidality, or unusual changes in behavior.

- Adolescents and children may be more susceptible to heart-related side effects of tricyclic antidepressants. Risk must be balanced with need. Blood levels and heart function should be monitored in children and adolescents taking tricyclic antidepressants.

SIDE EFFECTS

Not all side effects will occur. Many side effects will diminish with time. *However, some side effects may require attention from your doctor.* Check with your doctor immediately if you experience any of the following:

- Seizure, changes in blood pressure, irregular heart rate, shortness of breath, problems with urination (difficult or painful urination, unable to urinate), confusion, extreme sedation, excitation or mania, increased skin sensitivity to the sunlight, extreme constipation, yellow skin or eyes

Some side effects appear when you first start taking imipramine and go away for most people. If the following side effects continue, contact your doctor.

- Dizziness, blurred vision, dry mouth, mild to moderate constipation, increased appetite, weight gain, breast enlargement (men or women), discharge from the breast, sexual problems, tremor of the hands, persistent sore throat

DRUG INTERACTIONS

Imipramine can adversely interact with the following frequently prescribed medications:

- Cimetidine—can cause high imipramine levels
- SSRI antidepressants—can cause high imipramine levels
- MAOI antidepressants—severe reaction causing danger-

ously high blood pressure, high body temperature, seizures, or death
- Clonidine—if clonidine is being taken for high blood pressure, imipramine may cause clonidine to work less well
- Antipsychotics—may increase certain neurologic side effects
- Thyroid hormones—increased effects of both, especially excitation and changes in heart rate or rhythm
- Carbamazepine—can lower imipramine levels
- Bupropion—can increase imipramine levels
- Anticoagulants (blood thinners)—the effect of the anticoagulant can be increased
- Quinolones—increased risk of heart arrhythmias
- Amphetamines—increased blood pressure, irregular heart rate, or very high fever may result
- Drugs used during surgery—can cause increased blood pressure. Make sure your doctors are aware of upcoming planned surgeries.
- Drugs that depress certain functions of the nervous system, when combined with imipramine, cause extreme drowsiness and slowed reaction times. Examples of these medicines are antihistamines, narcotics, muscle relaxants, and barbiturates.

MEDICAL CONSIDERATIONS
If you have any of the following medical conditions, make sure your doctor is aware of it.
- Liver disease or alcoholism—imipramine levels may be higher than expected
- Kidney disease—imipramine levels may be higher than expected
- Glaucoma—imipramine can increase pressure inside the eye
- Heart problems—some heart problems can be made worse

by imipramine; imipramine should not be taken by some-one who has had a recent heart attack

- Urinary retention, prostate enlargement—urination may become more difficult
- Seizure disorder—imipramine can lower seizure threshold
- Diabetes mellitus (sugar diabetes)—blood sugar levels may be affected
- Thyroid disorders—imipramine may cause increased heart rate

ISOCARBOXAZID (iso-car-BOX-uh-zid)

Drug Category: Antidepressant, MAOI (monoamine oxidase inhibitor)

Requires prescription

COMMONLY USED BRAND-NAME PRODUCTS

Tablets

Marplan 10mg

GENERAL INFORMATION

Use to treat major depression and the depressed phase of bi-polar disorder.

BEFORE TAKING THIS MEDICATION

Talk to your doctor about the benefits and risks associated with isocarboxazid. Make sure you understand how to take it safely and effectively. You and your family members should be very familiar with the side effects and signs of having too much in your system. Make sure your doctor has the following in-formation in detail:

- Any allergic or bad reactions you have had to isocarboxazid or any other medication

- All prescription and over-the-counter medicines you are taking
- Your complete medical history
- If you are pregnant, could be pregnant, or are planning a pregnancy in the near future, isocarboxazid should not be taken
- If you are breast feeding, isocarboxazid can pass into breast milk and affect the baby

USUAL ADULT DOSAGE RANGE

10–40mg daily.

Older adults are more susceptible to side effects and will generally require lower dosages.

DIRECTIONS FOR PROPER USE

- *Take exactly as prescribed. Do not take more or less than prescribed. Accidental or intended overdoses of isocarboxazid can be potentially fatal.*
- *Follow the dietary instructions carefully while taking isocarboxazid. Not doing so can lead to dangerously high blood pressure.*
- *Check with your doctor or pharmacist before taking any other prescription or over-the-counter medicine.*
- Do not abruptly stop taking isocarboxazid unless instructed to do so by your doctor.
- It is advised that you check your blood pressure frequently while taking isocarboxazid.
- If you miss a bedtime dose, do not take it the next morning, since it may make you drowsy. Do not double doses.
- It may take several weeks before you feel the full benefits of isocarboxazid.

PRECAUTIONS

- Isocarboxazid can cause drowsiness and slowed reaction times. Be cautious when driving, operating machinery, or doing jobs requiring alertness.

- Alcohol can cause changes in mood and may interfere with isocarboxazid's effectiveness. Alcohol can cause extreme drowsiness when taken with isocarboxazid. *Alcohol should be avoided while taking isocarboxazid.*

- When taking isocarboxazid, stand up slowly after sitting or lying down, since it may cause your blood pressure to drop and cause faintness or dizziness. Stand up slowly from a seated or lying position, especially when you first start taking isocarboxazid.

- The amount of tyramine, or tryptophan, in your diet must be restricted while taking isocarboxazid. Tyramine is found in foods that have been aged, foods that have been preserved, and foods that have undergone protein breakdown. The amount of tyramine in food is NOT inactivated by cooking. These restrictions will need to be followed for 2 weeks after isocarboxazid has been stopped.

- *Antidepressants may increase the risk of suicidal thinking and behavior in adolescents and children. When considering an antidepressant in a child or adolescent, the risk must be balanced with the need. Children and adolescents taking antidepressants should be closely monitored for worsening of symptoms, suicidality, or unusual changes in behavior.*

SIDE EFFECTS

Not all side effects will occur. Many side effects will diminish with time. *However, some side effects may require attention from your doctor.* Check with your doctor immediately if you experience any of the following:

- Seizure, changes in blood pressure, severe headache, irregular heart rate, shortness of breath, problems with urination (difficult or painful urination, unable to urinate), confusion, extreme sedation, excitation or mania, extreme sweating, severe skin sensitivity to the sunlight (burning or blistering), extreme constipation, yellow skin or eyes

Some side effects appear when you first start taking isocarboxazid and go away for most people. If the following side effects continue, contact your doctor.

- Dizziness, blurred vision, dry mouth, mild to moderate constipation, increased appetite, weight gain, tremor of the hands

DRUG INTERACTIONS

Isocarboxazid can adversely interact with the following frequently prescribed medications. A severe reaction causing dangerously high blood pressure, high body temperature, seizures, or death is possible. These interactions are possible for up to 2 weeks even after isocarboxazid has been stopped. A washout period of up to 5 weeks after stopping some of the medications listed below may be necessary before starting isocarboxazid.

- SSRI antidepressants
- Cyclic antidepressants
- Stimulant drugs—amphetamines, methylphenidate (Ritalin), cocaine
- Ephedrine, pseudoephedrine—found in prescription and over-the-counter cough and cold medicines and asthma medicines
- Phenylephrine, phenylpropanolamine—found in prescription and over-the-counter cough and cold medicines and asthma medicines
- Levodopa

- Buspirone (Buspar)
- Buproprion
- Carbamazepine
- Dextromethorphan—found in prescription and over-the-counter cough syrups and lozenges
- Meperidine (Demerol)
- L-tryptophan
- Drugs used during surgery can cause increased blood pressure. Make sure your doctors are aware of upcoming planned surgeries.
- Drugs that depress certain functions of the nervous system, when combined with isocarboxazid, cause extreme drowsiness and slowed reaction times. Examples of these medicines are antihistamines, narcotics, muscle relaxants, and barbiturates.

MEDICAL CONSIDERATIONS

If you have any of the following medical conditions, make sure your doctor is aware of it.

- Liver disease or alcoholism—isocarboxazid levels may be higher than expected
- Kidney disease—isocarboxazid levels may be higher than expected
- Heart problems—some heart problems can be made worse by isocarboxazid; isocarboxazid should not be taken by someone who has had a recent heart attack
- High blood pressure—blood pressure may be increased
- Urinary retention, prostate enlargement—urination may become more difficult
- Seizure disorder—isocarboxazid can lower seizure threshold
- Diabetes mellitus (sugar diabetes)—blood sugar levels may be affected

- Thryoid disorders—isocarboxazid may cause increased heart rate
- Pheochromocytoma—can lead to high blood pressure

LAMOTRIGINE (lam-OH-tru-gene)

Drug Category: Mood stabilizer
Requires prescription

COMMONLY USED BRAND-NAME PRODUCTS

Tablets
Lamictal (and generic) 25mg, 100mg, 150mg, 200mg
Tablets, chewable, dispersible
Lamictal (and generic) 2mg, 5mg, 25mg

GENERAL INFORMATION

Used in treating the depressed phase of bipolar disorder.

BEFORE TAKING THIS MEDICATION

Talk to your doctor about the benefits and risks associated with lamotrigine. Make sure you understand how to take it safely and effectively. You and your family members should be very familiar with the side effects and signs of having too much in your system. Make sure your doctor has the following information in detail:

- Any allergic or bad reactions you have had to lamotrigine or any other medication
- All prescription and over-the-counter medicines you are taking
- Your complete medical history
- If you are pregnant, could be pregnant, or are planning a pregnancy in the near future, lamotrigine should not be taken

- If you are breast feeding, lamotrigine can pass into breast milk and affect the baby

DOSAGE

The starting dose of lamotrigine will be adjusted on the basis of your response and blood levels. You may require more lamotrigine during and immediately following an acute manic episode, than when your symptoms have stabilized.

Adults: 100–400mg daily. Careful dosage adjustments are required when adding or stopping other medicines.

Older adults are more susceptible to side effects and will generally require lower dosages.

DIRECTIONS FOR PROPER USE

- ***Take exactly as prescribed. Do not take more or less than prescribed. Lamotrigine levels that are too high can cause serious toxicity.***
- If you take lamotrigine regularly for an extended period of time, do not stop taking it unless told to do so by your doctor. It may be necessary to gradually reduce the dose before stopping completely.
- Laboratory tests are necessary to determine if the amount of lamotrigine in your bloodstream is in the correct range.

PRECAUTIONS

- Lamotrigine can cause drowsiness and slowed reaction times. Be cautious when driving, operating machinery, or doing jobs requiring alertness.
- Alcohol can cause changes in mood and may interfere with lamotrigine's effectiveness. Alcohol can cause extreme drowsiness when taken with lamotrigine. *Alcohol should be avoided while taking lamotrigine.*
- Tell your doctor if you plan to start or stop taking estrogen-containing birth control pills.

- *Serious rashes requiring hospitalization and stopping lamotrigine can occur. Sometimes these rashes are life-threatening. Not all rashes that occur with lamotrigine are serious. However, it is not possible to predict whether a rash will become serious. If you experience a rash with lamotrigine, immediately report it to your doctor and/or seek immediate care.*
- Lamotrigine may cause suicidal thoughts. Notify your doctor immediately if you notice changes in mood, behavior, or actions or have thoughts of harming yourself.

SIDE EFFECTS

Not all side effects will occur. Many side effects will diminish with time. *However, some side effects may be warning signs of toxicity and will require attention from your doctor.* Check with your doctor immediately if you experience any of the following:

- Rash, fever, shortness of breath or difficulty breathing, mood changes, suicidal thoughts, lack of coordination, bruising/bleeding, dark urine, fever

Some side effects appear when you first start taking lamotrigine and go away for most people. If the following side effects continue, contact your doctor.

- Dizziness, blurred or double vision, fatigue, insomnia, nausea, vomiting, dry mouth, headache

DRUG INTERACTIONS

Lamotrigine can adversely interact with the following frequently prescribed medications:

- Birth control pills containing estrogen—lamotrigine dosage adjustments may be necessary if birth control pills are started or stopped
- Valproic acid—causes lamotrigine levels to increase

- Phenytoin—causes lamotrigine levels to decrease
- Carbamazepine—causes lamotrigine levels to decrease
- Drugs that depress certain functions of the nervous system, when combined with lamotrigine, cause extreme drowsiness and slowed reaction times. Examples of these medicines are antihistamines, narcotics, muscle relaxants, and barbiturates.

MEDICAL CONSIDERATIONS

If you have any of the following medical conditions, make sure your doctor is aware of it.

- Liver disease, or alcoholism—lamotrigine levels may be higher than expected
- Kidney disease—lamotrigine levels may be higher than expected

LITHIUM (LITH-ee-um)
Drug Category: Mood stabilizer
Requires prescription

COMMONLY USED BRAND-NAME PRODUCTS
Tablets or capsules
Various products available: 150mg, 300mg, 600mg
Tablets, extended release
Eskalith CR 450mg tablets
Lithobid 300mg tablets
Syrup
Various generic products: 300mg/5ml

GENERAL INFORMATION
Used to treat bipolar disorder, especially the acute manic and hypomanic phases. Lithium has also been shown to reduce the

number and severity of subsequent episodes of both mania and depression. It can be used alone or in combination with other mood stabilizers in severe cases. Also used to treat schizoaffective disorder, usually in combination with other medications called antipsychotics. Lithium can increase the effectiveness of antidepressants and is sometimes given to people with major depression who have not responded to an antidepressant alone.

BEFORE TAKING THIS MEDICATION

Talk to your doctor about the benefits and risks associated with lithium. Make sure you understand how to take it safely and effectively. You and your family members should be very familiar with the side effects and signs of having too much in your system. Make sure your doctor has the following information in detail:

- Any allergic or bad reactions you have had to lithium or any other medication
- All prescription and over-the-counter medicines you are taking
- Your complete medical history
- If you are pregnant, could be pregnant, or are planning a pregnancy in the near future, lithium should not be taken
- If you are breast feeding, lithium can pass into breast milk and affect the baby

USUAL ADULT DOSAGE RANGE

The starting dose of lithium will be adjusted on the basis of your response and blood levels. You may require more lithium during and immediately following an acute manic episode than when your symptoms have stabilized.

Acute mania: 300–600mg three times daily. Maintenance dose: 300mg three to four times daily.

Older adults are more susceptible to side effects and will generally require lower dosages.

DIRECTIONS FOR PROPER USE
- *Take exactly as prescribed. Do not take more or less than prescribed. Lithium levels that are too high can cause serious toxicity.*
- If you take lithium regularly for an extended period of time, do not stop taking it unless told to do so by your doctor. It may be necessary to gradually reduce the dose before stopping completely.
- Take lithium with meals or a snack to reduce stomach upset and diarrhea.
- If you take the syrup form, mix your dose in fruit juice or another flavored beverage before taking.
- Drink lots of fluids throughout the day while taking lithium (2–3 quarts per day).
- Do not drink large amounts of coffee, tea, or colas. These beverages can cause increased urination and may also worsen hand tremor.
- Do not make drastic changes in your diet while taking lithium. It is important that your body not lose fluids or sodium when taking lithium. Use a normal amount of salt in your diet.
- If you miss a dose, take it as soon as possible. However, if the missed dose is within 4 hours of your next dose, skip the missed dose and resume with your next scheduled dose. Do not double the dose.

If you are taking the long-acting form:
- If you are taking the long-acting tablet form and you miss a dose, take it as soon as possible. However, if the missed dose is within 6 hours of your next dose, skip the missed dose and resume with your next scheduled dose.

- Long-acting tablets are not interchangeable with regular tablets, capsules, or liquid forms.
- Swallow tablets whole; do not crush, chew, or break.
- It may take several weeks before you feel the full benefits.
- Laboratory tests are necessary to determine if the amount of lithium in your bloodstream is in the correct range.

PRECAUTIONS

- Lithium can cause drowsiness and slowed reaction times. Be cautious when driving, operating machinery, or doing jobs requiring alertness. Alcohol can cause extreme drowsiness when taken with lithium.
- Alcohol can cause changes in mood and may interfere with lithium's effectiveness. It can also cause increased urination and may affect lithium levels. *Alcohol should be avoided while taking lithium.*

SIDE EFFECTS

Not all side effects will occur. Many side effects will diminish with time. *However, some side effects may be warning signs of toxicity and will require attention from your doctor.* Check with your doctor immediately if you experience any of the following:

- Seizure, severe diarrhea, loss of appetite, severe nausea, muscle weakness, trembling, slurred speech, clumsiness, confusion, significant drowsiness, blurred vision, irregular heartbeat, difficulty breathing, swelling of the hands or feet

Some side effects appear when you first start taking lithium and go away for most people. If the following side effects continue, contact your doctor.

- Mild hand tremor, mild nausea, mild diarrhea, thirst, increased frequency of urination, acne, weight gain, hair loss, sensitivity to cold

DRUG INTERACTIONS

Lithium can adversely interact with the following frequently prescribed medications:

- Diuretics (water pills)—can cause sodium loss leading to high lithium levels
  - Certain medications for high blood pressure
  - Calcium channel blockers—can cause high lithium levels
- ACE inhibitors—can cause high lithium levels
- Pain relievers known as nonsteroidal anti-inflammatory drugs (NSAIDs)—can cause lithium levels to increase
- Antipsychotics—may worsen certain neurological side effects
- Theophylline—can cause lithium levels to increase
- Serotonin-type antidepressants—when taken with lithium can worsen side effects such as agitation, confusion, dizziness, tremor, and diarrhea
- Drugs that depress certain functions of the nervous system, when combined with lithium, cause extreme drowsiness and slowed reaction times. Examples of these medicines are antihistamines, narcotics, muscle relaxants, and barbiturates.

MEDICAL CONSIDERATIONS

If you have any of the following medical conditions, make sure your doctor is aware of it.

- Kidney disease—lithium levels may be higher than expected
- Thyroid disorders—lithium may worsen certain thyroid conditions
- Heart problems—some heart problems can be worsened by lithium
- Diabetes mellitus (sugar diabetes)—blood sugar levels can be increased

- Dehydration—fluid and sodium may be lost, leading to increased lithium levels
- Severe infection (with fever, sweating, diarrhea, or vomiting)—can increase lithium levels
- Parkinson's disease—some Parkinson's symptoms may be worsened

LORAZEPAM (lor-AZ-e-pam)

Drug Category: Antianxiety medicine
Requires prescription, controlled substance, moderate potential for abuse

COMMONLY USED BRAND-NAME PRODUCTS

Tablets
Ativan (and generic) 0.5mg, 1mg, 2mg
Solution
Ativan (and generic) 2mg/ml

GENERAL INFORMATION

Used to treat anxiety and symptoms of alcohol withdrawal. *This medicine is not intended to help with the stress of everyday life. Even when taken as prescribed, lorazepam may cause psychological and/or physical dependence.*

BEFORE TAKING THIS MEDICATION

Talk to your doctor about the benefits and risks associated with lorazepam. Make sure you understand how to take it safely and effectively. You and your family members should be very familiar with the side effects and signs of having too much in your system. Make sure your doctor has the following information in detail:

- Any allergic or bad reactions you have had to lorazepam or any other medication
- All prescription and over-the-counter medicines you are taking
- Your complete medical history, including mental health conditions
- If you are pregnant, could be pregnant, or are planning a pregnancy in the near future, lorazepam should not be taken
- If you are breast feeding, lorazepam can pass into breast milk and affect the baby

USUAL ADULT DOSAGE RANGE

0.5–2 mg two to three times a day.

Older adults are more susceptible to side effects and will generally require lower dosages.

DIRECTIONS FOR PROPER USE

- *Take exactly as prescribed. Do not take more or less than prescribed. Lorazepam levels that are too high can cause serious toxicity.*
- If you take lorazepam regularly for an extended period of time, do not stop taking it unless told to do so by your doctor. It may be necessary to gradually reduce the dose before stopping completely. If the medicine is stopped too quickly, your condition could become worse, or you could experience serious side effects, such as seizures.
- May be taken with food to decrease stomach upset.
- If you miss a dose, take it as soon as possible. However, if the missed dose is within 4 hours of your next dose, skip the missed dose and resume with your next scheduled dose. Do not double the dose.
- If you are taking the liquid form, the dose should be mixed in water, soda, applesauce, or pudding.

PRECAUTIONS

- Lorazepam can cause drowsiness and slowed reaction times. Be cautious when driving, operating machinery, or doing jobs requiring alertness.
- Alcohol can cause extreme drowsiness when taken with lorazepam. *Alcohol should be avoided while taking lorazepam.*

SIDE EFFECTS

Not all side effects will occur. Many side effects will diminish with time. *However, some side effects may be warning signs of toxicity and will require attention from your doctor.* Check with your doctor immediately if you experience any of the following:

- Confusion, severe drowsiness, slurred speech, severe weakness, unusual thoughts, shortness of breath, excitement, hyperactivity, memory problems

Some side effects appear when you first start taking lorazepam and go away for most people. If the following side effects continue, contact your doctor.

- Dizziness, lightheadedness, drowsiness, blurred vision, stomach problems

DRUG INTERACTIONS

Lorazepam can adversely interact with the following frequently prescribed medications or foods:

- Cimetidine (Tagamet)—can cause high lorazepam levels
- Disulfiram (Antabuse)—can cause high lorazepam levels
- Birth control pills—can cause high lorazepam levels
- Levodopa—decreased effectiveness of levodopa
- Macrolide antibiotics (e.g., erythromycin)—can cause high lorazepam levels
- Oral antifungal agents—can cause high lorazepam levels

- HIV protease inhibitors—can cause high lorazepam levels
- Calcium channel blockers—can cause high lorazepam levels
- Serotonin-type antidepressants—can cause high lorazepam levels
- Digoxin—lorazepam can cause high digoxin levels
- Valproic acid—can cause high lorazepam levels
- Isoniazid—can cause high lorazepam levels
- Beta blockers—can cause high lorazepam levels
- Propoxyphene—can cause high lorazepam levels
- Carbamazepine—can lower lorazepam levels
- Grapefruit juice—can cause high lorazepam levels
- Drugs that depress certain functions of the nervous system, when combined with lorazepam, cause extreme drowsiness and slowed reaction times. Examples of these medicines are antihistamines, narcotics, muscle relaxants, and barbiturates.

MEDICAL CONSIDERATIONS

If you have any of the following medical conditions, make sure your doctor is aware of it.

- Liver disease or alcoholism—lorazepam levels may be higher than expected
- Kidney disease—lorazepam levels may be higher than expected
- Drug or alcohol dependence—dependence on lorazepam may occur
- Seizure disorder—stopping lorazepam abruptly may cause seizures
- Chronic lung disease—lorazepam may make breathing more difficult
- Glaucoma—lorazepam may worsen your condition
- Sleep apnea—lorazepam may worsen your condition

LOXAPINE (LOX-uh-peen)
Drug Category: Neuroleptic; Antipsychotic
Requires prescription

COMMONLY USED BRAND-NAME PRODUCTS
Capsules
Loxitane (and generic) 5mg, 10mg, 25mg, 50mg

GENERAL INFORMATION
Used to treat psychotic symptoms, such as hallucinations and delusions. These symptoms occur in schizophrenia, schizoaffective disorder, bipolar disorder, or major depression with psychotic features. Loxapine can be used for short-term management of aggressive, out-of-control behaviors or feelings of anger and rage.

BEFORE TAKING THIS MEDICATION
Talk to your doctor about the benefits and risks associated with loxapine. Make sure you understand how to take it safely and effectively. You and your family members should be very familiar with its side effects. Make sure your doctor has the following information in detail:
- Any allergic or bad reactions you have had to loxapine or any other medication
- All prescription and over-the-counter medicines you are taking
- Your complete medical history
- If you are pregnant, could be pregnant, or are planning a pregnancy in the near future, loxapine has not been shown to be absolutely safe
- If you are breast feeding, loxapine can pass into breast milk and affect the baby

USUAL ADULT DOSAGE RANGE

25–250mg daily. There is a wide effective dosage range.
Older adults are *extremely* susceptible to side effects and will generally require lower dosages.

DIRECTIONS FOR PROPER USE

- **Take exactly as prescribed. Do not take more or less than prescribed. Loxapine levels that are too high can cause serious toxicity.**
- If you miss a dose, take it as soon as possible. However, if the missed dose is within 4 hours of your next dose, skip the missed dose and resume with your next scheduled dose. Do not double the dose.
- If you take the solution form, the dose must be mixed in orange or grapefruit juice before being taken.
- If you are taking the liquid form, use the dropper that comes with the bottle to measure out the dose.
- It may be several weeks before you feel the full benefits.

PRECAUTIONS

- Loxapine can cause drowsiness and slowed reaction times. Be cautious when driving, operating machinery, or doing jobs requiring alertness.
- Alcohol can cause extreme drowsiness when taken with loxapine. **Alcohol should be avoided while taking loxapine.**
- Loxapine may cause your body temperature to increase and could result in heat stroke. Be extra careful in hot weather, when exercising, or when taking hot baths or saunas not to become overheated.
- Loxapine may cause your skin and eyes to be more sensitive to sunlight. Exposure to sunlight may cause a rash, skin discoloration, or sunburn. Limit direct exposure to sunlight, and use sunscreen when in direct sunlight. Avoid

tanning booths and beds. Wear UV-blocking sunglasses when outdoors.

- When taking loxapine, stand up slowly after sitting or lying down, since it may cause your blood pressure to drop and cause faintness or dizziness. Stand up slowly from a seated or lying position, especially when you first start taking loxapine.

SIDE EFFECTS

Not all side effects will occur. Many side effects will diminish with time. *However, some side effects may be warning signs of toxicity and will require attention from your doctor.* Check with your doctor immediately if you experience any of the following:

- Seizure; high fever; fast or irregular heartbeat; very low blood pressure; faintness; any abnormal movements of the mouth, tongue, neck, arms or legs; difficulty speaking or swallowing; imbalance or difficulty walking normally; severe muscle stiffness; discoloration of the skin or eyes; confusion; significant drowsiness; restlessness; difficulty urinating; sexual problems; vomiting; diarrhea; unusual bruising or bleeding; serious skin reaction to sunlight (burning or blistering); severe constipation; breast pain or enlargement

Some side effects appear when you first start taking loxapine and go away for most people. If the following side effects continue, contact your doctor.

- Dry mouth, mild to moderate constipation, dizziness, hand tremor, stuffy nose, weight gain

DRUG INTERACTIONS

Loxapine can adversely interact with the following frequently prescribed medications:

- Lithium—increased neurologic side effects
- Levodopa—decreased effectiveness of levodopa

- Amphetamines—increased psychotic symptoms are possible
- Anticonvulsants—decreased loxapine levels
- Tricyclic antidepressants—increased TCA levels
- Serotonin-type antidepressants—can cause high loxapine levels
- Beta blockers—can cause high loxapine levels
- HIV protease inhibitors—can cause high loxapine levels
- Drugs that depress certain functions of the nervous system, when combined with loxapine, cause extreme drowsiness and slowed reaction times. Examples of these medicines are antihistamines, narcotics, muscle relaxants, and barbiturates.

MEDICAL CONSIDERATIONS

If you have any of the following medical conditions, make sure your doctor is aware of it.

- Kidney disease—loxapine levels may be higher than expected
- Liver disease—loxapine levels may be higher than expected
- Heart problems—some heart problems can be made worse by loxapine
- Seizure disorder—loxapine can lower seizure threshold
- Urinary retention, prostate enlargement—urination may be more difficult
- Glaucoma—loxapine can increase pressure inside the eye
- Parkinson's disease—some Parkinson's symptoms may be worsened
- Breast cancer—may increase risk of cancer progression

MAPROTILINE (ma-PROE-ti-leen)

Drug Category: Antidepressant, tetracyclic
Requires prescription.

COMMONLY USED BRAND-NAME PRODUCTS

Tablets
Ludiomil (and generic) 25mg, 50mg, 75mg

GENERAL INFORMATION

Used in treating major depression and the depressed phase of bipolar disorder.

BEFORE TAKING THIS MEDICATION

Talk to your doctor about the benefits and risks associated with maprotiline. Make sure you understand how to take it safely and effectively. You and your family members should be very familiar with the side effects and signs of having too much in your system. Make sure your doctor has the following information in detail:

- Any allergic or bad reactions you have had to maprotiline or any other medication
- All prescription and over-the-counter medicines you are taking
- Your complete medical history
- If you are pregnant, could be pregnant, or are planning a pregnancy in the near future, maprotiline should not be taken
- If you are breast feeding, maprotiline can pass into breast milk and affect the baby

USUAL ADULT DOSAGE RANGE

Starting dose 25–50mg at bedtime. Increased to 150–225 mg at bedtime over 2 to 3 weeks.

Older adults are more susceptible to side effects and will generally require lower dosages.

DIRECTIONS FOR PROPER USE

- *Take exactly as prescribed. Do not take more or less than prescribed. Accidental or intended overdoses of maprotiline can be potentially fatal.*
- Do not abruptly stop taking maprotiline unless instructed to do so by your doctor. Gradually reducing the dose can help prevent mood changes, headache, or diarrhea.
- If you miss a bedtime dose, do not take it the next morning, since it may make you drowsy. Do not double doses.
- It may take several weeks before you feel the full benefits of maprotiline.

PRECAUTIONS

- Maprotiline can cause drowsiness and slowed reaction times. Be cautious when driving, operating machinery, or doing jobs requiring alertness.
- Alcohol can cause changes in mood and may interfere with maprotiline's effectiveness. Alcohol can cause extreme drowsiness when taken with maprotiline. *Alcohol should be avoided while taking maprotiline.*
- Maprotiline may cause your skin and eyes to be more sensitive to sunlight. Exposure to sunlight may cause a rash, skin discoloration, or sunburn. Limit direct exposure to sunlight, and use sunscreen when in direct sunlight. Avoid tanning booths and beds. Wear UV-blocking sunglasses when outdoors.
- *Antidepressants may increase the risk of suicidal thinking and behavior in adolescents and children. When considering an antidepressant in a child or adolescent, the risk must be balanced with the need. Children and adolescents*

taking antidepressants should be closely monitored for worsening of symptoms, suicidality, or unusual changes in behavior.

SIDE EFFECTS

Not all side effects will occur. Many side effects will diminish with time. *However, some side effects may require attention from your doctor.* Check with your doctor immediately if you experience any of the following:

- Seizure, changes in blood pressure, irregular heart rate, shortness of breath, problems with urination (difficult or painful urination, unable to urinate), confusion, extreme sedation, excitement or mania, increased skin sensitivity to the sunlight, extreme constipation, yellow skin or eyes

Some side effects appear when you first start taking maprotiline and go away for most people. If the following side effects continue, contact your doctor.

- Dizziness, blurred vision, dry mouth, mild to moderate constipation, increased appetite, weight gain, breast enlargement (men or women), discharge from the breast, sexual problems, tremor of the hands, persistent sore throat

DRUG INTERACTIONS

Maprotiline can adversely interact with the following frequently prescribed medications:

- Cimetidine—can cause high maprotiline levels
- SSRI antidepressants—can cause high maprotiline levels
- MAOI antidepressants—severe reaction causing dangerously high blood pressure, high body temperature, seizures, or death
- Clonidine—if clonidine is being taken for high blood pressure, maprotiline may cause clonidine to work less well
- Antipsychotics—may increase certain neurologic side effects

- Thyroid hormones—increased effects of both, especially excitation and changes in heart rate or rhythm
- Drugs used during surgery—can cause increased blood pressure. Make sure your doctors are aware of upcoming planned surgeries.
- Drugs that depress certain functions of the nervous system, when combined with maprotiline, cause extreme drowsiness and slowed reaction times. Examples of these medicines are antihistamines, narcotics, muscle relaxants, and barbiturates.

MEDICAL CONSIDERATIONS

If you have any of the following medical conditions, make sure your doctor is aware of it.

- Liver disease or alcoholism—maprotiline levels may be higher than expected
- Kidney disease—maprotiline levels may be higher than expected
- Glaucoma—maprotiline can increase pressure inside the eye
- Heart problems—some heart problems can be made worse by maprotiline; maprotiline should not be taken by someone who has had a recent heart attack
- Urinary retention, prostate enlargement—urination may become more difficult
- Seizure disorder—maprotiline can lower seizure threshold
- Diabetes mellitus (sugar diabetes)—blood sugar levels may be affected
- Thyroid disorders—maprotiline may cause increased heart rate

METHYLPHENIDATE (meth-ill-PHEN-i-date)

Drug Category: Stimulant

Requires prescription, controlled substance, high potential for abuse, requires special prescription (triplicate, nonrefillable)

COMMONLY USED BRAND-NAME PRODUCTS

Brand names include Ritalin, Methylin, Metadate, Concerta, Daytrana, and generic products. Dosage forms include tablets, extended-release tablets, extended-release capsules, oral solution, and topical patches

GENERAL INFORMATION

Used to treat Attention Deficit Hyperactivity Disorder, as part of a total program that includes psychological, educational, and social components. Sometimes used in the treatment of major depression in select patients when traditional antidepressants cannot be used.

BEFORE TAKING THIS MEDICATION

Talk to your doctor about the benefits and risks associated with methylphenidate. Make sure you understand how to take it safely and effectively. You and your family members should be very familiar with the side effects and signs of having too much in your system. Make sure your doctor has the following information in detail:

- Any allergic or bad reactions you have had to methylphenidate or any other medication
- All prescription and over-the-counter medicines you are taking
- Your complete medical history
- If you are pregnant, could be pregnant, or are planning a pregnancy in the near future, methylphenidate should not be taken

- If you are breast feeding, methylphenidate can pass into breast milk and affect the baby

DOSAGE

Adults and children over 6: Dosages are highly individualized, depending on response, age, and dosage form. For regular tablets, dosages can range from 5mg to 20mg at intervals of two to three times daily. For long-acting products, dosages can range from 20mg to 72mg daily at intervals of one to two times daily.

Older adults are more susceptible to side effects and will generally require lower dosages.

DIRECTIONS FOR PROPER USE

- *Take exactly as prescribed. Do not take more or less than prescribed. Accidental or intended overdoses of methylphenidate are very serious.*
- If you take methylphenidate regularly for an extended period of time, do not stop taking it unless told to do so by your doctor. It may be necessary to gradually reduce the dose before stopping completely.
- If you miss a dose of the regular tablets, take it as soon as possible, unless it is within 3 hours of your next scheduled dose; then skip the missed dose and resume with your next scheduled dose. Do not double the dose. If you miss a dose of the long-acting tablets, skip the dose and resume with your next scheduled dose.
- To prevent trouble sleeping, do not take the last dose later than 6 pm for regular tablets and 3 pm for long-acting forms, unless otherwise directed by your doctor.
- If you are taking a long-acting form, swallow whole; do not crush, chew, or break. Some long-acting capsules can be sprinkled over food. Make sure you are aware of how to take the particular medication prescribed for you.

- The chewable form should be taken with at least 8 ounces of water.
- Treatment with these medications may last for months to years. Your doctor may discuss the option of "drug holidays." These are planned periods of time when you may not take the medicine—for example, during summer holidays from school.

PRECAUTIONS

Methylphenidate can mask some of the effects of alcohol. Routine alcohol use, or alcohol withdrawal, can increase the chance of seizures, as can methylphenidate. *Alcohol should be avoided while taking methylphenidate.*

SIDE EFFECTS

Not all side effects will occur. Many side effects will diminish with time. *However, some side effects may be warning signs of toxicity and will require attention from your doctor.* Check with your doctor immediately if you experience any of the following:

- Seizures; increased blood pressure; fast or irregular heartbeat; shortness of breath; confusion; agitation; excitement or mania; persistent throbbing headache; muscle twitches; tics or movement problems; unusual behavior; depressed mood; soreness of the mouth, gums, or throat; skin rash or itching; swelling of the face; any unusual bruising or bleeding; appearance of splotchy purplish darkening of the skin; vomiting; fatigue; weakness; fever or flulike symptoms; yellow tinge of the eyes or skin; dark-colored urine

Some side effects appear when you first start taking methylphenidate and go away for most people. If the following side effects continue, contact your doctor.

- Dizziness, nervousness, blurred vision, difficulty sleeping, decreased appetite, weight loss, headache, nausea, dry mouth

DRUG INTERACTIONS

Methylphenidate can adversely interact with the following frequently prescribed medications:

- Anticoagulants (blood thinners)—the effect of the anticoagulant can be increased
- MAOI antidepressants—severe reaction causing dangerously high blood pressure, high body temperature, seizures, or death
- Other stimulant medications such as decongestants, diet pills, some asthma medications, caffeine—can worsen side effects, especially nervousness, insomnia, high blood pressure
- Serotonin-type antidepressants—can worsen side effects, especially nervousness, insomnia, high blood pressure
- Tricyclic antidepressants—methylphenidate can increase tricyclic levels
- Digoxin—additive effects on the heart resulting in irregular heartbeat
- Anticonvulsants—methylphenidate can increase anticonvulsant levels
- Pimozide—methylphenidate may worsen tics
- Clonidine and other medications used to treat high blood pressure—methylphenidate may make these drugs less effective

MEDICAL CONSIDERATIONS

If you have any of the following medical conditions, make sure your doctor is aware of it.

- Liver disease or alcoholism—methylphenidate levels may be higher than expected

- Kidney disease—methylphenidate levels may be higher than expected
- Drug or alcohol dependence—dependence on methylphenidate may occur
- Seizure disorder—stopping methylphenidate abruptly may cause seizures
- Heart problems—some heart problems can be worsened by methylphenidate
- High blood pressure—methylphenidate may increase blood pressure
- Glaucoma—methylphenidate may worsen your condition
- Tourette's syndrome—methylphenidate may worsen tics
- Hyperthyroidism—thyroid hormone levels may increase

MIRTAZAPINE (mur-TAZ-a-peen)

Drug Category: Antidepressant, tetracyclic
Requires prescription

COMMONLY USED BRAND-NAME PRODUCTS

Tablets
Remeron (and generic) 7.5mg, 15mg, 30mg, 45mg
Tablets, oral disintegrating
Remeron (and generic) 15mg, 30mg, 45mg

GENERAL INFORMATION

Used to treat major depression and the depressed phase of bipolar disorder.

BEFORE TAKING THIS MEDICATION

Talk to your doctor about the benefits and risks associated with mirtazapine. Make sure you understand how to take it safely and effectively. You and your family members should be very familiar with the side effects and signs of having too much in your system. Make sure your doctor has the following information in detail:

- Any allergic or bad reactions you have had to mirtazapine or any other medication
- All prescription and over-the-counter medicines you are taking
- Your complete medical history
- If you are pregnant, could be pregnant, or are planning a pregnancy in the near future, mirtazapine should not be taken
- If you are breast feeding, mirtazapine can pass into breast milk and affect the baby

USUAL ADULT DOSAGE RANGE

Starting dose 15mg daily, usually at bedtime, increased over 2–3 weeks up to 45mg.

Older adults are more susceptible to side effects and will generally require lower dosages.

DIRECTIONS FOR PROPER USE

- *Take exactly as prescribed. Do not take more or less than prescribed. Accidental or intended overdoses of mirtazapine are potentially fatal.*
- Do not abruptly stop taking mirtazapine unless instructed to do so by your doctor. Gradually reducing the dose can help prevent mood changes, headache, or diarrhea.
- If you miss a dose, skip the missed dose and resume with your next scheduled dose. Do not double doses.
- If you are taking the oral disintegrating form, place the tablet in your mouth, allow it to dissolve, and swallow. Water is not required. Keep the tablets in the original package until right before you take a tablet. Any rapidly dissolving tablets that have been exposed to air should be discarded.

- It may take several weeks before you feel the full benefits of mirtazapine.

PRECAUTIONS

- Mirtazapine can cause drowsiness and slowed reaction times. Be cautious when driving, operating machinery, or doing jobs requiring alertness.
- Alcohol can cause changes in mood and may interfere with mirtazapine's effectiveness. Alcohol can cause extreme drowsiness when taken with mirtazapine. *Alcohol should be avoided while taking mirtazapine.*
- Mirtazapine may cause your skin and eyes to be more sensitive to sunlight. Exposure to sunlight may cause a rash, skin discoloration, or sunburn. Limit direct exposure to sunlight, and use sunscreen when in direct sunlight. Avoid tanning booths and beds. Wear UV-blocking sunglasses when outdoors.
- When taking mirtazapine, stand up slowly after sitting or lying down, since it may cause your blood pressure to drop and cause faintness or dizziness. Stand up slowly from a seated or lying position, especially when you first start taking mirtazapine.
- *Antidepressants may increase the risk of suicidal thinking and behavior in adolescents and children. When considering an antidepressant in a child or adolescent, the risk must be balanced with the need. Children and adolescents taking antidepressants should be closely monitored for worsening of symptoms, suicidality, or unusual changes in behavior.*

SIDE EFFECTS

Not all side effects will occur. Many side effects will diminish with time. *However, some side effects may require attention from your doctor.* Check with your doctor immediately if you experience any of the following:

- Extreme drowsiness, decreased blood pressure, decreased heart rate, skin rash or hives, shortness of breath, chills or fever, swelling of the hands or feet, seizures

Some side effects appear when you first start taking mirtazapine and go away for most people. If the following side effects continue, contact your doctor.

- Dizziness, increased appetite, weight gain, dry mouth, constipation

DRUG INTERACTIONS

Mirtazapine can adversely interact with the following frequently prescribed medications or foods:

- Anticoagulants (blood thinners)—the effect of the anticoagulant can be increased
- Some nonsedating antihistamines—cardiac (heart) toxicity
- Diet pills—severe reaction causing dangerously high blood pressure, high body temperature, seizures, or death
- Products containing L-tryptophan—severe reaction causing dangerously high blood pressure, high body temperature, seizures, or death
- Cimetidine—can cause high mirtazapine levels
- TCA antidepressants—can cause high mirtazapine levels
- MAOI antidepressants—severe reaction causing dangerously high blood pressure, high body temperature, seizures, or death
- Antipsychotics—may increase certain neurologic side effects
- Lithium—increased lithium levels causing possible confusion, dizziness, tremor
- Anticonvulsants—increased anticonvulsant levels or decreased mirtazapine levels

- Drugs that depress certain functions of the nervous system, when combined with mirtazapine, cause extreme drowsiness and slowed reaction times. Examples of these medicines are antihistamines, narcotics, muscle relaxants, and barbiturates.

MEDICAL CONSIDERATIONS
If you have any of the following medical conditions, make sure your doctor is aware of it.

- Liver disease or alcoholism—mirtazapine levels may be higher than expected
- Kidney disease—mirtazapine levels may be higher than expected
- Seizure disorder—mirtazapine can lower seizure threshold
- Diabetes mellitus (sugar diabetes)—blood sugar levels may be affected

MOLINDONE (moe-LIN-doan)
Drug Category: Neuroleptic; Antipsychotic
Requires prescription

COMMONLY USED BRAND-NAME PRODUCTS
Tablets
Moban 5mg, 10mg, 25mg, 50mg

GENERAL INFORMATION
Used to treat psychotic symptoms such as hallucinations and delusions. These symptoms occur in schizophrenia, schizoaffective disorder, bipolar disorder, or major depression with psychotic features.

BEFORE TAKING THIS MEDICATION

Talk to your doctor about the benefits and risks associated with molindone. Make sure you understand how to take it safely and effectively. You and your family members should be very familiar with its side effects. Make sure your doctor has the following information in detail:

- Any allergic or bad reactions you have had to molindone or any other medication
- All prescription and over-the-counter medicines you are taking
- Your complete medical history
- If you are pregnant, could be pregnant, or are planning a pregnancy in the near future, molindone has not been shown to be absolutely safe
- If you are breast feeding, molindone can pass into breast milk and affect the baby

USUAL ADULT DOSAGE RANGE

50–225mg daily. There is a wide effective dosage range.
Older adults are *extremely* susceptible to side effects and will generally require lower dosages.

DIRECTIONS FOR PROPER USE

- *Take exactly as prescribed. Do not take more or less than prescribed. Molindone levels that are too high can cause serious toxicity.*
- If you miss a dose, take it as soon as possible. However, if the missed dose is within 4 hours of your next dose skip the missed dose and resume with your next scheduled dose. Do not double the dose.
- It may be several weeks before you feel the full benefits.

PRECAUTIONS

- Molindone can cause drowsiness and slowed reaction times. Be cautious when driving, operating machinery, or doing jobs requiring alertness.
- Alcohol can cause extreme drowsiness when taken with molindone. *Alcohol should be avoided while taking molindone.*
- Molindone may cause your body temperature to increase and could result in heat stroke. Be extra careful in hot weather, when exercising, or when taking hot baths or saunas not to become overheated.
- Molindone may cause your skin and eyes to be more sensitive to sunlight. Exposure to sunlight may cause a rash, skin discoloration, or sunburn. Limit direct exposure to sunlight, and use sunscreen when in direct sunlight. Avoid tanning booths and beds. Wear UV-blocking sunglasses when outdoors.
- When taking molindone, stand up slowly after sitting or lying down, since it may cause your blood pressure to drop and cause faintness or dizziness. Stand up slowly from a seated or lying position, especially when you first start taking molindone.

SIDE EFFECTS

Not all side effects will occur. Many side effects will diminish with time. *However, some side effects may be warning signs of toxicity and will require attention from your doctor.* Check with your doctor immediately if you experience any of the following:

- Seizure; high fever; fast or irregular heartbeat; very low blood pressure; faintness; any abnormal movements of the mouth, tongue, neck, arms, or legs; difficulty speaking or swallowing, imbalance or difficulty walking normally; severe muscle stiffness; discoloration of the skin or eyes; confusion; significant drowsiness; restlessness; difficulty urinating; sexual problems; vomiting; diarrhea; unusual bruising or bleeding; serious skin reaction to sunlight (burning or blistering); severe constipation; breast pain or enlargement

Some side effects appear when you first start taking molindone and go away for most people. If the following side effects continue, contact your doctor.

- Dry mouth, mild to moderate constipation, dizziness, hand tremor, stuffy nose, weight gain

DRUG INTERACTIONS

Molindone can adversely interact with the following frequently prescribed medications:

- Lithium—increased neurologic side effects
- Levodopa—decreased effectiveness of levodopa
- Amphetamines—increased psychotic symptoms are possible
- Anticonvulsants—decreased molindone levels
- Tricyclic antidepressants—increased TCA levels
- Serotonin-type antidepressants—can cause high molindone levels
- Beta blockers—can cause high molindone levels
- HIV protease inhibitors—can cause high molindone levels
- Drugs that depress certain functions of the nervous system, when combined with molindone, cause extreme drowsiness and slowed reaction times. Examples of these medicines are antihistamines, narcotics, muscle relaxants, and barbiturates.

MEDICAL CONSIDERATIONS

If you have the following medical conditions, make sure your doctor is aware of it.

- Kidney disease—molindone levels may be higher than expected
- Liver disease—molindone levels may be higher than expected
- Heart problems—some heart problems can be made worse by molindone
- Seizure disorder—molindone can lower seizure threshold
- Urinary retention, prostate enlargement—urination may be more difficult
- Glaucoma—molindone can increase pressure inside the eye
- Parkinson's disease—some Parkinson's symptoms may be worsened
- Breast cancer—may increase risk of cancer progression

NORTRIPTYLINE (nor-TRIP-ti-leen)

Drug Category: Antidepressant, tricyclic
Requires prescription

COMMONLY USED BRAND-NAME PRODUCTS

Capsules
Pamelor, Aventyl (and generic), 10mg, 25mg, 50mg, 75mg
Solution
Pamelor, Aventyl (and generic) 10mg/5ml (contains alcohol)

GENERAL INFORMATION

Used to treat major depression and the depressed phase of bipolar disorder. Because of its sedative effects, it is sometimes given in low doses to help with insomnia. Also used to treat certain chronic pain disorders, such as migraine headache and diabetic neuropathy.

BEFORE TAKING THIS MEDICATION

Talk to your doctor about the benefits and risks associated with nortriptyline. Make sure you understand how to take it safely and effectively. You and your family members should be very familiar with the side effects and signs of having too much in your system. Make sure your doctor has the following information in detail:

- Any allergic or bad reactions you have had to nortriptyline or any other medication
- All prescription and over-the-counter medicines you are taking
- Your complete medical history
- If you are pregnant, could be pregnant, or are planning a pregnancy in the near future, nortriptyline should not be taken
- If you are breast feeding, nortriptyline can pass into breast milk and affect the baby

USUAL ADULT DOSAGE RANGE

The starting dose of nortriptyline will be low and will gradually be increased. Sometimes blood levels are tested to ensure that the dose you are taking is in the safe and effective range.

Depression: Starting dose 10–25mg at bedtime. Increased to 75–150mg at bedtime over 2–3 weeks.

Insomnia: 10–25mg at bedtime.

Chronic pain syndrome: 10–50mg daily.

Older adults are more susceptible to side effects and will generally require lower dosages.

DIRECTIONS FOR PROPER USE

- *Take exactly as prescribed. Do not take more or less than prescribed. Accidental or intended overdoses of nortriptyline are potentially fatal.*

- Do not abruptly stop taking nortriptyline unless instructed to do so by your doctor. Gradually reducing the dose can help prevent mood changes, headache, or diarrhea.
- If you miss a bedtime dose, do not take it the next morning, since it may make you drowsy. Do not double doses.
- It may take several weeks before you feel the full benefits.

PRECAUTIONS

- Nortriptyline can cause drowsiness and slowed reaction times. Be cautious when driving, operating machinery, or doing jobs requiring alertness.
- Alcohol can cause changes in mood and may interfere with nortriptyline's effectiveness. Alcohol can cause extreme drowsiness when taken with nortriptyline. *Alcohol should be avoided while taking nortriptyline.*
- Nortriptyline may cause your skin and eyes to be more sensitive to sunlight. Exposure to sunlight may cause a rash, skin discoloration, or sunburn. Limit direct exposure to sunlight, and use sunscreen when in direct sunlight. Avoid tanning booths and beds. Wear UV-blocking sunglasses when outdoors.
- When taking nortriptyline, stand up slowly after sitting or lying down, since it may cause your blood pressure to drop and cause faintness or dizziness. Stand up slowly from a seated or lying position, especially when you first start taking nortriptyline.
- *Antidepressants may increase the risk of suicidal thinking and behavior in adolescents and children. When considering an antidepressant in a child or adolescent, the risk must be balanced with the need. Children and adolescents taking antidepressants should be closely monitored for worsening of symptoms, suicidality, or unusual changes in behavior.*

- Adolescents and children may be more susceptible to heart-related side effects of tricyclic antidepressants. Risk must be balanced with need. Blood levels and heart function should be monitored in children and adolescents taking tricyclic antidepressants.

SIDE EFFECTS

Not all side effects will occur. Many side effects will diminish with time. *However, some side effects may require attention from your doctor.* Check with your doctor immediately if you experience any of the following:

- Seizure, changes in blood pressure, irregular heart rate, shortness of breath, problems with urination (difficult or painful urination, unable to urinate), confusion, extreme sedation, excitement or mania, increased skin sensitivity to the sunlight, extreme constipation, yellow skin or eyes

Some side effects appear when you first start taking nortriptyline and go away for most people. If the following side effects continue, contact your doctor.

- Dizziness, blurred vision, dry mouth, mild to moderate constipation, increased appetite, weight gain, breast enlargement (men or women), discharge from the breast, sexual problems, tremor of the hands, persistent sore throat

DRUG INTERACTIONS

Nortriptyline can adversely interact with the following frequently prescribed medications:

- Cimetidine—can cause high nortriptyline levels
- SSRI antidepressants—can cause high nortriptyline levels
- MAOI antidepressants—severe reaction causing dangerously high blood pressure, high body temperature, seizures, or death
- Clonidine—if clonidine is being taken for high blood pressure, nortriptyline may cause clonidine to work less well

- Antipsychotics—may increase certain neurologic side effects
- Thyroid hormones—increased effects of both, especially excitation and changes in heart rate or rhythm
- Carbamazepine—can lower nortriptyline levels
- Bupropion—can increase nortriptyline levels
- Anticoagulants (blood thinners)—the effect of the anticoagulant can be increased
- Quinolones—increased risk of heart arrhythmias
- Amphetamines—increased blood pressure, irregular heart rate, or very high fever may result
- Drugs used during surgery—can cause increased blood pressure. Make sure your doctors are aware of upcoming planned surgeries
- Drugs that depress certain functions of the nervous system, when combined with nortriptyline, cause extreme drowsiness and slowed reaction times. Examples of these medicines are antihistamines, narcotics, muscle relaxants, and barbiturates.

MEDICAL CONSIDERATIONS
If you have any of the following medical conditions, make sure your doctor is aware of it.

- Liver disease, or alcoholism—nortriptyline levels may be higher than expected
- Kidney disease—nortriptyline levels may be higher than expected
- Glaucoma—nortriptyline can increase pressure inside the eye
- Heart problems—some heart problems can be made worse by nortriptyline; nortriptyline should not be taken by someone who has had a recent heart attack

- Urinary retention, prostate enlargement—urination may become more difficult
- Seizure disorder—nortriptyline can lower seizure threshold
- Diabetes mellitus (sugar diabetes)—blood sugar levels may be affected
- Thyroid disorders—nortriptyline may cause increased heart rate

OLANZAPINE (oh-LANZ-un-peen)
Drug Category: Neuroleptic; Antipsychotic
Requires prescription

COMMONLY USED BRAND-NAME PRODUCTS
Tablets
Zyprexa 2.5mg, 5mg, 7.5mg, 10mg, 15mg, 20mg
Tablets, oral disintegrating
Zyprexa, Zydis 5mg, 10mg, 15mg, 20mg

GENERAL INFORMATION
Used to treat psychotic symptoms such as hallucinations and delusions. These symptoms occur in schizophrenia, schizoaffective disorder, bipolar disorder, or major depression with psychotic features. Olanzapine can be used for short-term management of aggressive, out-of-control behaviors or feelings of anger and rage. Because of its mood stabilizing properties, may be used in the treatment of bipolar disorder, especially manic episodes. For difficult-to-treat depression, may be used in combination with an antidepressant.

BEFORE TAKING THIS MEDICATION

Talk to your doctor about the benefits and risks associated with olanzapine. Make sure you understand how to take it safely and effectively. You and your family members should be very familiar with its side effects. *Your doctor may periodically monitor your weight, blood pressure, blood sugar, and blood lipid levels while you are taking olanzapine.* Make sure your doctor has the following information in detail:

- Any allergic or bad reactions you have had to olanzapine or any other medication
- All prescription and over-the-counter medicines you are taking
- Your complete medical history
- If you are pregnant, could be pregnant, or are planning a pregnancy in the near future, olanzapine has not been shown to be absolutely safe
- If you are breast feeding, olanzapine can pass into breast milk and affect the baby

USUAL ADULT DOSAGE RANGE

5–20mg daily.

Older adults are *extremely* susceptible to side effects and will generally require lower dosages. *Should not be used in elderly patients to treat dementia-related psychosis or behavioral disturbances.*

DIRECTIONS FOR PROPER USE

- *Take exactly as prescribed. Do not take more or less than prescribed. Olanzapine levels that are too high can cause serious toxicity.*
- If you miss a dose, take it as soon as possible. However, if the missed dose is within 4 hours of your next dose, skip the missed dose and resume with your next scheduled dose. Do not double the dose.

- If you are taking the oral disintegrating form, place the tablet in your mouth, allow it to dissolve, and swallow. Water is not required. Keep the tablets in the original package until right before you take a tablet. Any rapidly dissolving tablets that have been exposed to air should be discarded.
- It may be several weeks before you feel the full benefits.

PRECAUTIONS

- Olanzapine can cause drowsiness and slowed reaction times. Be cautious when driving, operating machinery, or doing jobs requiring alertness.
- Alcohol can cause extreme drowsiness when taken with olanzapine. *Alcohol should be avoided while taking olanzapine.*
- Olanzapine may cause your body temperature to increase and could result in heat stroke. Be extra careful in hot weather, when exercising, or when taking hot baths or saunas not to become overheated.
- When taking olanzapine, stand up slowly after sitting or lying down, since it may cause your blood pressure to drop and cause faintness or dizziness. Stand up slowly from a seated or ying position, especially when you first start taking olanzapine.

SIDE EFFECTS

Not all side effects will occur. Many side effects will diminish with time. *However, some side effects may be warning signs of toxicity and will require attention from your doctor.* Check with your doctor immediately if you experience any of the following:

- Seizure; high fever; fast or irregular heartbeat; very low blood pressure; faintness; any abnormal movements of the mouth, tongue, neck, arms, or legs; difficulty speaking or swallowing; imbalance or difficulty walking normally; severe muscle stiffness; discoloration of the skin or eyes; confusion; significant drowsiness; restlessness; difficulty urinating; sexual problems; vomiting; diarrhea; unusual bruising or bleeding; serious skin reaction to sunlight (burning or blistering); severe constipation; breast pain or enlargement

Some side effects appear when you first start taking olanzapine and go away for most people. If the following side effects continue, contact your doctor.

- Dry mouth, mild to moderate constipation, dizziness, hand tremor, stuffy nose, weight gain

DRUG INTERACTIONS

Olanzapine can adversely interact with the following frequently prescribed medications or foods:

- Lithium—increased neurologic side effects
- Levodopa—decreased effectiveness of levodopa
- Amphetamines—increased psychotic symptoms are possible
- Anticonvulsants—decreased olanzapine levels
- Tricyclic antidepressants—increased TCA levels
- Macrolide antibiotics (e.g., erythromycin)—can cause high olanzapine levels
- Oral antifungal agents—can cause high olanzapine levels
- HIV protease inhibitors—can cause high olanzapine levels
- Cimetidine—can cause high olanzapine levels
- Serotonin-type antidepressants—can cause high olanzapine levels
- Caffeine—can cause high olanzapine levels
- Drugs that depress certain functions of the nervous system, when combined with olanzapine, cause extreme drowsiness and slowed reaction times. Examples of these medi-

cines are antihistamines, narcotics, muscle relaxants, and barbiturates.

MEDICAL CONSIDERATIONS

If you have any of the following medical conditions, make sure your doctor is aware of it.

- Kidney disease—olanzapine levels may be higher than expected
- Liver disease—olanzapine levels may be higher than expected
- Heart problems—some heart problems can be made worse by olanzapine
- Seizure disorder—olanzapine can lower seizure threshold
- Urinary retention, prostate enlargement—urination may be more difficult
- Glaucoma—olanzapine can increase pressure inside the eye
- Parkinson's disease—some Parkinson's symptoms may be worsened
- Breast cancer—may increase risk of cancer progression
- Overweight/obesity—olanzapine can cause weight gain
- Diabetes—olanzapine can make this condition worse
- Elevated lipid (cholesterol and triglycerides) levels—olanzapine can make this condition worse
- High blood pressure—olanzapine can make this condition worse

OXAZEPAM (ox-AZ-e-pam)

Drug Category: Antianxiety medicine
Requires prescription, controlled substance, moderate potential for abuse

COMMONLY USED BRAND-NAME PRODUCTS
Capsules and Tablets
Serax (and generic) 10mg, 15mg, 30mg

GENERAL INFORMATION
Used to treat anxiety and symptoms of alcohol withdrawal. *This medicine is not intended to help with the stress of everyday life. Even when taken as prescribed, oxazepam may cause psychological and/or physical dependence.*

BEFORE TAKING THIS MEDICATION
Talk to your doctor about the benefits and risks associated with oxazepam. Make sure you understand how to take it safely and effectively. You and your family members should be very familiar with the side effects and signs of having too much in your system. Make sure your doctor has the following information in detail:

- Any allergic or bad reactions you have had to oxazepam or any other medication
- All prescription and over-the-counter medicines you are taking
- Your complete medical history, including mental health conditions
- If you are pregnant, could be pregnant, or are planning a pregnancy in the near future, oxazepam should not be taken
- If you are breast feeding, oxazepam can pass into breast milk and affect the baby

USUAL ADULT DOSAGE RANGE
10–60mg daily, in divided doses.
Older adults are more susceptible to side effects and will generally require lower dosages.

DIRECTIONS FOR PROPER USE

- *Take exactly as prescribed. Do not take more or less than prescribed. Oxazepam levels that are too high can cause serious toxicity.*
- If you take oxazepam regularly for an extended period of time, do not stop taking it unless told to do so by your doctor. It may be necessary to gradually reduce the dose before stopping completely. If the medicine is stopped too quickly, your condition could become worse, or you could experience serious side effects, such as seizures.
- May be taken with food to decrease stomach upset.
- If you miss a dose, take it as soon as possible. However, if the missed dose is within 4 hours of your next dose skip the missed dose and resume with your next scheduled dose. Do not double the dose.
- If you are taking the liquid form, the dose should be mixed in water, soda, applesauce, or pudding.

PRECAUTIONS

- Oxazepam can cause drowsiness and slowed reaction times. Be cautious when driving, operating machinery, or doing jobs requiring alertness.
- Alcohol can cause extreme drowsiness when taken with oxazepam. *Alcohol should be avoided while taking oxazepam.*

SIDE EFFECTS

Not all side effects will occur. Many side effects will diminish with time. *However, some side effects may be warning signs of toxicity and will require attention from your doctor.* Check with your doctor immediately if you experience any of the following:

- Confusion, severe drowsiness, slurred speech, severe weakness, unusual thoughts, shortness of breath, excitement, hyperactivity, memory problems

Some side effects appear when you first start taking oxazepam and go away for most people. If the following side effects continue, contact your doctor.

- Dizziness, lightheadedness, drowsiness, blurred vision, stomach problems

DRUG INTERACTIONS

Oxazepam can adversely interact with the following frequently prescribed medications or foods

- Cimetidine (Tagamet)—can cause high oxazepam levels
- Disulfiram (Antabuse)—can cause high oxazepam levels
- Birth control pills—can cause high oxazepam levels
- Levodopa—decreased effectiveness of levodopa
- Macrolide antibiotics (e.g., erythromycin)—can cause high oxazepam levels
- Oral antifungal agents—can cause high oxazepam levels
- HIV protease inhibitors—can cause high oxazepam levels
- Calcium channel blockers—can cause high oxazepam levels
- Serotonin-type antidepressants—can cause high oxazepam levels
- Valproic acid—can cause high oxazepam levels
- Isoniazid—can cause high oxazepam levels
- Beta blockers—can cause high oxazepam levels
- Propoxyphene—can cause high oxazepam levels
- Carbamazepine—can lower oxazepam levels
- Digoxin—oxazepam can cause high digoxin levels
- Grapefruit juice—can cause high oxazepam levels
- Drugs that depress certain functions of the nervous system, when combined with oxazepam, cause extreme drowsiness and slowed reaction times. Examples of these medicines are antihistamines, narcotics, muscle relaxants, and barbiturates.

MEDICAL CONSIDERATIONS

If you have any of the following medical conditions, make sure your doctor is aware of it.

- Liver disease or alcoholism—oxazepam levels may be higher than expected
- Kidney disease—oxazepam levels may be higher than expected
- Drug or alcohol dependence—dependence on oxazepam may occur
- Seizure disorder—stopping oxazepam abruptly may cause seizures
- Chronic lung disease—oxazepam may make breathing more difficult
- Glaucoma—oxazepam may worsen your condition
- Sleep apnea—oxazepam may worsen your condition

PALIPERIDONE (pal-ih-PAIR-ah-doan)

Drug Category: Neuroleptic; Antipsychotic

Requires prescription

COMMONLY USED BRAND-NAME PRODUCTS

Tablets, extended release

Invega 3mg, 6mg, 9mg

GENERAL INFORMATION

Used to treat psychotic symptoms, such as hallucinations and delusions. These symptoms occur in schizophrenia, schizoaffective disorder, bipolar disorder, or major depression with psychotic features. Because of its mood stabilizing properties, may be used in the treatment of bipolar disorder. For difficult-to-treat depression, may be used in combination with an antidepressant.

BEFORE TAKING THIS MEDICATION

Talk to your doctor about the benefits and risks associated with paliperidone. Make sure you understand how to take it safely and effectively. You and your family members should be very familiar with its side effects. *Your doctor may periodically monitor your weight, blood pressure, blood sugar, and blood lipid levels while you are taking paliperidone.* Make sure your doctor has the following information in detail:

- Any allergic or bad reactions you have had to paliperidone or any other medication
- All prescription and over-the-counter medicines you are taking
- Your complete medical history
- If you are pregnant, could be pregnant, or are planning a pregnancy in the near future, paliperidone has not been shown to be absolutely safe
- If you are breast feeding, paliperidone can pass into breast milk and affect the baby

USUAL ADULT DOSAGE RANGE

6–12mg daily.

Older adults are *extremely* susceptible to side effects and will generally require lower dosages. *Should not be used in elderly patients to treat dementia-related psychosis or behavioral disturbances.*

DIRECTIONS FOR PROPER USE

- *Take exactly as prescribed. Do not take more or less than prescribed. Paliperidone levels that are too high can cause serious toxicity.*
- If you miss a dose, take it as soon as possible. If within 1 to 2 hours of your next dose, skip the missed dose and resume with your next scheduled dose. Do not double the dose.
- Tablets must be swallowed whole and taken with liquids.

Tablets should not be chewed, divided, or crushed. The medication is absorbed from the tablet shell, which is eliminated from the body. Do not be concerned if you occasionally see the tablet shell in the stool.

- It may be several weeks before you feel the full benefits.

PRECAUTIONS

- Paliperidone can cause drowsiness and slowed reaction times. Be cautious when driving, operating machinery, or doing jobs requiring alertness.
- Alcohol can cause extreme drowsiness when taken with paliperidone. *Alcohol should be avoided while taking paliperidone.*
- Paliperidone may cause your body temperature to increase and could result in heat stroke. Be extra careful in hot weather, when exercising, or when taking hot baths or saunas not to become overheated.
- When taking paliperidone, stand up slowly after sitting or lying down, since it may cause your blood pressure to drop and cause faintness or dizziness. Stand up slowly from a seated or lying position, especially when you first start taking paliperidone.

SIDE EFFECTS

Not all side effects will occur. Many side effects will diminish with time. *However, some side effects may be warning signs of toxicity and will require attention from your doctor.* Check with your doctor immediately if you experience any of the following:

- Seizure; high fever; fast or irregular heartbeat; very low blood pressure; faintness; any abnormal movements of the mouth, tongue, neck, arms, or legs; difficulty speaking or swallowing; imbalance or difficulty walking normally; severe muscle stiffness; discoloration of the skin or eyes;

confusion; significant drowsiness; restlessness; difficulty urinating; sexual problems; vomiting; diarrhea; unusual bruising or bleeding; serious skin reaction to sunlight (burning or blistering); severe constipation; breast pain or enlargement

Some side effects appear when you first start taking paliperidone and go away for most people. If the following side effects continue, contact your doctor.

- Dry mouth, mild to moderate constipation, dizziness, hand tremor, stuffy nose, weight gain

DRUG INTERACTIONS

Paliperidone can adversely interact with the following frequently prescribed medications or foods:

- Lithium—increased neurologic side effects
- Levodopa—decreased effectiveness of levodopa
- Amphetamines—increased psychotic symptoms are possible
- Anticonvulsants—decreased paliperidone levels
- Tricyclic antidepressants—increased TCA levels
- Macrolide antibiotics (e.g., erythromycin)—can cause high paliperidone levels
- Oral antifungal agents—can cause high paliperidone levels
- HIV protease inhibitors—can cause high paliperidone levels
- Cimetidine—can cause high paliperidone levels
- Serotonin-type antidepressants—can cause high paliperidone levels
- Antiarrhythmics or other drugs that can affect the heartbeat—when taken with paliperidone can cause serious disturbances of heart rhythm
- Caffeine—can cause high paliperidone levels
- Drugs that depress certain functions of the nervous system,

when combined with paliperidone, cause extreme drowsiness and slowed reaction times. Examples of these medicines are antihistamines, narcotics, muscle relaxants, and barbiturates.

MEDICAL CONSIDERATIONS

If you have any of the following medical conditions, make sure your doctor is aware of it.

- Kidney disease—paliperidone levels may be higher than expected
- Liver disease—paliperidone levels may be higher than expected
- Heart problems—some heart problems can be made worse by paliperidone
- Seizure disorder—paliperidone can lower seizure threshold
- Urinary retention, prostate enlargement—urination may be more difficult
- Glaucoma—paliperidone can increase pressure inside the eye
- Parkinson's disease—some Parkinson's symptoms may be worsened
- Breast cancer—may increase risk of cancer progression
- Overweight/obesity—paliperidone can cause weight gain
- Diabetes—paliperidone can make this condition worse
- Elevated lipid (cholesterol and triglycerides) levels—paliperidone can make this condition worse
- High blood pressure—paliperidone can make this condition worse

PAROXETINE (pair-OX-a-teen)

Drug Category: Antidepressant, SSRI (serotonin specific reuptake inhibitor)

Requires prescription

COMMONLY USED BRAND-NAME PRODUCTS

Tablets

Paxil (and generic) 20mg, 30mg, 40mg

Tablets, controlled release

Paxil CR 12.5mg, 25mg, 37.5mg

Suspension

Paxil (and generic) 10mg/5ml

GENERAL INFORMATION

Used to treat major depression and the depressed phase of bipolar disorder. Also used to treat obsessive compulsive disorder (OCD), panic disorder, generalized anxiety disorder, social anxiety disorder, premenstrual dysphoric disorder (PMDD), and post-traumatic stress disorder (PTSD)

BEFORE TAKING THIS MEDICATION

Talk to your doctor about the benefits and risks associated with paroxetine. Make sure you understand how to take it safely and effectively. You and your family members should be very familiar with the side effects and signs of having too much in your system. Make sure your doctor has the following information in detail:

- Any allergic or bad reactions you have had to paroxetine or any other medication
- All prescription and over-the-counter medicines you are taking
- Your complete medical history

- If you are pregnant, could be pregnant, or are planning a pregnancy in the near future, paroxetine should not be taken
- If you are breast feeding, paroxetine can pass into breast milk and affect the baby

USUAL ADULT DOSAGE RANGE

10–40mg daily. Dosage increases should not be more often than every 1 to 2 weeks.
OCD: 20–50mg daily.
Older adults are more susceptible to side effects and will generally require lower dosages.

DIRECTIONS FOR PROPER USE

- *Take exactly as prescribed. Do not take more or less than prescribed.*
- Do not abruptly stop taking paroxetine unless instructed to do so by your doctor.
- May be taken with food or meals to lessen stomach upset.
- If you are taking the long-acting tablet form and you miss a dose, take it as soon as possible within 1 to 2 hours of the missed dose. However, if it is more than 2 hours after the missed dose, skip the missed dose and resume with your next scheduled dose. Swallow tablets whole; do not crush, chew, or break.
- If you miss a dose, do not try to make it up. Wait and take your next scheduled dose. Do not double doses.
- It may take several weeks before you feel the full benefits.

PRECAUTIONS

- Paroxetine can cause drowsiness and slowed reaction times. Be cautious when driving, operating machinery, or doing jobs requiring alertness.
- Alcohol can cause changes in mood and may interfere with paroxetine's effectiveness. Alcohol can cause extreme drowsiness when taken with paroxetine. *Alcohol should be avoided while taking paroxetine.*
- Paroxetine may cause your skin and eyes to be more sensitive to sunlight. Exposure to sunlight may cause a rash, skin discoloration, or sunburn. Limit direct exposure to sunlight, and use sunscreen when in direct sunlight. Avoid tanning booths and beds. Wear UV-blocking sunglasses when outdoors.
- *Antidepressants may increase the risk of suicidal thinking and behavior in adolescents and children. When considering an antidepressant in a child or adolescent, the risk must be balanced with the need. Children and adolescents taking antidepressants should be closely monitored for worsening of symptoms, suicidality, or unusual changes in behavior.*

SIDE EFFECTS

Not all side effects will occur. Many side effects will diminish with time. *However, some side effects may require attention from your doctor.* Check with your doctor immediately if you experience any of the following:

- Skin rash or hives, shortness of breath, chills or fever, swelling of the hands or feet, seizures, bleeding or bruising

Some side effects appear when you first start taking paroxetine and go away for most people. If the following side effects continue, contact your doctor.

- Agitation, anxiety, insomnia, dizziness, sexual problems,

sweating, blurred vision, dry mouth, mild to moderate constipation, change in appetite, change in weight, tremor of the hands

DRUG INTERACTIONS

Paroxetine can adversely interact with the following frequently prescribed medications or foods:

- Anticoagulants (blood thinners)—the effect of the anticoagulant can be increased
- Some nonsedating antihistamines—cardiac (heart) toxicity
- Diet pills—severe reaction causing dangerously high blood pressure, high body temperature, seizures, or death
- Products containing L-tryptophan—severe reaction causing dangerously high blood pressure, high body temperature, seizures, or death
- Cimetidine—can cause high paroxetine levels
- Bupropion—dosage adjustment of one or both drugs may be necessary
- Amphetamines—increased blood pressure, irregular heart rate, or very high fever may result
- TCA antidepressants—can cause high TCA levels
- MAOI antidepressants—severe reaction causing dangerously high blood pressure, high body temperature, seizures, or death
- Antipsychotics—may increase certain neurologic side effects
- Lithium—increased lithium levels causing possible confusion, dizziness, tremor
- Anticonvulsants—increased anticonvulsant levels or decreased paroxetine levels
- Antiarrhythmic drugs—increased risk of arrhythmias
- Benzodiazepines—paroxetine can increase benzodiazepine levels

- Beta blockers—paroxetine can increase levels of beta blockers
- Aspirin, NSAIDs—increased chance of bleeding
- HIV protease inhibitors—paroxetine can increase levels of protease inhibitors
- Drugs that depress certain functions of the nervous system, when combined with paroxetine, cause extreme drowsiness and slowed reaction times. Examples of these medicines are antihistamines, narcotics, muscle relaxants, and barbiturates.

MEDICAL CONSIDERATIONS
If you have any of the following medical conditions, make sure your doctor is aware of it.
- Liver disease or alcoholism—paroxetine levels may be higher than expected
- Kidney disease—paroxetine levels may be higher than expected
- Seizure disorder—paroxetine can lower seizure threshold
- Diabetes mellitus (sugar diabetes)—blood sugar levels may be affected
- Low sodium—paroxetine may worsen this condition
- Bleeding disorder—paroxetine may worsen this condition

PERPHENAZINE (pur-FEN-uh-zeen)
Drug Category: Neuroleptic; Antipsychotic
Requires prescription

COMMONLY USED BRAND-NAME PRODUCTS
Tablets
Trilafon (and generic) 2mg, 4mg, 8mg, 16mg

Liquid
Trilafon (and generic) solution 16mg/5ml (contains alcohol)

GENERAL INFORMATION

Used to treat psychotic symptoms such as hallucinations and delusions. These symptoms occur in schizophrenia, schizo-affective disorder, bipolar disorder, or major depression with psychotic features. Can be used for short-term management of aggressive, out-of-control behaviors or feelings of anger and rage.

BEFORE TAKING THIS MEDICATION

Talk to your doctor about the benefits and risks associated with perphenazine. Make sure you understand how to take it safely and effectively. You and your family members should be very familiar with its side effects. Make sure your doctor has the following information in detail:

- Any allergic or bad reactions you have had to perphenazine or any other medication
- All prescription and over-the-counter medicines you are taking
- Your complete medical history
- If you are pregnant, could be pregnant, or are planning a pregnancy in the near future, perphenazine has not been shown to be absolutely safe
- If you are breast feeding, perphenazine can pass into breast milk and affect the baby

USUAL ADULT DOSAGE RANGE

4–64mg daily. There is a wide effective dosage range.
Older adults are *extremely* susceptible to side effects and will generally require lower dosages.

DIRECTIONS FOR PROPER USE

- *Take exactly as prescribed. Do not take more or less than prescribed. Perphenazine levels that are too high can cause serious toxicity.*
- If you miss a dose, take it as soon as possible. However, if the missed dose is within 4 hours of your next dose, skip the missed dose and resume with your next scheduled dose. Do not double the dose.
- If you are taking a liquid form, it must be diluted before swallowing. It may be diluted in water, milk, tomato juice, or fruit juices, except apple juice. It should not be mixed with coffee, tea, or colas. The dose should be measured carefully.
- If you are taking the solution form, avoid contacting the skin with the medicine. Irritation can result by the medicine coming in contact with skin. Do not use the liquid form if the medicine becomes very discolored (dark yellow) or has a sediment at the bottom of the bottle.
- It may be several weeks before you feel the full benefits.

PRECAUTIONS

- Perphenazine can cause drowsiness and slowed reaction times. Be cautious when driving, operating machinery, or doing jobs requiring alertness.
- Alcohol can cause extreme drowsiness when taken with perphenazine. *Alcohol should be avoided while taking perphenazine.*
- Perphenazine may cause your body temperature to increase and could result in heat stroke. Be extra careful in hot weather, when exercising, or when taking hot baths or saunas not to become overheated.
- Perphenazine may cause your skin and eyes to be more sensitive to sunlight. Exposure to sunlight may cause a

rash, skin discoloration, or sunburn. Limit direct exposure to sunlight, and use sunscreen when in direct sunlight. Avoid tanning booths and beds. Wear UV-blocking sunglasses when outdoors.

- When taking perphenazine, stand up slowly after sitting or lying down, since it may cause your blood pressure to drop and cause faintness or dizziness. Stand up slowly from a seated or lying position, especially when you first start taking perphenazine.

SIDE EFFECTS

Not all side effects will occur. Many side effects will diminish with time. *However, some side effects may be warning signs of toxicity and will require attention from your doctor.* Check with your doctor immediately if you experience any of the following:

- Seizure; high fever; fast or irregular heartbeat; very low blood pressure; faintness; any abnormal movements of the mouth, tongue, neck, arms, or legs; difficulty speaking or swallowing; imbalance or difficulty walking normally; severe muscle stiffness; discoloration or the skin or eyes; confusion; significant drowsiness; restlessness; difficulty urinating; sexual problems; vomiting; diarrhea; unusual bruising or bleeding; serious skin reaction to sunlight (burning or blistering); severe constipation; breast pain or enlargement

Some side effects appear when you first start taking perphenazine and go away for most people. If the following side effects continue, contact your doctor.

- Dry mouth, mild to moderate constipation, dizziness, hand tremor, stuffy nose, weight gain

DRUG INTERACTIONS

Perphenazine can adversely interact with the following frequently prescribed medications:

- Lithium—increased neurologic side effects
- Levodopa—decreased effectiveness of levodopa
- Amphetamines—increased psychotic symptoms are possible
- Anticonvulsants—decreased perphenazine levels
- Tricyclic antidepressants—increased TCA levels
- Serotonin-type antidepressants—can cause high perphenazine levels
- Beta blockers—can cause high perphenazine levels
- HIV protease inhibitors—can cause high perphenazine levels
- Drugs that depress certain functions of the nervous system, when combined with perphenazine, cause extreme drowsiness and slowed reaction times. Examples of these medicines are antihistamines, narcotics, muscle relaxants, and barbiturates.

MEDICAL CONSIDERATIONS

If you have any of the following medical conditions, make sure your doctor is aware of it.

- Kidney disease—perphenazine levels may be higher than expected
- Liver disease—perphenazine levels may be higher than expected
- Heart problems—some heart problems can be made worse by perphenazine
- Seizure disorder—perphenazine can lower seizure threshold
- Urinary retention, prostate enlargement—urination may be more difficult
- Glaucoma—perphenazine can increase pressure inside the eye

- Parkinson's disease—Some Parkinson's symptoms may be worsened
- Breast cancer—may increase risk of cancer progression

PHENELZINE (fen-EL-zeen)

Drug Category: Antidepressant, MAOI (monoamine oxidase inhibitor)

Requires prescription

COMMONLY USED BRAND-NAME PRODUCTS

Tablets

Nardil 15mg

GENERAL INFORMATION

Used to treat major depression and the depressed phase of bipolar disorder.

BEFORE TAKING THIS MEDICATION

Talk to your doctor about the benefits and risks associated with phenelzine. Make sure you understand how to take it safely and effectively. You and your family members should be very familiar with the side effects and signs of having too much in your system. Make sure your doctor has the following information in detail:

- Any allergic or bad reactions you have had to phenelzine or any other medication
- All prescription and over-the-counter medicines you are taking
- Your complete medical history
- If you are pregnant, could be pregnant, or are planning a pregnancy in the near future, phenelzine should not be taken

- If you are breast feeding, phenelzine can pass into breast milk and affect the baby

USUAL ADULT DOSAGE RANGE
30–60mg daily.
Older adults are more susceptible to side effects and will generally require lower dosages.

DIRECTIONS FOR PROPER USE
- *Take exactly as prescribed. Do not take more or less than prescribed. Accidental or intended overdoses of phenelzine can be potentially fatal.*
- *Follow the dietary instructions carefully while taking phenelzine. Not doing so can lead to dangerously high blood pressure.*
- *Check with your doctor or pharmacist before taking any other prescription or over-the-counter medicine.*
- Do not abruptly stop taking phenelzine unless instructed to do so by your doctor.
- It is advised that you check your blood pressure frequently while taking phenelzine.
- If you miss a bedtime dose, do not take it the next morning, since it may make you drowsy. Do not double doses.
- It may take several weeks before you feel the full benefits of phenelzine.

PRECAUTIONS
- Phenelzine can cause drowsiness and slowed reaction times. Be cautious when driving, operating machinery, or doing jobs requiring alertness.
- Alcohol can cause changes in mood and may interfere with phenelzine's effectiveness. Alcohol can cause extreme drowsiness when taken with phenelzine. *Alcohol should be avoided while taking phenelzine.*

- When taking phenelzine, stand up slowly after sitting or lying down, since it may cause your blood pressure to drop and cause faintness or dizziness. Stand up slowly from a seated or lying position, especially when you first start taking phenelzine.
- The amount of tyramine, or tryptophan, in your diet must be restricted while taking phenelzine. Tyramine is found in foods that have been aged, foods that have been preserved, and foods that have undergone protein breakdown. The amount of tyramine in food is NOT inactivated by cooking. These restrictions will need be followed for 2 weeks after phenelzine has been stopped.
- *Antidepressants may increase the risk of suicidal thinking and behavior in adolescents and children. When considering an antidepressant in a child or adolescent, the risk must be balanced with the need. Children and adolescents taking antidepressants should be closely monitored for worsening of symptoms, suicidality, or unusual changes in behavior.*

SIDE EFFECTS

Not all side effects will occur. Many side effects will diminish with time. *However, some side effects may require attention from your doctor.* Check with your doctor immediately if you experience any of the following:

- Seizure, changes in blood pressure, severe headache, irregular heart rate, shortness of breath, problems with urination (difficult or painful urination, unable to urinate), confusion, extreme sedation, excitement or mania, extreme sweating, severe skin sensitivity to the sunlight (burning or blistering), extreme constipation, yellow skin or eyes

Some side effects appear when you first start taking phenelzine and go away for most people. If the following side effects continue, contact your doctor.

- Dizziness, blurred vision, dry mouth, mild to moderate constipation, increased appetite, weight gain, tremor of the hands

DRUG INTERACTIONS

Phenelzine can adversely interact with the following frequently prescribed medications. A severe reaction causing dangerously high blood pressure, high body temperature, seizures, or death is possible. These interactions are possible for up to 2 weeks even after phenelzine has been stopped. A washout period of up to 5 weeks after stopping some of the medications listed below may be necessary before starting phenelzine.

- SSRI antidepressants
- Cyclic antidepressants
- Stimulant drugs—amphetamines, methylphenidate (Ritalin), cocaine
- Ephedrine, pseudoephedrine—found in prescription and over-the-counter cough and cold medicines and asthma medicines
- Phenylephrine, phenylpropanolamine—found in prescription and over-the-counter cough and cold medicines and asthma medicines
- Levodopa
- Buspirone (Buspar)
- Buproprion
- Carbamazepine
- Dextromethorphan—found in prescription and over-the-counter cough syrups and lozenges
- Meperidine (Demerol)
- L-trytophan
- Drugs used during surgery—can cause increased blood

pressure. Make sure your doctors are aware of upcoming planned surgeries.

- Drugs that depress certain functions of the nervous system, when combined with phenelzine, cause extreme drowsiness and slowed reaction times. Examples of these medicines are antihistamines, narcotics, muscle relaxants, and barbiturates.

MEDICAL CONSIDERATIONS

If you have any of the following medical conditions, make sure your doctor is aware of it.

- Liver disease or alcoholism—phenelzine levels may be higher than expected
- Kidney disease—phenelzine levels may be higher than expected
- Heart problems—some heart problems can be made worse by phenelzine; phenelzine should not be taken by someone who has had a recent heart attack
- High blood pressure—blood pressure may be increased
- Urinary retention, prostate enlargement—urination may become more difficult
- Seizure disorder—phenelzine can lower seizure threshold
- Diabetes mellitus (sugar diabetes)—blood sugar levels may be affected
- Thyroid disorders—phenelzine may cause increased heart rate
- Pheochromocytoma—can lead to high blood pressure

PIMOZIDE (PIM-o-zide)

Drug Category: Neuroleptic; Antipsychotic
Requires prescription

COMMONLY USED BRAND-NAME PRODUCTS

Tablets
Orap 1mg, 2mg

GENERAL INFORMATION

Used to treat Tourette's syndrome to help reduce motor tics
and vocalizations.

BEFORE TAKING THIS MEDICATION

Talk to your doctor about the benefits and risks associated
with pimozide. Make sure you understand how to take it safely
and effectively. You and your family members should be very
familiar with its side effects. Make sure your doctor has the
following information in detail:

- Any allergic or bad reactions you have had to pimozide or
  any other medication
- All prescription and over-the-counter medicines you are
  taking
- Your complete medical history
- If you are pregnant, could be pregnant, or are planning a
  pregnancy in the near future, pimozide has not been shown
  to be absolutely safe
- If you are breast feeding, pimozide can pass into breast
  milk and affect the baby

DOSAGE

Adults and adolescents: 1–10mg daily. There is a wide effective
dosage range. The starting dose will be small and will be gradually increased.

Older adults are *extremely* susceptible to side effects and will generally require lower dosages.

Children under 12: Dosages in this age group have not been established.

DIRECTIONS FOR PROPER USE

- *Take exactly as prescribed. Do not take more or less than prescribed. Pimozide levels that are too high can cause serious toxicity.*
- If you miss a dose, take it as soon as possible. However, if the missed dose is within 4 hours of your next dose, skip the missed dose and resume with your next scheduled dose. Do not double the dose.
- It may be several weeks before you feel the full benefits.

PRECAUTIONS

- Pimozide can cause drowsiness and slowed reaction times. Be cautious when driving, operating machinery, or doing jobs requiring alertness.
- Alcohol can cause extreme drowsiness when taken with pimozide. *Alcohol should be avoided while taking pimozide.*
- Pimozide may cause your body temperature to increase and could result in heat stroke. Be extra careful in hot weather, when exercising, or when taking hot baths or saunas not to become overheated.
- Pimozide may cause your skin and eyes to be more sensitive to sunlight. Exposure to sunlight may cause a rash, skin discoloration, or sunburn. Limit direct exposure to sunlight, and use sunscreen when in direct sunlight. Avoid tanning booths and beds. Wear UV-blocking sunglasses when outdoors.
- When taking pimozide, stand up slowly after sitting or lying down, since it may cause your blood pressure to drop

and cause faintness or dizziness. Stand up slowly from a seated or lying position, especially when you first start taking pimozide.

SIDE EFFECTS

Not all side effects will occur. Many side effects will diminish with time. *However, some side effects may be warning signs of toxicity and will require attention from your doctor.* Check with your doctor immediately if you experience any of the following:

- Seizure; high fever; fast or irregular heartbeat; very low blood pressure; faintness; any abnormal movements of the mouth, tongue, neck, arms, or legs; difficulty speaking or swallowing; imbalance or difficulty walking normally; severe muscle stiffness; discoloration of the skin or eyes; confusion; significant drowsiness; restlessness; difficulty urinating; sexual problems; vomiting; diarrhea; unusual bruising or bleeding; serious skin reaction to sunlight (burning or blistering); severe constipation; breast pain or enlargement

Some side effects appear when you first start taking pimozide and go away for most people. If the following side effects continue, contact your doctor.

- Dry mouth, mild to moderate constipation, dizziness, hand tremor, stuffy nose, weight gain

DRUG INTERACTIONS

Pimozide can adversely interact with the following frequently prescribed medications or foods:

- Lithium—increased neurologic side effects
- Levodopa—decreased effectiveness of levodopa
- Amphetamines—increased psychotic symptoms are possible
- Anticonvulsants—decreased pimozide levels
- Tricyclic antidepressants—increased TCA levels

- Serotonin-type antidepressants—can cause high pimozide levels
- Beta blockers—can cause high pimozide levels
- HIV protease inhibitors—can cause high pimozide levels
- Macrolide antibiotics (e.g., erythromycin)—can cause high pimozide levels
- Oral antifungal agents—can cause high pimozide levels
- Grapefruit juice—can cause high pimozide levels
- Drugs that depress certain functions of the nervous system, when combined with pimozide, cause extreme drowsiness and slowed reaction times. Examples of these medicines are antihistamines, narcotics, muscle relaxants, and barbiturates.

MEDICAL CONSIDERATIONS

If you have any of the following medical conditions, make sure your doctor is aware of it.

- Kidney disease—pimozide levels may be higher than expected
- Liver disease—pimozide levels may be higher than expected
- Heart problems—some heart problems can be made worse by pimozide
- Seizure disorder—pimozide can lower seizure threshold
- Urinary retention, prostate enlargement—urination may be more difficult
- Glaucoma—pimozide can increase pressure inside the eye
- Parkinson's disease—some Parkinson's symptoms may be worsened
- Breast cancer—may increase risk of cancer progression

PROTRIPTYLINE (pro-TRIP-ti-leen)

Drug Category: Antidepressant, tricyclic
Requires prescription

COMMONLY USED BRAND-NAME PRODUCTS

Tablets
Vivactil (and generic) 5mg, 10mg

GENERAL INFORMATION

Used to treat major depression and the depressed phase of
bipolar disorder. If used to treat the depressed phase of bipolar
disorder, watch for signs of mania or hypomania.

BEFORE TAKING THIS MEDICATION

Talk to your doctor about the benefits and risks associated
with protriptyline. Make sure you understand how to take it
safely and effectively. You and your family members should be
very familiar with the side effects and signs of having too much
in your system. Make sure your doctor has the following information in detail:

- Any allergic or bad reactions you have had to protriptyline
  or any other medication
- All prescription and over-the-counter medicines you are
  taking
- Your complete medical history
- If you are pregnant, could be pregnant, or are planning a
  pregnancy in the near future, protriptyline should not be
  taken
- If you are breast feeding, protriptyline can pass into breast
  milk and affect the baby

USUAL ADULT DOSAGE RANGE

The starting dose of protriptyline will be low and will gradually be increased. Sometimes blood levels are tested to en-

sure that the dose you are taking is in the safe and effective range.

Depression: Starting dose 5–10mg daily. Increased up to 45–60mg daily over 2 to 3 weeks. Because protriptyline can be activating, some people may need to avoid taking the dose near bedtime as it could cause difficulty sleeping.

Older adults are more susceptible to side effects and will generally require lower dosages.

DIRECTIONS FOR PROPER USE

- *Take exactly as prescribed. Do not take more or less than prescribed. Accidental or intended overdoses of protriptyline are potentially fatal.*
- Do not abruptly stop taking protriptyline unless instructed to do so by your doctor. Gradually reducing the dose can help prevent mood changes, headache, or diarrhea.
- If you miss a bedtime dose, do not take it the next morning, since it may make you drowsy. Do not double doses.
- It may take several weeks before you feel the full benefits.

PRECAUTIONS

- Protriptyline can cause drowsiness and slowed reaction times. Be cautious when driving, operating machinery, or doing jobs requiring alertness.
- Alcohol can cause changes in mood and may interfere with protriptyline's effectiveness. Alcohol can cause extreme drowsiness when taken with protriptyline. *Alcohol should be avoided with taking protriptyline.*
- Protriptyline may cause your skin and eyes to be more sensitive to sunlight. Exposure to sunlight may cause a rash, skin discoloration, or sunburn. Limit direct exposure to sunlight, and use sunscreen when in direct sunlight. Avoid

tanning booths and beds. Wear UV-blocking sunglasses when outdoors.

- When taking protriptyline, stand up slowly after sitting or lying down, since it may cause your blood pressure to drop and cause faintness or dizziness. Stand up slowly from a seated or lying position, especially when you first start taking protriptyline.

- *Antidepressants may increase the risk of suicidal thinking and behavior in adolescents and children. When considering an antidepressant in a child or adolescent, the risk must be balanced with the need. Children and adolescents taking antidepressants should be closely monitored for worsening of symptoms, suicidality, or unusual changes in behavior.*

- Adolescents and children may be more susceptible to heart-related side effects of tricyclic antidepressants. Risk must be balanced with need. Blood levels and heart function should be monitored in children and adolescents taking tricyclic antidepressants.

SIDE EFFECTS

Not all side effects will occur. Many side effects will diminish with time. *However, some side effects may require attention from your doctor.* Check with your doctor immediately if you experience any of the following:

- Seizure, changes in blood pressure, irregular heart rate, shortness of breath, problems with urination (difficult or painful urination, unable to urinate), confusion, extreme sedation, excitement or mania, increased skin sensitivity to the sunlight, extreme constipation, yellow skin or eyes

Some side effects appear when you first start taking protriptyline and go away for most people. If the following side effects continue, contact your doctor.

- Dizziness, blurred vision, dry mouth, mild to moderate constipation, increased appetite, weight gain, breast enlargement (men or women), discharge from the breast, sexual problems, tremor of the hands, persistent sore throat

DRUG INTERACTIONS

Protriptyline can adversely interact with the following frequently prescribed medications:

- Cimetidine—can cause high protriptyline levels
- SSRI antidepressants—can cause high protriptyline levels
- MAOI antidepressants—severe reaction causing dangerously high blood pressure, high body temperature, seizures, or death
- Clonidine—if clonidine is being taken for high blood pressure, protriptyline may cause clonidine to work less well
- Antipsychotics—may increase certain neurologic side effects
- Thyroid hormones—increased effects of both, especially excitation and changes in heart rate or rhythm
- Carbamazepine—can lower protriptyline levels
- Bupropion—can increase protriptyline levels
- Anticoagulants (blood thinners)—the effect of the anticoagulant can be increased
- Quinolones—increased risk of heart arrhythmias
- Amphetamines—increased blood pressure, irregular heart rate, or very high fever may result
- Drugs used during surgery—can cause increased blood pressure. Make sure your doctors are aware of upcoming planned surgeries.
- Drugs that depress certain functions of the nervous system, when combined with protriptyline, cause extreme drowsiness and slowed reaction times. Examples of these medi-

cines are antihistamines, narcotics, muscle relaxants, and barbiturates.

MEDICAL CONSIDERATIONS

If you have the following medical conditions, make sure your doctor is aware of it.

- Liver disease or alcoholism—protriptyline levels may be higher than expected
- Kidney disease—protriptyline levels may be higher than expected
- Glaucoma—protriptyline can increase pressure inside the eye
- Heart problems—some heart problems can be made worse by protriptyline; protriptyline should not be taken by someone who has had a recent heart attack
- Urinary retention, prostate enlargement—urination may become more difficult
- Seizure disorder—protriptyline can lower seizure threshold
- Diabetes mellitus (sugar diabetes)—blood sugar levels may be affected
- Thyroid disorders—protriptyline may cause increased heart rate

QUAZEPAM (KWAY-ze-pam)

Drug Category: Insomnia medicine
Requires prescription, controlled substance, moderate potential for abuse

COMMONLY USED BRAND-NAME PRODUCTS

Tablets
Doral 7.5mg, 15mg

GENERAL INFORMATION

Used to treat insomnia. *Even when taken as prescribed, quaze-pam may cause psychological and/or physical dependence. Not intended for long-term use.*

BEFORE TAKING THIS MEDICATION

Talk to your doctor about the benefits and risks associated with quazepam. Make sure you understand how to take it safely and effectively. You and your family members should be very familiar with the side effects and signs of having too much in your system. Make sure your doctor has the following information in detail:

- Any allergic or bad reactions you have had to quazepam or any other medication
- All prescription and over-the-counter medicines you are taking
- Your complete medical history, including mental health conditions
- If you are pregnant, could be pregnant, or are planning a pregnancy in the near future, quazepam should not be taken
- If you are breast feeding, quazepam can pass into breast milk and affect the baby

USUAL ADULT DOSAGE RANGE

7.5–15mg at bedtime.
Older adults are more susceptible to side effects and will generally require lower dosages.

DIRECTIONS FOR PROPER USE

- *Take exactly as prescribed. Do not take more or less than prescribed. Quazepam levels that are too high can cause serious toxicity.*
- If you take quazepam regularly for an extended period of

time, do not stop taking it unless told to do so by your doctor. It may be necessary to gradually reduce the dose before stopping completely.

- If you miss a dose, take it as soon as possible if it is within 1 hour of the scheduled time. However, quazepam should be taken only if you are sure you will get a full night's sleep of at least 7 to 8 hours.

PRECAUTIONS

- Quazepam can cause drowsiness and slowed reaction times. Be cautious when driving, operating machinery, or doing jobs requiring alertness.
- Alcohol can cause extreme drowsiness when taken with quazepam. *Alcohol should be avoided while taking quazepam.*
- Quazepam may cause a severe allergic reaction and/or severe facial swelling, which can occur as early as the first dose.
- Quazepam can cause complex sleep-related behaviors, which may include sleep-driving, making phone calls, and preparing and eating food (while asleep).

SIDE EFFECTS

Not all side effects will occur. Many side effects will diminish with time. *However, some side effects may be warning signs of toxicity and will require attention from your doctor.* Check with your doctor immediately if you experience any of the following:

- Confusion, severe drowsiness, slurred speech, severe weakness, unusual thoughts, shortness of breath, excitement, hyperactivity, memory problems

Some side effects appear when you first start taking quazepam and go away for most people. If the following side effects continue, contact your doctor.

- Dizziness, lightheadedness, daytime drowsiness, blurred vision

DRUG INTERACTIONS

Quazepam can adversely interact with the following frequently prescribed medications or foods:

- Cimetidine (Tagamet)—can cause high quazepam levels
- Disulfiram (Antabuse)—can cause high quazepam levels
- Birth control pills—can cause high quazepam levels
- Levodopa—decreased effectiveness of levodopa
- Macrolide antibiotics (e.g., erythromycin)—can cause high quazepam levels
- Oral antifungal agents—can cause high quazepam levels
- HIV protease inhibitors—can cause high quazepam levels
- Calcium channel blockers—can cause high quazepam levels
- Serotonin-type antidepressants—can cause high quazepam levels
- Digoxin—quazepam can cause high digoxin levels
- Valproic acid—can cause high quazepam levels
- Isoniazid—can cause high quazepam levels
- Beta blockers—can cause high quazepam levels
- Propoxyphene—can cause high quazepam levels
- Carbamazepine—can lower quazepam levels
- Grapefruit juice—can cause high quazepam levels
- Drugs that depress certain functions of the nervous system, when combined with quazepam, cause extreme drowsiness and slowed reaction times. Examples of these medicines are antihistamines, narcotics, muscle relaxants, and barbiturates

MEDICAL CONSIDERATIONS

If you have any of the following medical conditions, make sure your doctor is aware of it.

- Liver disease or alcoholism—quazepam levels may be higher than expected
- Kidney disease—quazepam levels may be higher than expected
- Drug or alcohol dependence—dependence on quazepam may occur
- Seizure disorder—stopping quazepam abruptly may cause seizures
- Chronic lung disease—quazepam may make breathing more difficult
- Glaucoma—quazepam may worsen your condition
- Sleep apnea—quazepam may worsen your condition

QUETIAPINE (kwe-TIE-uh-peen)
Drug Category: Neuroleptic; Antipsychotic
Requires prescription

COMMONLY USED BRAND-NAME PRODUCTS
Tablets
Seroquel 25mg, 100mg, 200mg, 300mg, 400mg
Tablets, extended release
Seroquel XR 400mg, 600mg, 800mg

GENERAL INFORMATION
Used to treat psychotic symptoms such as hallucinations and delusions. These symptoms occur in schizophrenia, schizoaffective disorder, bipolar disorder, or major depression with psychotic features. Quetiapine can be used for short-term management of aggressive, out-of-control behaviors or feelings of anger and rage. Also indicated for acute manic epi-

sodes and depressive episodes associated with bipolar disorder. For difficult-to-treat depression, may be used in combination with an antidepressant.

BEFORE TAKING THIS MEDICATION

Talk to your doctor about the benefits and risks associated with quetiapine. Make sure you understand how to take it safely and effectively. You and your family members should be very familiar with its side effects. *Your doctor may periodically monitor your weight, blood pressure, blood sugar, and blood lipid levels while you are taking quetiapine.* Make sure your doctor has the following information in detail:

- Any allergic or bad reactions you have had to quetiapine or any other medication
- All prescription and over-the-counter medicines you are taking
- Your complete medical history
- If you are pregnant, could be pregnant, or are planning a pregnancy in the near future, quetiapine has not been shown to be absolutely safe
- If you are breast feeding, quetiapine can pass into breast milk and affect the baby

DOSAGE
Adults and Adolescents
Psychotic symptoms: 150–750mg daily.
Acute mania: 400–800mg daily.
Depression associated with bipolar disorder: 300–600mg daily.
Older adults are *extremely* susceptible to side effects and will generally require lower dosages. ***Should not be used in elderly patients to treat dementia-related psychosis or behavioral disturbances.***
Children: Not approved for use in children.

DIRECTIONS FOR PROPER USE

- *Take exactly as prescribed. Do not take more or less than prescribed. Quetiapine levels that are too high can cause serious toxicity.*
- If you miss a dose of the regular tablet, take it as soon as possible. However, if the missed dose is within 4 hours of your next dose, skip the missed dose and resume with your next scheduled dose. Do not double the dose.
- If you are taking the long-acting tablet form and you miss a dose, take it as soon as possible within 1 to 2 hours of the missed dose. However, if it is more than 2 hours after the missed dose, skip the missed dose and resume with your next scheduled dose. Swallow tablets whole; do not crush, chew, or break.
- It may be several weeks before you feel the full benefits.

PRECAUTIONS

- Quetiapine can cause drowsiness and slowed reaction times. Be cautious when driving, operating machinery, or doing jobs requiring alertness.
- Alcohol can cause extreme drowsiness when taken with quetiapine. *Alcohol should be avoided while taking quetiapine.*
- Quetiapine may cause your body temperature to increase and could result in heat stroke. Be extra careful in hot weather, when exercising, or when taking hot baths or saunas not to become overheated.
- When taking quetiapine, stand up slowly after sitting or lying down, since it may cause your blood pressure to drop and cause faintness or dizziness. Stand up slowly from a seated or lying position, especially when you first start taking quetiapine.

SIDE EFFECTS

Not all side effects will occur. Many side effects will diminish with time. *However, some side effects may be warning signs of toxicity and will require attention from your doctor.* Check with your doctor immediately if you experience any of the following:

- Seizure; high fever; fast or irregular heartbeat; very low blood pressure; faintness; any abnormal movements of the mouth, tongue, neck, arms, or legs; difficulty speaking or swallowing; imbalance or difficulty walking normally; severe muscle stiffness; discoloration or the skin or eyes; confusion; significant drowsiness; restlessness; difficulty urinating; sexual problems; vomiting; diarrhea; unusual bruising or bleeding; serious skin reaction to sunlight (burning or blistering); severe constipation; breast pain or enlargement

Some side effects appear when you first start taking quetiapine and go away for most people. If the following side effects continue, contact your doctor.

- Dry mouth, mild to moderate constipation, dizziness, hand tremor, stuffy nose, weight gain

DRUG INTERACTIONS

Quetiapine can adversely interact with the following frequently prescribed medications:

- Lithium—increased neurologic side effects
- Levodopa—decreased effectiveness of levodopa
- Amphetamines—increased psychotic symptoms are possible
- Anticonvulsants—decreased quetiapine levels
- Tricyclic antidepressants—increased TCA levels
- Macrolide antibiotics (e.g., erythromycin)—can cause high quetiapine levels

- Oral antifungal agents—can cause high quetiapine levels
- HIV protease inhibitors—can cause high quetiapine levels
- Cimetidine—can cause high quetiapine levels
- Caffeine—can cause high quetiapine levels
- Serotonin-type antidepressants—can cause high quetiapine levels
- Drugs that depress certain functions of the nervous system, when combined with quetiapine, cause extreme drowsiness and slowed reaction times. Examples of these medicines are antihistamines, narcotics, muscle relaxants, and barbiturates.

MEDICAL CONSIDERATIONS

If you have any of the following medical conditions, make sure your doctor is aware of it.

- Kidney disease—quetiapine levels may be higher than expected
- Liver disease—quetiapine levels may be higher than expected
- Heart problems—some heart problems can be made worse by quetiapine
- Seizure disorder—quetiapine can lower seizure threshold
- Urinary retention, prostate enlargement—urination may be more difficult
- Glaucoma—quetiapine can increase pressure inside the eye
- Parkinson's disease—some Parkinson's symptoms may be worsened
- Breast cancer—may increase risk of cancer progression
- Overweight/obesity—quetiapine can cause weight gain
- Diabetes—quetiapine can make this condition worse
- Elevated lipid (cholesterol and triglycerides) levels—quetiapine can make this condition worse

- High blood pressure—quetiapine can make this condition worse

RAMELTEON (ram-EL-tee-on)

Drug Category: Insomnia medicine
Requires prescription

COMMONLY USED BRAND-NAME PRODUCTS
Tablets
Rozerem 8mg

GENERAL INFORMATION
Used to treat insomnia. *Even when taken as prescribed, ramelteon may cause psychological and/or physical dependence. Not intended for long-term use.*

BEFORE TAKING THIS MEDICATION
Talk to your doctor about the benefits and risks associated with ramelteon. Make sure you understand how to take it safely and effectively. You and your family members should be very familiar with the side effects and signs of having too much in your system. Make sure your doctor has the following information in detail:

- Any allergic or bad reactions you have had to ramelteon or any other medication
- All prescription and over-the-counter medicines you are taking
- Your complete medical history, including mental health conditions
- If you are pregnant, could be pregnant, or are planning a pregnancy in the near future, ramelteon should not be taken

- If you are breast feeding, ramelteon can pass into breast milk and affect the baby

USUAL ADULT DOSAGE RANGE
8mg at bedtime.
Older adults are more susceptible to side effects and will generally require lower dosages.

DIRECTIONS FOR PROPER USE
- *Take exactly as prescribed. Do not take more or less than prescribed. Ramelteon levels that are too high can cause serious toxicity.*
- If you take ramelteon regularly for an extended period of time, do not stop taking it unless told to do so by your doctor. It may be necessary to gradually reduce the dose before stopping completely.
- Do not take with or immediately after a high-fat meal.
- Take immediately before bedtime and only if you are sure you will get a full night's sleep of at least 7 to 8 hours.

PRECAUTIONS
- Ramelteon can cause drowsiness and slowed reaction times. Be cautious when driving, operating machinery, or doing jobs requiring alertness.
- Alcohol can cause extreme drowsiness when taken with ramelteon. *Alcohol should be avoided while taking ramelteon.*
- Ramelteon may cause a severe allergic reaction and/or severe facial swelling, which can occur as early as the first dose.
- Ramelteon can cause complex sleep-related behaviors, which may include sleep-driving, making phone calls, and preparing and eating food (while asleep).

SIDE EFFECTS

Not all side effects will occur. Many side effects will diminish with time. *However, some side effects may be warning signs of toxicity and will require attention from your doctor.* Check with your doctor immediately if you experience any of the following:

- Confusion, severe drowsiness, slurred speech, severe weakness, unusual thoughts, shortness of breath, excitement, hyperactivity, memory problems, abnormal addictive behaviors

Some side effects appear when you first start taking ramelteon and go away for most people. If the following side effects continue, contact your doctor.

- Dizziness, lightheadedness, daytime drowsiness, blurred vision, change in menstrual periods

DRUG INTERACTIONS

Ramelteon can adversely interact with the following frequently prescribed medications:

- Oral antifungal agents—can cause high ramelteon levels
- Fluvoxamine—can cause high ramelteon levels
- Drugs that depress certain functions of the nervous system, when combined with ramelteon, cause extreme drowsiness and slowed reaction times. Examples of these medicines are antihistamines, narcotics, muscle relaxants, and barbiturates.

MEDICAL CONSIDERATIONS

If you have any of the following medical conditions, make sure your doctor is aware of it.

- Liver disease or alcoholism—ramelteon levels may be higher than expected
- Kidney disease—ramelteon levels may be higher than expected

- Drug or alcohol dependence—dependence on ramelteon may occur
- Chronic lung disease—ramelteon may make breathing more difficult

RISPERIDONE (ris-PAIR-ih-doan)

Drug Category: Neuroleptic; Antipsychotic

Requires prescription

COMMONLY USED BRAND-NAME PRODUCTS

Tablets

Risperdal 0.25mg, 0.5mg, 1mg, 2mg, 3mg, 4mg

Tablets, rapidly disintegrating

Risperdal M-Tab 0.5mg, 1mg, 2mg, 3mg, 4mg

Solution

Risperdal 1mg/ml

Injection, extended release

Risperdal Consta 12.5mg, 25mg, 37.5mg, 50mg

GENERAL INFORMATION

Used to treat psychotic symptoms such as hallucinations and delusions. These symptoms occur in schizophrenia, schizoaffective disorder, bipolar disorder, or major depression with psychotic features. Risperidone can be used for short-term management of aggressive, out-of-control behaviors or feelings of anger and rage. Because of its mood stabilizing properties, may be used in the treatment of bipolar disorder, especially manic episodes. For difficult-to-treat depression, may be used in combination with another antidepressant.

BEFORE TAKING THIS MEDICATION

Talk to your doctor about the benefits and risks associated with risperidone. Make sure you understand how to take it safely and effectively. You and your family members should be very familiar with its side effects. *Your doctor may periodically monitor your weight, blood pressure, blood sugar, and blood lipid levels while you are taking risperidone.* Make sure your doctor has the following information in detail:

- Any allergic or bad reactions you have had to risperidone or any other medication
- All prescription and over-the-counter medicines you are taking
- Your complete medical history
- If you are pregnant, could be pregnant, or are planning a pregnancy in the near future, risperidone has not been shown to be absolutely safe
- If you are breast feeding, risperidone can pass into breast milk and affect the baby

USUAL ADULT DOSAGE RANGE

Psychotic symptoms: 2–16mg daily.

Mania: 1–6mg daily.

Older adults are *extremely* susceptible to side effects and will generally require lower dosages. *Should not be used in elderly patients to treat dementia-related psychosis or behavioral disturbances.*

DIRECTIONS FOR PROPER USE

- *Take exactly as prescribed. Do not take more or less than prescribed. Risperidone levels that are too high can cause serious toxicity.*
- If you miss a dose, take it as soon as possible. However, if the missed dose is within 4 hours of your next dose, skip

the missed dose and resume with your next scheduled dose. Do not double the dose.

- If you are taking a liquid form, use the pipette provided to measure the dose, and then stir completely in 3 to 4 ounces of water, coffee, orange juice, or low-fat milk. Do not mix with cola or tea.
- If you are taking the oral disintegrating form, place the tablet in your mouth, allow it to dissolve, and swallow. Water is not required. Keep the tablets in the original package until right before you take a tablet. Any rapidly dissolving tablets that have been exposed to air should be discarded.
- It may be several weeks before you feel the full benefits.

PRECAUTIONS

- Risperidone can cause drowsiness and slowed reaction times. Be cautious when driving, operating machinery, or doing jobs requiring alertness.
- Alcohol can cause extreme drowsiness when taken with risperidone. *Alcohol should be avoided while taking risperidone.*
- Risperidone may cause your body temperature to increase and could result in heat stroke. Be extra careful in hot weather, when exercising, or when taking hot baths or saunas not to become overheated.
- When taking risperidone, stand up slowly after sitting or lying down, since it may cause your blood pressure to drop and cause faintness or dizziness. Stand up slowly from a seated or lying position, especially when you first start taking risperidone.

SIDE EFFECTS

Not all side effects will occur. Many side effects will diminish with time. *However, some side effects may be warning signs of toxicity and will require attention from your doctor.* Check with your doctor immediately if you experience any of the following:

- Seizure; high fever; fast or irregular heartbeat; very low blood pressure; faintness; any abnormal movements of the mouth, tongue, neck, arms, or legs; difficulty speaking or swallowing; imbalance or difficulty walking normally; severe muscle stiffness; discoloration or the skin or eyes; confusion; significant drowsiness; restlessness; difficulty urinating; sexual problems; vomiting; diarrhea; unusual bruising or bleeding; serious skin reaction to sunlight (burning or blistering); severe constipation; breast pain or enlargement

Some side effects appear when you first start taking risperidone and go away for most people. If the following side effects continue, contact your doctor.

- Dry mouth, mild to moderate constipation, dizziness, hand tremor, stuffy nose, weight gain

DRUG INTERACTIONS

Risperidone can adversely interact with the following frequently prescribed medications or foods:

- Lithium—increased neurologic side effects
- Levodopa—decreased effectiveness of levodopa
- Amphetamines—increased psychotic symptoms are possible
- Anticonvulsants—decreased risperidone levels
- Tricyclic antidepressants—increased TCA levels
- Macrolide antibiotics (e.g., erythromycin)—can cause high risperidone levels
- Oral antifungal agents—can cause high risperidone levels
- HIV protease inhibitors—can cause high risperidone levels
- Cimetidine—can cause high risperidone levels

- Serotonin-type antidepressants—can cause high risperidone levels
- Caffeine—can cause high risperidone levels
- Drugs that depress certain functions of the nervous system, when combined with risperidone, cause extreme drowsiness and slowed reaction times. Examples of these medicines are antihistamines, narcotics, muscle relaxants, and barbiturates.

MEDICAL CONSIDERATIONS

If you have any of the following medical conditions, make sure your doctor is aware of it.

- Kidney disease—risperidone levels may be higher than expected
- Liver disease—risperidone levels may be higher than expected
- Heart problems—some heart problems can be made worse by risperidone
- Seizure disorder—risperidone can lower seizure threshold
- Urinary retention, prostate enlargement—urination may be more difficult
- Glaucoma—risperidone can increase pressure inside the eye
- Parkinson's disease—some Parkinson's symptoms may be worsened
- Breast cancer—may increase risk of cancer progression
- Overweight/obesity—risperidone can cause weight gain
- Diabetes—risperidone can make this condition worse
- Elevated lipid (cholesterol and triglycerides) levels—risperidone can make this condition worse
- High blood pressure—risperidone can make this condition worse

SERTRALINE (sur-TRA-leen)

Drug Category: Antidepressant, SSRI (serotonin specific reuptake inhibitor)

Requires prescription

COMMONLY USED BRAND-NAME PRODUCTS

Tablets

Zoloft (and generic) 25mg, 50mg, 100mg

Liquid

20mg/ml

GENERAL INFORMATION

Used to treat major depression and the depressed phase of bipolar disorder. Also used to treat obsessive compulsive disorder (OCD), panic disorder, social anxiety disorder, premenstrual dysphoric disorder (PMDD) and post-traumatic stress disorder (PTSD).

BEFORE TAKING THIS MEDICATION

Talk to your doctor about the benefits and risks associated with sertraline. Make sure you understand how to take it safely and effectively. You and your family members should be very familiar with the side effects and signs of having too much in your system. Make sure your doctor has the following information in detail:

- Any allergic or bad reactions you have had to sertraline or any other medication
- All prescription and over-the-counter medicines you are taking
- Your complete medical history
- If you are pregnant, could be pregnant, or are planning a pregnancy in the near future, sertraline should not be taken

- If you are breast feeding, sertraline can pass into breast milk and affect the baby

USUAL ADULT DOSAGE RANGE

Depression, panic disorder: 50–200mg daily. Dosage increases should not be more often than every 1 to 2 weeks.

OCD: 100–200mg daily.

Older adults are more susceptible to side effects and will generally require lower dosages.

DIRECTIONS FOR PROPER USE

- *Take exactly as prescribed. Do not take more or less than prescribed.*
- Do not abruptly stop taking sertraline unless instructed to do so by your doctor.
- May be taken with food or meals to lessen stomach upset.
- If you miss a dose, do not try to make it up. Wait and take your next scheduled dose. Do not double doses.
- It may take several weeks before you feel the full benefits.

PRECAUTIONS

- Sertraline can cause drowsiness and slowed reaction times. Be cautious when driving, operating machinery, or doing jobs requiring alertness.
- Alcohol can cause changes in mood and may interfere with sertraline's effectiveness. Alcohol can cause extreme drowsiness when taken with sertraline. *Alcohol should be avoided while taking sertraline.*
- Sertraline may cause your skin and eyes to be more sensitive to sunlight. Exposure to sunlight may cause a rash, skin discoloration, or sunburn. Limit direct exposure to sunlight, and use sunscreen when in direct sunlight. Avoid tanning booths and beds. Wear UV-blocking sunglasses when outdoors.

- *Antidepressants may increase the risk of suicidal thinking and behavior in adolescents and children. When considering an antidepressant in a child or adolescent, the risk must be balanced with the need. Children and adolescents taking antidepressants should be closely monitored for worsening of symptoms, suicidality, or unusual changes in behavior.*

SIDE EFFECTS

Not all side effects will occur. Many side effects will diminish with time. *However, some side effects may require attention from your doctor.* Check with your doctor immediately if you experience any of the following:

- Skin rash or hives, shortness of breath, chills or fever, swelling of the hands or feet, seizures, bleeding or bruising

Some side effects appear when you first start taking sertraline and go away for most people. If the following side effects continue, contact your doctor.

- Agitation, anxiety, insomnia, dizziness, sexual problems, sweating, blurred vision, dry mouth, mild to moderate constipation, change in appetite, change in weight, tremor of the hands

DRUG INTERACTIONS

Sertraline can adversely interact with the following frequently prescribed medications or foods:

- Anticoagulants (blood thinners)—the effect of the anticoagulant can be increased
- Some nonsedating antihistamines—cardiac (heart) toxicity
- Diet pills—severe reaction causing dangerously high blood pressure, high body temperature, seizures, or death
- Products containing L-tryptophan—severe reaction causing dangerously high blood pressure, high body temperature, seizures, or death

- Cimetidine—can cause high sertraline levels
- Amphetamines—increased blood pressure, irregular heart rate, or very high fever may result
- Bupropion—dosage adjustment of one or both drugs may be necessary
- TCA antidepressants—can cause high TCA levels
- MAOI antidepressants—severe reaction causing dangerously high blood pressure, high body temperature, seizures, or death
- Antipsychotics—may increase certain neurologic side effects
- Lithium—increased lithium levels causing possible confusion, dizziness, tremor
- Anticonvulsants—increased anticonvulsant levels or decreased sertraline levels
- Antiarrhythmic drugs—increased risk of arrhythmias
- Benzodiazepines—sertraline can increase benzodiazepine levels
- Beta blockers—sertraline can increase beta blocker levels
- Aspirin, NSAIDs—increased chance of bleeding
- HIV protease inhibitors—sertraline can increase levels of protease inhibitors
- Drugs that depress certain functions of the nervous system, when combined with sertraline, cause extreme drowsiness and slowed reaction times. Examples of these medicines are antihistamines, narcotics, muscle relaxants, and barbiturates.

MEDICAL CONSIDERATIONS

If you have any of the following medical conditions, make sure your doctor is aware of it.

- Liver disease or alcoholism—sertraline levels may be higher than expected

- Kidney disease—sertraline levels may be higher than expected
- Seizure disorder—sertraline can lower seizure threshold
- Diabetes mellitus (sugar diabetes)—blood sugar levels may be affected
- Low sodium—sertraline may worsen this condition
- Bleeding disorder—sertraline may worsen this condition

TEMAZEPAM (tem-AZ-e-pam)

Drug Category: Insomnia medicine
Requires prescription, controlled substance, moderate potential for abuse

COMMONLY USED BRAND-NAME PRODUCTS
Capsules
Restoril (and generic) 7.5mg, 15mg, 30mg

GENERAL INFORMATION
Used to treat insomnia. *Even when taken as prescribed, temazepam may cause psychological and/or physical dependence. Not intended for long-term use.*

BEFORE TAKING THIS MEDICATION
Talk to your doctor about the benefits and risks associated with temazepam. Make sure you understand how to take it safely and effectively. You and your family members should be very familiar with the side effects and signs of having too much in your system. Make sure your doctor has the following information in detail:

- Any allergic or bad reactions you have had to temazepam or any other medication

- All prescription and over-the-counter medicines you are taking
- Your complete medical history, including mental health conditions
- If you are pregnant, could be pregnant, or are planning a pregnancy in the near future, temazepam should not be taken
- If you are breast feeding, temazepam can pass into breast milk and affect the baby

USUAL ADULT DOSAGE RANGE

7.5–30mg at bedtime.
Older adults are more susceptible to side effects and will generally require lower dosages.

DIRECTIONS FOR PROPER USE

- ***Take exactly as prescribed. Do not take more or less than prescribed. Temazepam levels that are too high can cause serious toxicity.***
- If you take temazepam regularly for an extended period of time, do not stop taking it unless told to do so by your doctor. It may be necessary to gradually reduce the dose before stopping completely.
- If you miss a dose, take it as soon as possible if it is within 1 hour of the scheduled time. However, temazepam should be taken only if you are sure you will get a full night's sleep of at least 7 to 8 hours.

PRECAUTIONS

- Temazepam can cause drowsiness and slowed reaction times. Be cautious when driving, operating machinery, or doing jobs requiring alertness.
- Alcohol can cause extreme drowsiness when taken with

temazepam. *Alcohol should be avoided while taking temazepam.*

- Temazepam may cause a severe allergic reaction and/or severe facial swelling, which can occur as early as the first dose.
- Temazepam can cause complex sleep-related behaviors, which may include sleep-driving, making phone calls, and preparing and eating food (while asleep).

SIDE EFFECTS

Not all side effects will occur. Many side effects will diminish with time. *However, some side effects may be warning signs of toxicity and will require attention from your doctor.* Check with your doctor immediately if you experience any of the following:

- Confusion, severe drowsiness, slurred speech, severe weakness, unusual thoughts, shortness of breath, excitement, hyperactivity, memory problems

Some side effects appear when you first start taking temazepam and go away for most people. If the following side effects continue, contact your doctor.

- Dizziness, lightheadedness, daytime drowsiness, blurred vision

DRUG INTERACTIONS

Temazepam can adversely interact with the following frequently prescribed medications or foods:

- Cimetidine (Tagamet)—can cause high temazepam levels
- Disulfiram (Antabuse)—can cause high temazepam levels
- Birth control pills—can cause high temazepam levels
- Levodopa—decreased effectiveness of levodopa
- Macrolide antibiotics (e.g., erythromycin)—can cause high temazepam levels

- Oral antifungal agents—can cause high temazepam levels
- HIV protease inhibitors—can cause high temazepam levels
- Calcium channel blockers—can cause high temazepam levels
- Serotonin-type antidepressants—can cause high temazepam levels
- Digoxin—temazepam can cause high digoxin levels
- Valproic acid—can cause high temazepam levels
- Isoniazid—can cause high temazepam levels
- Beta blockers—can cause high temazepam levels
- Propoxyphene—can cause high temazepam levels
- Grapefruit juice—can cause high temazepam levels
- Carbamazepine—can lower temazepam levels
- Drugs that depress certain functions of the nervous system, when combined with temazepam, cause extreme drowsiness and slowed reaction times. Examples of these medicines are antihistamines, narcotics, muscle relaxants, and barbiturates.

MEDICAL CONSIDERATIONS

If you have any of the following medical conditions, make sure your doctor is aware of it.

- Liver disease or alcoholism—temazepam levels may be higher than expected
- Kidney disease—temazepam levels may be higher than expected
- Drug or alcohol dependence—dependence on temazepam may occur
- Seizure disorder—stopping temazepam abruptly may cause seizures
- Chronic lung disease—temazepam may make breathing more difficult

- Glaucoma—temazepam may worsen your condition
- Sleep apnea—temazepam may worsen your condition

THIORIDAZINE (thi-o-RID-uh-zeen)
Drug Category: Neuroleptic; Antipsychotic
Requires prescription

COMMONLY USED BRAND-NAME PRODUCTS
Tablets
Mellaril (and generic) 10mg, 15mg, 25mg, 50mg, 100mg, 150mg, 200mg

GENERAL INFORMATION
Used to treat schizophrenia only when other antipsychotics have failed. *Thioridazine has been shown to cause potentially life-threatening heart arrhythmias, so its use is reserved.*

BEFORE TAKING THIS MEDICATION
Talk to your doctor about the benefits and risks associated with thioridazine. Make sure you understand how to take it safely and effectively. You and your family members should be very familiar with its side effects. Make sure your doctor has the following information in detail:

- Any allergic or bad reactions you have had to thioridazine or any other medication
- All prescription and over-the-counter medicines you are taking
- Your complete medical history
- If you are pregnant, could be pregnant, or are planning a pregnancy in the near future, thioridazine has not been shown to be absolutely safe

- If you are breast feeding, thioridazine can pass into breast milk and affect the baby

USUAL ADULT DOSAGE RANGE
50–800mg daily. There is a wide effective dosage range.
Older adults are *extremely* susceptible to side effects and will generally require lower dosages.

DIRECTIONS FOR PROPER USE
- *Take exactly as prescribed. Do not take more or less than prescribed. Thioridazine levels that are too high can cause serious toxicity.*
- If you miss a dose, take it as soon as possible. However, if the missed dose is within 4 hours of your next dose, skip the missed dose and resume with your next scheduled dose. Do not double the dose.
- It may be several weeks before you feel the full benefits.

PRECAUTIONS
- Thioridazine can cause drowsiness and slowed reaction times. Be cautious when driving, operating machinery, or doing jobs requiring alertness.
- Alcohol can cause extreme drowsiness when taken with thioridazine. *Alcohol should be avoided while taking thioridazine.*
- Thioridazine may cause your body temperature to increase and could result in heat stroke. Be extra careful in hot weather, when exercising, or when taking hot baths or saunas not to become overheated.
- Thioridazine may cause your skin and eyes to be more sensitive to sunlight. Exposure to sunlight may cause a rash, skin discoloration, or sunburn. Limit direct exposure to sunlight, and use sunscreen when in direct sunlight. Avoid

tanning booths and beds. Wear UV-blocking sunglasses when outdoors.

- When taking thioridazine, stand up slowly after sitting or lying down, since it may cause your blood pressure to drop and cause faintness or dizziness. Stand up slowly from a seated or lying position, especially when you first start taking thioridazine.

SIDE EFFECTS

Not all side effects will occur. Many side effects will diminish with time. *However, some side effects may be warning signs of toxicity and will require attention from your doctor.* Check with your doctor immediately if you experience any of the following:

- Seizure; high fever; fast or irregular heartbeat; very low blood pressure; faintness, any abnormal movements of the mouth, tongue, neck, arms, or legs; difficulty speaking or swallowing; imbalance or difficulty walking normally; severe muscle stiffness; discoloration or the skin or eyes; confusion; significant drowsiness; restlessness; difficulty urinating; sexual problems; vomiting; diarrhea; unusual bruising or bleeding; serious skin reaction to sunlight (burning or blistering); severe constipation; breast pain or enlargement

Some side effects appear when you first start taking thioridazine and go away for most people. If the following side effects continue, contact your doctor.

- Dry mouth, mild to moderate constipation, dizziness, hand tremor, stuffy nose, weight gain

DRUG INTERACTIONS

Thioridazine can adversely interact with the following frequently prescribed medications:

- Lithium—increased neurologic side effects
- Levodopa—decreased effectiveness of levodopa

- Amphetamines—increased psychotic symptoms are possible
- Anticonvulsants—decreased thioridazine levels
- Tricyclic antidepressants—increased TCA levels
- Serotonin-type antidepressants—can cause high thioridazine levels
- Beta blockers—can cause high thioridazine levels
- HIV protease inhibitors—can cause high thioridazine levels
- Drugs that depress certain functions of the nervous system, when combined with thioridazine, cause extreme drowsiness and slowed reaction times. Examples of these medicines are antihistamines, narcotics, muscle relaxants, and barbiturates.

MEDICAL CONSIDERATIONS

If you have any of the following medical conditions, make sure your doctor is aware of it.

- Kidney disease—thioridazine levels may be higher than expected
- Liver disease—thioridazine levels may be higher than expected
- Heart problems—some heart problems can be made worse by thioridazine
- Seizure disorder—thioridazine can lower seizure threshold
- Urinary retention, prostate enlargement—urination may be more difficult
- Glaucoma—thioridazine can increase pressure inside the eye
- Parkinson's disease—some Parkinson's symptoms may be worsened
- Breast cancer—may increase risk of cancer progression

TRANYLCYPROMINE (tran-el-SIP-ro-meen)

Drug Category: Antidepressant, MAOI (monoamine oxidase inhibitor)

Requires prescription

COMMONLY USED BRAND-NAME PRODUCTS

Tablets

Parnate (and generic) 10mg

GENERAL INFORMATION

Used to treat major depression and the depressed phase of bipolar disorder.

BEFORE TAKING THIS MEDICATION

Talk to your doctor about the benefits and risks associated with tranylcypromine. Make sure you understand how to take it safely and effectively. You and your family members should be very familiar with the side effects and signs of having too much in your system. Make sure your doctor has the following information in detail:

- Any allergic or bad reactions you have had to tranylcypromine or any other medication
- All prescription and over-the-counter medicines you are taking
- Your complete medical history
- If you are pregnant, could be pregnant, or are planning a pregnancy in the near future, tranylcypromine should not be taken
- If you are breast feeding, tranylcypromine can pass into breast milk and affect the baby

USUAL ADULT DOSAGE RANGE

20–40mg daily.

Older adults are more susceptible to side effects and will generally require lower dosages.

DIRECTIONS FOR PROPER USE

- *Take exactly as prescribed. Do not take more or less than prescribed. Accidental or intended overdoses of tranylcypromine can be potentially fatal.*
- *Follow the dietary instructions carefully while taking tranylcypromine. Not doing so can lead to dangerously high blood pressure.*
- *Check with your doctor or pharmacist before taking any other prescription or over-the-counter medicine.*
- Do not abruptly stop taking tranylcypromine unless instructed to do so by your doctor.
- It is advised that you check your blood pressure frequently while taking tranylcypromine.
- If you miss a bedtime dose, do not take it the next morning, since it may make you drowsy. Do not double doses.
- It may take several weeks before you feel the full benefits of tranylcypromine.

PRECAUTIONS

- Tranylcypromine can cause drowsiness and slowed reaction times. Be cautious when driving, operating machinery, or doing jobs requiring alertness.
- Alcohol can cause changes in mood and may interfere with tranylcypromine's effectiveness. Alcohol can cause extreme drowsiness when taken with tranylcypromine. *Alcohol should be avoided while taking tranylcypromine.*
- When taking tranylcypromine, stand up slowly after sitting or lying down, since it may cause your blood pressure to drop and cause faintness or dizziness. Stand up slowly from a seated or lying position, especially when you first start taking tranylcypromine.

- The amount of tyramine, or tryptophan, in your diet must be restricted while taking tranylcypromine. Tyramine is found in foods that have been aged, foods that have been preserved, and foods that have undergone protein breakdown. The amount of tyramine in food is NOT inactivated by cooking. These restrictions will need be followed for 2 weeks after tranylcypromine has been stopped.
- *Antidepressants may increase the risk of suicidal thinking and behavior in adolescents and children. When considering an antidepressant in a child or adolescent, the risk must be balanced with the need. Children and adolescents taking antidepressants should be closely monitored for worsening of symptoms, suicidality, or unusual changes in behavior.*

SIDE EFFECTS

Not all side effects will occur. Many side effects will diminish with time. *However, some side effects may require attention from your doctor.* Check with your doctor immediately if you experience any of the following:

- Seizure, changes in blood pressure, severe headache, irregular heart rate, shortness of breath, problems with urination (difficult or painful urination, unable to urinate), confusion, extreme sedation, excitement or mania, extreme sweating, severe skin sensitivity to the sunlight (burning or blistering), extreme constipation, yellow skin or eyes

Some side effects appear when you first start taking tranylcypromine and go away for most people. If the following side effects continue, contact your doctor.

- Dizziness, blurred vision, dry mouth, mild to moderate constipation, increased appetite, weight gain, tremor of the hands

DRUG INTERACTIONS

Tranylcypromine can adversely interact with the following frequently prescribed medications. A severe reaction causing dangerously high blood pressure, high body temperature, seizures, or death is possible. These interactions are possible for up to 2 weeks even after tranylcypromine has been stopped. A washout period of up to 5 weeks after stopping some of the medications listed below may be necessary before starting tranylcypromine.

- SSRI antidepressants
- Cyclic antidepressants
- Stimulant drugs—amphetamines, methylphenidate (Ritalin), cocaine
- Ephedrine, pseudoephedrine—found in prescription and over-the-counter cough and cold medicines and asthma medicines
- Phenylephrine, phenylpropanolamine—found in prescription and over-the-counter cough and cold medicines and asthma medicines
- Levodopa
- Buspirone (Buspar)
- Buproprion
- Carbamazepine
- Dextromethorphan—found in prescription and over-the-counter cough syrups and lozenges
- Meperidine (Demerol)
- L-tryptophan
- Drugs used during surgery—can cause increased blood pressure. Make sure your doctors are aware of upcoming planned surgeries.
- Drugs that depress certain functions of the nervous system, when combined with tranylcypromine, cause extreme

drowsiness and slowed reaction times. Examples of these medicines are antihistamines, narcotics, muscle relaxants, and barbiturates.

MEDICAL CONSIDERATIONS

If you have any of the following medical conditions, make sure your doctor is aware of it.

- Liver disease or alcoholism—tranylcypromine levels may be higher than expected
- Kidney disease—tranylcypromine levels may be higher than expected
- Heart problems—some heart problems can be made worse by tranylcypromine; tranylcypromine should not be taken by someone who has had a recent heart attack
- High blood pressure—blood pressure may be increased
- Urinary retention, prostate enlargement—urination may become more difficult
- Seizure disorder—tranylcypromine can lower seizure threshold
- Diabetes mellitus (sugar diabetes)—blood sugar levels may be affected
- Thyroid disorders—tranylcypromine may cause increase heart rate
- Pheochromocytoma—can lead to high blood pressure

TRAZODONE (TRAZ-oh-doan)

Drug Category: Antidepressant, SSRI (serotonin specific reuptake inhibitor)

Requires prescription

COMMONLY USED BRAND-NAME PRODUCTS

Tablets

Desyrel (and generic) 50mg, 100mg, 150mg, 300mg

GENERAL INFORMATION

Used to treat major depression and the depressed phase of bipolar disorder. Because of its sedative effects, it is often given in low doses to help with insomnia.

BEFORE TAKING THIS MEDICATION

Talk to your doctor about the benefits and risks associated with trazodone. Make sure you understand how to take it safely and effectively. You and your family members should be very familiar with the side effects and signs of having too much in your system. Make sure your doctor has the following information in detail:

- Any allergic or bad reactions you have had to trazodone or any other medication
- All prescription and over-the-counter medicines you are taking
- Your complete medical history
- If you are pregnant, could be pregnant, or are planning a pregnancy in the near future, trazodone should not be taken
- If you are breast feeding, trazodone can pass into breast milk and affect the baby

USUAL ADULT DOSAGE RANGE

Depression: Starting dose 50mg at bedtime. Increased to 75–500mg at bedtime over 2 to 3 weeks.

Insomnia: 50–100mg at bedtime.

Older adults are more susceptible to side effects and will generally require lower dosages.

DIRECTIONS FOR PROPER USE

- *Take exactly as prescribed. Do not take more or less than prescribed.*
- Do not abruptly stop taking trazodone unless instructed to do so by your doctor. Gradually reducing the dose can help prevent mood changes, headache, or diarrhea.
- May be taken with food or meals to lessen stomach upset.
- If you miss a bedtime dose, do not take it the next morning, since it may make you drowsy. Do not double doses.
- It may take several weeks before you feel the full benefits.

PRECAUTIONS

- Trazodone can cause drowsiness and slowed reaction times. Be cautious when driving, operating machinery, or doing jobs requiring alertness.
- Alcohol can cause changes in mood and may interfere with trazodone's effectiveness. Alcohol can cause extreme drowsiness when taken with trazodone. *Alcohol should be avoided while taking trazodone.*
- Trazodone may cause your skin and eyes to be more sensitive to sunlight. Exposure to sunlight may cause a rash, skin discoloration, or sunburn. Limit direct exposure to sunlight, and use sunscreen when in direct sunlight. Avoid tanning booths and beds. Wear UV-blocking sunglasses when outdoors.
- *Antidepressants may increase the risk of suicidal thinking and behavior in adolescents and children. When considering an antidepressant in a child or adolescent, the risk must be balanced with the need. Children and adolescents taking antidepressants should be closely monitored for worsening of symptoms, suicidality, or unusual changes in behavior.*

SIDE EFFECTS

Not all side effects will occur. Many side effects will diminish with time. ***However, some side effects may require attention from your doctor.*** Check with your doctor immediately if you experience any of the following:

- Seizure, prolonged erection of the penis, changes in blood pressure, irregular heart rate, shortness of breath, problems with urination (difficult or painful urination, unable to urinate), confusion, extreme sedation, excitement or mania, increased skin sensitivity to the sunlight, extreme constipation, yellow skin or eyes

Some side effects appear when you first start taking trazodone and go away for most people. If the following side effects continue, contact your doctor.

- Dizziness, blurred vision, dry mouth, mild to moderate constipation, increased appetite, weight gain, breast enlargement (men or women), discharge from the breast, sexual problems, tremor of the hands, persistent sore throat

DRUG INTERACTIONS

Trazodone can adversely interact with the following frequently prescribed medications or foods:

- SSRI antidepressants—can cause high trazodone levels
- MAOI antidepressants—severe reaction causing dangerously high blood pressure, high body temperature, seizures, or death
- Clonidine—if clonidine is being taken for high blood pressure, trazodone may cause clonidine to work less well
- Antipsychotics—may increase certain neurologic side effects
- Drugs used during surgery—can cause increased blood pressure; make sure your doctors are aware of upcoming planned surgeries

- Anticoagulants (blood thinners)—the effect of the anticoagulant can be increased
- HIV protease inhibitors—can cause high trazodone levels
- Some nonsedating antihistamines—cardiac (heart) toxicity
- Drugs that depress certain functions of the nervous system, when combined with trazodone, cause extreme drowsiness and slowed reaction times. Examples of these medicines are antihistamines, narcotics, muscle relaxants, and barbiturates.

MEDICAL CONSIDERATIONS
If you have any of the following medical conditions, make sure your doctor is aware of it.
- Liver disease or alcoholism—trazodone levels may be higher than expected
- Kidney disease—trazodone levels may be higher than expected
- Seizure disorder—trazodone can lower seizure threshold
- Diabetes mellitus (sugar diabetes)—blood sugar levels may be affected

TRIAZOLAM (try-AZ-o-lam)
Drug Category: Insomnia medicine
Requires prescription, controlled substance, moderate potential for abuse

COMMONLY USED BRAND-NAME PRODUCTS
Tablets
Halcion 0.125mg, 0.25mg

GENERAL INFORMATION

Highly effective in treating insomnia. *Even when taken as prescribed, triazolam may cause psychological and/or physical dependence. Not intended for long-term use.*

BEFORE TAKING THIS MEDICATION

Talk to your doctor about the benefits and risks associated with triazolam. Make sure you understand how to take it safely and effectively. You and your family members should be very familiar with the side effects and signs of having too much in your system. Make sure your doctor has the following information in detail:

- Any allergic or bad reactions you have had to triazolam or any other medication
- All prescription and over-the-counter medicines you are taking
- Your complete medical history, including mental health conditions
- If you are pregnant, could be pregnant, or are planning a pregnancy in the near future, triazolam should not be taken
- If you are breast feeding, triazolam can pass into breast milk and affect the baby

DOSAGE

Adults: 0.125–0.25mg at bedtime.

Older adults are more susceptible to side effects and will generally require lower dosages.

Children under 18: Safe use has not been established in this age group.

DIRECTIONS FOR PROPER USE

- *Take exactly as prescribed. Do not take more or less than prescribed. Triazolam levels that are too high can cause serious toxicity.*

- If you take triazolam regularly for an extended period of time, do not stop taking it unless told to do so by your doctor. It may be necessary to gradually reduce the dose before stopping completely.
- If you miss a dose, take it as soon as possible if it is within 1 hour of the scheduled time. However, triazolam should be taken only if you are sure you will get a full night's sleep of at least 7 to 8 hours.

PRECAUTIONS

- Triazolam can cause drowsiness and slowed reaction times. Be cautious when driving, operating machinery, or doing jobs requiring alertness.
- Triazolam may cause a severe allergic reaction and/or severe facial swelling, which can occur as early as the first dose.
- Alcohol can cause extreme drowsiness when taken with triazolam. *Alcohol should be avoided while taking triazolam.*
- Triazolam can cause complex sleep-related behaviors, which may include sleep-driving, making phone calls, and preparing and eating food (while asleep).

SIDE EFFECTS

Not all side effects will occur. Many side effects will diminish with time. *However, some side effects may be warning signs of toxicity and will require attention from your doctor.* Check with your doctor immediately if you experience any of the following:

- Confusion, severe drowsiness, slurred speech, severe weakness, unusual thoughts, shortness of breath, excitement, hyperactivity, memory problems

Some side effects appear when you first start taking triazolam and go away for most people. If the following side effects continue, contact your doctor.

- Dizziness, lightheadedness, daytime drowsiness, blurred vision

DRUG INTERACTIONS

Triazolam can adversely interact with the following frequently prescribed medications or foods:

- Cimetidine (Tagamet)—can cause high triazolam levels
- Disulfiram (Antabuse)—can cause high triazolam levels
- Birth control pills—can cause high triazolam levels
- Levodopa—decreased effectiveness of levodopa
- Macrolide antibiotics (e.g., erythromycin)—can cause high triazolam levels
- Oral antifungal agents—can cause high triazolam levels
- HIV protease inhibitors—can cause high triazolam levels
- Calcium channel blockers—can cause high triazolam levels
- Serotonin-type antidepressants—can cause high triazolam levels
- Digoxin—triazolam can cause high digoxin levels
- Valproic acid—can cause high triazolam levels
- Isoniazid—can cause high triazolam levels
- Beta blockers—can cause high triazolam levels
- Propoxyphene—can cause high triazolam levels
- Carbamazepine—can lower triazolam levels
- Grapefruit juice—can cause high triazolam levels
- Drugs that depress certain functions of the nervous system, when combined with triazolam, cause extreme drowsiness and slowed reaction times. Examples of these medicines are antihistamines, narcotics, muscle relaxants, and barbiturates.

MEDICAL CONSIDERATIONS

If you have any of the following medical conditions, make sure your doctor is aware of it.

- Liver disease or alcoholism—triazolam levels may be higher than expected

- Kidney disease—triazolam levels may be higher than expected
- Drug or alcohol dependence—dependence on triazolam may occur
- Seizure disorder—stopping triazolam abruptly may cause seizures
- Chronic lung disease—triazolam may make breathing more difficult
- Glaucoma—triazolam may worsen your condition
- Sleep apnea—triazolam may worsen your condition

TRIMIPRAMINE (trim-IP-ra-meen)

Drug Category: Antidepressant, tricyclic
Requires prescription

COMMONLY USED BRAND-NAME PRODUCTS

Capsules
Surmontil (and generic) 25mg, 50mg, 100mg

GENERAL INFORMATION

Used to treat major depression and the depressed phase of bipolar disorder.

BEFORE TAKING THIS MEDICATION

Talk to your doctor about the benefits and risks associated with trimipramine. Make sure you understand how to take it safely and effectively. You and your family members should be very familiar with the side effects and signs of having too much in your system. Make sure your doctor has the following information in detail:

- Any allergic or bad reactions you have had to trimipramine or any other medication

- All prescription and over-the-counter medicines you are taking
- Your complete medical history
- If you are pregnant, could be pregnant, or are planning a pregnancy in the near future, trimipramine should not be taken
- If you are breast feeding, trimipramine can pass into breast milk and affect the baby

USUAL ADULT DOSAGE RANGE

The starting dose of trimipramine will be low and will gradually be increased. Sometimes blood levels are tested to ensure that the dose you are taking is in the safe and effective range. Starting dose 25–50mg at bedtime. Increased to 75–300 mg at bedtime over 2 to 3 weeks.

Older adults are more susceptible to side effects and will generally require lower dosages.

DIRECTIONS FOR PROPER USE

- *Take exactly as prescribed. Do not take more or less than prescribed. Accidental or intended overdoses of trimipramine are potentially fatal.*
- Do not abruptly stop taking trimipramine unless instructed to do so by your doctor. Gradually reducing the dose can help prevent mood changes, headache, or diarrhea.
- If you miss a bedtime dose, do not take it the next morning, since it may make you drowsy. Do not double doses.
- It may take several weeks before you feel the full benefits.

PRECAUTIONS

- Trimipramine can cause drowsiness and slowed reaction times. Be cautious when driving, operating machinery, or doing jobs requiring alertness.

- Alcohol can cause changes in mood and may interfere with trimipramine's effectiveness. Alcohol can cause extreme drowsiness when taken with trimipramine. *Alcohol should be avoided while taking trimipramine.*

- Trimipramine may cause your skin and eyes to be more sensitive to sunlight. Exposure to sunlight may cause a rash, skin discoloration, or sunburn. Limit direct exposure to sunlight, and use sunscreen when in direct sunlight. Avoid tanning booths and beds. Wear UV-blocking sunglasses when outdoors.

- When taking trimipramine, stand up slowly after sitting or lying down, since it may cause your blood pressure to drop and cause faintness or dizziness. Stand up slowly from a seated or lying position, especially when you first start taking trimipramine.

- *Antidepressants may increase the risk of suicidal thinking and behavior in adolescents and children. When considering an antidepressant in a child or adolescent, the risk must be balanced with the need. Children and adolescents taking antidepressants should be closely monitored for worsening of symptoms, suicidality, or unusual changes in behavior.*

- Adolescents and children may be more susceptible to heart-related side effects of tricyclic antidepressants. Risk must be balanced with need. Blood levels and heart function should be monitored in children and adolescents taking tricyclic antidepressants.

SIDE EFFECTS

Not all side effects will occur. Many side effects will diminish with time. *However, some side effects may require attention from your doctor.* Check with your doctor immediately if you experience any of the following:

- Seizure, changes in blood pressure, irregular heart rate, shortness of breath, problems with urination (difficult or painful urination, unable to urinate), confusion, extreme sedation, excitement or mania, increased skin sensitivity to the sunlight, extreme constipation, yellow skin or eyes

Some side effects appear when you first start taking trimipramine and go away for most people. If the following side effects continue, contact your doctor.

- Dizziness, blurred vision, dry mouth, mild to moderate constipation, increased appetite, weight gain, breast enlargement (men or women), discharge from the breast, sexual problems, tremor of the hands, persistent sore throat

DRUG INTERACTIONS ·

Trimipramine can adversely interact with the following frequently prescribed medications:

- Cimetidine—can cause high trimipramine levels
- SSRI antidepressants—can cause high trimipramine levels
- MAOI antidepressants—severe reaction causing dangerously high blood pressure, high body temperature, seizures, or death
- Clonidine—if clonidine is being taken for high blood pressure, trimipramine may cause clonidine to work less well
- Antipsychotics—may increase certain neurologic side effects
- Thyroid hormones—increased effects of both, especially excitation and changes in heart rate or rhythm
- Carbamazepine—can lower trimipramine levels
- Bupropion—can increase trimipramine levels

- Anticoagulants (blood thinners)—the effect of the anticoagulant can be increased
- Quinolones—increased risk of heart arrhythmias
- Amphetamines—increased blood pressure, irregular heart rate, or very high fever may result
- Drugs used during surgery—can cause increased blood pressure. Make sure your doctors are aware of upcoming planned surgeries.
- Drugs that depress certain functions of the nervous system, when combined with trimipramine, cause extreme drowsiness and slowed reaction times. Examples of these medicines are antihistamines, narcotics, muscle relaxants, and barbiturates.

MEDICAL CONSIDERATIONS

If you have any of the following medical conditions, make sure your doctor is aware of it.

- Liver disease or alcoholism—trimipramine levels may be higher than expected
- Kidney disease—trimipramine levels may be higher than expected
- Glaucoma—trimipramine can increase pressure inside the eye
- Heart problems—some heart problems can be made worse by trimipramine; trimipramine should not be taken by someone who has had a recent heart attack
- Urinary retention, prostate enlargement—urination may become more difficult
- Seizure disorder—trimipramine can lower seizure threshold
- Diabetes mellitus (sugar diabetes)—blood sugar levels may be affected
- Thyroid disorders—trimipramine may cause increased heart rate

VALPROATE (val-PRO-ate)

Drug Category: Mood stabilizer

Requires prescription

COMMONLY USED BRAND-NAME PRODUCTS

Capsules, as valproic acid
Depakene (also as generic) 250mg
Capsules, sprinkle
Depakote 125mg
Tablets, delayed release, as divalproex sodium
Depakote 125mg, 250mg, 500mg
Liquid, as valproate sodium
Depakene (and generic) 250mg/teaspoon

GENERAL INFORMATION

Used to treat bipolar disorder, especially acute manic and hypomanic phases. Has also been shown to reduce the number and severity of subsequent episodes of both mania and depression. Can be used alone or in combination with other mood stabilizers in severe cases. Also used to treat schizoaffective disorder, usually in combination with other medications called antipsychotics.

BEFORE TAKING THIS MEDICATION

Talk to your doctor about the benefits and risks associated with valproate. Make sure you understand how to take it safely and effectively. You and your family members should be very familiar with the side effects and signs of having too much in your system. Make sure your doctor has the following information in detail:

- Any allergic or bad reactions you have had to valproate or any other medication

- All prescription and over-the-counter medicines you are taking
- Your complete medical history
- If you are pregnant, could be pregnant, or are planning a pregnancy in the near future, valproate should not be taken
- If you are breast feeding, valproate can pass into breast milk and affect the baby

USUAL ADULT DOSAGE RANGE

The starting dose of valproate will be adjusted on the basis of your response and blood levels. You may require more valproate during and immediately following an acute manic episode than when your symptoms have stabilized.

Mania: 500–1500mg per day, divided in two to four doses.

Older adults are more susceptible to side effects and will generally require lower dosages.

DIRECTIONS FOR PROPER USE

- *Take exactly as prescribed. Do not take more or less than prescribed. Valproate levels that are too high can cause serious toxicity.*
- If you take valproate regularly for an extended period of time, do not stop taking it unless told to do so by your doctor. It may be necessary to gradually reduce the dose before stopping completely.
- If you miss a dose, take it as soon as possible. However, if the missed dose is within 6 hours of your next dose, skip the missed dose and resume with your next scheduled dose. Do not double doses.
- It may take several weeks before you feel the full benefits of valproate.
- Laboratory tests are necessary to determine if the amount of valproate in your bloodstream is in the correct range.

- Valproate can cause stomach upset. Taking it with food or meals can lessen this effect. See below for specific directions about the form of valproate you are taking, so you can take certain precautions as necessary.

If you are taking the regular capsule form:

- Swallow the capsule whole. Breaking or chewing the capsule can cause irritation of the mouth and throat.

If you are taking the long-acting tablet form:

- Swallow the tablet whole. Do not crush, split, or chew the tablet.
- Take with food or meals, but do not take the long-acting tablet form with milk. Milk will cause the special coating to dissolve too soon and cause stomach upset.
- Long-acting tablets are not interchangeable with regular capsules or liquid forms.

If you are taking the liquid form:

- The liquid form can be mixed with liquids, except carbonated beverages, or added to food, to improve the taste.

If you are taking the sprinkle capsule form:

- The capsule contains coated particles of the medicine. The contents of the capsule may be sprinkled over about a teaspoonful of semisolid food, such as pudding or applesauce. This mixture should not be chewed. It should not be saved and used at a later time. The sprinkle capsule may also be swallowed whole.

PRECAUTIONS

- Valproate can cause drowsiness and slowed reaction times. Be cautious when driving, operating machinery, or doing jobs requiring alertness.
- Alcohol can cause changes in mood and may interfere with valproate's effectiveness. Alcohol can cause extreme drows-

iness when taken with valproate. *Alcohol should be avoided while taking valproate.*

- **Valproate may cause suicidal thoughts. Notify your doctor immediately if you notice changes in mood, behavior, or actions or have thoughts of harming yourself.**

SIDE EFFECTS

Not all side effects will occur. Many side effects will diminish with time. *However, some side effects may be warning signs of toxicity and will require attention from your doctor.* Check with your doctor immediately if you experience any of the following:

- Unusual bleeding or bruising, confusion, significant drowsiness, yellow eyes or skin, severe abdominal pain

Some side effects appear when you first start taking valproate and go away for most people. If the following side effects continue, contact your doctor.

- Mild hand tremor, mild nausea, mild dizziness, diarrhea or constipation, unusual weight gain or loss, hair loss

DRUG INTERACTIONS

Valproate can adversely interact with the following frequently prescribed medications or foods:

- Anticoagulants (blood thinners)—the effect of the anticoagulant can be increased
- Aspirin or nonsteriodal anti-inflammatory drugs—when taken in moderate to high doses on a regular basis, can cause increased valproate levels. There is also the possibility of increased bleeding with this combination.
- Anticonvulsants—dosage adjustments may be necessary of valproate and/or other anticonvulsants
- Drugs that depress certain functions of the nervous system,

when combined with valproate, cause extreme drowsiness and slowed reaction times. Examples of these medicines are antihistamines, narcotics, muscle relaxants, and barbiturates.

MEDICAL CONSIDERATIONS

If you have any of the following medical conditions, make sure your doctor is aware of it.

- Liver disease or alcoholism—valproate levels may be higher than expected
- Kidney disease—valproate levels may be higher than expected
- Anemia or other blood problems—these conditions can be made worse by valproate
- Pancreatitis—this condition may be worsened by valproate

VENLAFAXINE (ven-la-FAX-een)

Drug Category: Antidepressant, SNRI (serotonin, norepinephrine reuptake inhibitor)

Requires prescription

COMMONLY USED BRAND-NAME PRODUCTS

Tablets

Effexor (and generic) 25mg, 37.5mg, 50mg, 75mg, 100mg

Capsules, extended release

Effexor 37.5mg, 75mg, 150mg

GENERAL INFORMATION

Used to treat major depression and the depressed phase of bipolar disorder. Also used to treat generalized anxiety disorder and social anxiety disorder.

BEFORE TAKING THIS MEDICATION

Talk to your doctor about the benefits and risks associated with venlafaxine. Make sure you understand how to take it safely and effectively. You and your family members should be very familiar with the side effects and signs of having too much in your system. Make sure your doctor has the following information in detail:

- Any allergic or bad reactions you have had to venlafaxine or any other medication
- All prescription and over-the-counter medicines you are taking
- Your complete medical history
- If you are pregnant, could be pregnant, or are planning a pregnancy in the near future, venlafaxine should not be taken
- If you are breast feeding, venlafaxine can pass into breast milk and affect the baby

DOSAGE

Adults: 75–350mg daily. When you first start taking venlafaxine, your initial dose will be lower, and it will be gradually increased depending on how you are doing and the side effects you might be experiencing.

Older adults are more susceptible to side effects and will generally require lower dosages.

DIRECTIONS FOR PROPER USE

- *Take exactly as prescribed. Do not take more or less than prescribed.*
- Do not abruptly stop taking venlafaxine unless instructed to do so by your doctor.
- If you miss a dose, take it as soon as possible unless it is within 6 hours of your next scheduled dose, then skip the

missed dose and resume with your next scheduled dose. Do not double doses.

- If you are taking the long-acting capsule form and you miss a dose, take it as soon as possible within 1 to 2 hours of the missed dose. However, if it is more than 2 hours after the missed dose, skip the missed dose and resume with your next scheduled dose. Swallow capsules whole; do not crush, chew, or break.
- It may take several weeks before you feel the full benefits of venlafaxine.

PRECAUTIONS

- Venlafaxine can cause drowsiness and slowed reaction times. Be cautious when driving, operating machinery, or doing jobs requiring alertness.
- Alcohol can cause changes in mood and may interfere with venlafaxine's effectiveness. Alcohol can cause extreme drowsiness when taken with venlafaxine. *Alcohol should be avoided while taking venlafaxine.*
- *Antidepressants may increase the risk of suicidal thinking and behavior in adolescents and children. When considering an antidepressant in a child or adolescent, the risk must be balanced with the need. Children and adolescents taking antidepressants should be closely monitored for worsening of symptoms, suicidality, or unusual changes in behavior.*

SIDE EFFECTS

Not all side effects will occur. Many side effects will diminish with time. *However, some side effects may require attention from your doctor.* Check with your doctor immediately if you experience any of the following:

- Increased blood pressure, increased heart rate, skin rash or hives, shortness of breath, chills or fever, swelling of the hands or feet, seizures

Some side effects appear when you first start taking venlafaxine and go away for most people. If the following side effects continue, contact your doctor.

- Agitation, anxiety, insomnia, dizziness, sexual problems, sweating, blurred vision, dry mouth, mild to moderate constipation, change in appetite, change in appetite, change in weight, tremor of the hands

DRUG INTERACTIONS

Venlafaxine can adversely interact with the following frequently prescribed medications or foods:

- Anticoagulants (blood thinners)—the effect of the anticoagulant can be increased
- Some nonsedating antihistamines—cardiac (heart) toxicity
- Diet pills—severe reaction causing dangerously high blood pressure, high body temperature, seizures, or death
- Products containing L-tryptophan or with serotonin activity—severe reaction causing dangerously high blood pressure, high body temperature, seizures, or death
- Cimetidine—can cause high venlafaxine levels
- TCA antidepressants—can cause high TCA levels
- MAOI antidepressants—severe reaction causing dangerously high blood pressure, high body temperature, seizures, or death
- Antipsychotics—may increase certain neurologic side effects
- Lithium—increased lithium levels causing possible confusion, dizziness, tremor
- Anticonvulsants—increased anticonvulsant levels or decreased venlafaxine levels
- Drugs that depress certain functions of the nervous system, when combined with venlafaxine, cause extreme drowsiness and slowed reaction times. Examples of these medi-

cines are antihistamines, narcotics, muscle relaxants, and barbiturates.

MEDICAL CONSIDERATIONS

If you have any of the following medical conditions, make sure your doctor is aware of it.

- Liver disease or alcoholism—venlafaxine levels may be higher than expected
- Kidney disease—venlafaxine levels may be higher than expected
- Seizure disorder—venlafaxine can lower seizure threshold
- Diabetes mellitus (sugar diabetes)—blood sugar levels may be affected

ZALEPLON (ZAL-e-plon)

Drug Category: Insomnia medicine
Requires prescription, controlled substance, moderate potential for abuse

COMMONLY USED BRAND-NAME PRODUCTS

Capsules
Sonata 5mg, 10mg

GENERAL INFORMATION

Used to treat insomnia. *Even when taken as prescribed, zaleplon may cause psychological and/or physical dependence. Not intended for long-term use.*

BEFORE TAKING THIS MEDICATION

Talk to your doctor about the benefits and risks associated with zaleplon. Make sure you understand how to take it safely and effectively. You and your family members should be very familiar with the side effects and signs of having too much in your system. Make sure your doctor has the following information in detail:

- Any allergic or bad reactions you have had to zaleplon or any other medication
- All prescription and over-the-counter medicines you are taking
- Your complete medical history, including mental health conditions
- If you are pregnant, could be pregnant, or are planning a pregnancy in the near future, zaleplon should not be taken
- If you are breast feeding, zaleplon can pass into breast milk and affect the baby

USUAL ADULT DOSAGE RANGE

5–10mg at bedtime.

Older adults are more susceptible to side effects and will generally require lower dosages.

DIRECTIONS FOR PROPER USE

- ***Take exactly as prescribed. Do not take more or less than prescribed. Zaleplon levels that are too high can cause serious toxicity.***
- If you take zaleplon regularly for an extended period of time, do not stop taking it unless told to do so by your doctor. It may be necessary to gradually reduce the dose before stopping completely.
- Do not take with or immediately after a high-fat meal.
- Take immediately before bedtime and only if you are sure you will get a full night's sleep of at least 8 hours.

PRECAUTIONS

- Zaleplon can cause drowsiness and slowed reaction times. Be cautious when driving, operating machinery, or doing jobs requiring alertness.
- Alcohol can cause extreme drowsiness when taken with zaleplon. *Alcohol should be avoided while taking zaleplon.*
- Zaleplon may cause a severe allergic reaction and/or severe facial swelling, which can occur as early as the first dose.
- Zaleplon can cause complex sleep-related behaviors which may include sleep-driving, making phone calls, and preparing and eating food (while asleep).

SIDE EFFECTS

Not all side effects will occur. Many side effects will diminish with time. *However, some side effects may be warning signs of toxicity and will require attention from your doctor.* Check with your doctor immediately if you experience any of the following:

- Confusion, severe drowsiness, slurred speech, severe weakness, unusual thoughts, shortness of breath, excitement, hyperactivity, memory problems, abnormal addictive behaviors

Some side effects appear when you first start taking zaleplon and go away for most people. If the following side effects continue, contact your doctor.

- Dizziness, lightheadedness, daytime drowsiness, blurred vision

DRUG INTERACTIONS

Zaleplon can adversely interact with the following frequently prescribed medications:

- Cimetidine—can cause high zaleplon levels
- Macrolide antibiotics (e.g., erythromycin)—can cause high zaleplon levels

- Oral antifungal agents—can cause high zaleplon levels
- HIV protease inhibitors—can cause high zaleplon levels
- Anticonvulsants—can cause lower zaleplon levels
- Drugs that depress certain functions of the nervous system, when combined with zaleplon, cause extreme drowsiness and slowed reaction times. Examples of these medicines are antihistamines, narcotics, muscle relaxants, and barbiturates.

MEDICAL CONSIDERATIONS

If you have any of the following medical conditions, make sure your doctor is aware of it.

- Liver disease or alcoholism—zaleplon levels may be higher than expected
- Kidney disease—zaleplon levels may be higher than expected
- Drug or alcohol dependence—dependence on zaleplon may occur
- Chronic lung disease—zaleplon may make breathing more difficult

ZIPRASIDONE (zi-PRAZ-ih-doan)

Drug Category: Neuroleptic; Antipsychotic
Requires prescription

COMMONLY USED BRAND-NAME PRODUCTS

Capsules

Geodon 20mg, 40mg, 60mg, 80mg

Used to treat psychotic symptoms such as hallucinations and delusions. These symptoms occur in schizophrenia, schizoaffective disorder, bipolar disorder, or major depression with psychotic features. Ziprasidone can be used for short-term management of aggressive, out-of-control behaviors or feelings of anger and rage. Because of its mood stabilizing properties, may be used in the treatment of bipolar disorder, especially manic episodes. For difficult-to-treat depression, may be used in combination with an antidepressant.

BEFORE TAKING THIS MEDICATION

Talk to your doctor about the benefits and risks associated with ziprasidone. Make sure you understand how to take it safely and effectively. You and your family members should be very familiar with its side effects. *Your doctor may periodically monitor your weight, blood pressure, blood sugar, and blood lipid levels while you are taking ziprasidone.* Make sure your doctor has the following information in detail:

- Any allergic or bad reactions you have had to ziprasidone or any other medication
- All prescription and over-the-counter medicines you are taking
- Your complete medical history
- If you are pregnant, could be pregnant, or are planning a pregnancy in the near future, ziprasidone has not been shown to be absolutely safe
- If you are breast feeding, ziprasidone can pass into breast milk and affect the baby

USUAL ADULT DOSAGE RANGE

60–160mg daily.

Older adults are *extremely* susceptible to side effects and will generally require lower dosages. *Should not be used in elderly patients to treat dementia-related psychosis or behavioral disturbances.*

DIRECTIONS FOR PROPER USE

- *Take exactly as prescribed. Do not take more or less than prescribed. Ziprasidone levels that are too high can cause serious toxicity.*
- If you miss a dose, take it as soon as possible. However, if the missed dose is within 4 hours of your next dose, skip the missed dose and resume with your next scheduled dose. Do not double the dose.
- Take with food.
- It may be several weeks before you feel the full benefits.

PRECAUTIONS

- Ziprasidone can cause drowsiness and slowed reaction times. Be cautious when driving, operating machinery, or doing jobs requiring alertness.
- Alcohol can cause extreme drowsiness when taken with ziprasidone. *Alcohol should be avoided while taking ziprasidone.*
- Ziprasidone may cause your body temperature to increase and could result in heat stroke. Be extra careful in hot weather, when exercising, or when taking hot baths or saunas not to become overheated.
- When taking ziprasidone, stand up slowly after sitting or lying down, since it may cause your blood pressure to drop and cause faintness or dizziness. Stand up slowly from a seated or lying position, especially when you first start taking ziprasidone.
- **Ziprasidone may cause potentially life-threatening heart arrhythmias. Careful consideration should be given to this risk before starting ziprasidone.**

SIDE EFFECTS

Not all side effects will occur. Many side effects will diminish with time. *However, some side effects may be warning signs of*

toxicity and will require attention from your doctor. Check with your doctor immediately if you experience any of the following:

- Seizure; high fever; fast or irregular heartbeat; very low blood pressure; faintness; any abnormal movements of the mouth, tongue, neck, arms, or legs; difficulty speaking or swallowing; imbalance or difficulty walking normally; severe muscle stiffness; discoloration or the skin or eyes; confusion; significant drowsiness; restlessness; difficulty urinating; sexual problems; vomiting; diarrhea; unusual bruising or bleeding; serious skin reaction to sunlight (burning or blistering); severe constipation; breast pain or enlargement

Some side effects appear when you first start taking ziprasidone and go away for most people. If the following side effects continue, contact your doctor.

- Dry mouth, mild to moderate constipation, dizziness, hand tremor, stuffy nose, weight gain

DRUG INTERACTIONS

Ziprasidone can adversely interact with the following frequently prescribed medications or foods:

- Lithium—increased neurologic side effects
- Levodopa—decreased effectiveness of levodopa
- Amphetamines—increased psychotic symptoms are possible
- Anticonvulsants—decreased ziprasidone levels
- Tricyclic antidepressants—increased TCA levels
- Macrolide antibiotics (e.g., erythromycin)—can cause high ziprasidone levels
- Oral antifungal agents—can cause high ziprasidone levels
- HIV protease inhibitors—can cause high ziprasidone levels
- Cimetidine—can cause high ziprasidone levels

- Serotonin-type antidepressants—can cause high ziprasidone levels
- Antiarrhythmics or other drugs that can affect the heartbeat—when taken with ziprasidone can cause serious disturbances of heart rhythm
- Caffeine—can cause high ziprasidone levels
- Drugs that depress certain functions of the nervous system, when combined with ziprasidone, cause extreme drowsiness and slowed reaction times. Examples of these medicines are antihistamines, narcotics, muscle relaxants, and barbiturates.

MEDICAL CONSIDERATIONS

If you have any of the following medical conditions, make sure your doctor is aware of it.

- Kidney disease—ziprasidone levels may be higher than expected
- Liver disease—ziprasidone levels may be higher than expected
- Heart problems—some heart problems can be made worse by ziprasidone
- Seizure disorder—ziprasidone can lower seizure threshold
- Urinary retention, prostate enlargement—urination may be more difficult
- Glaucoma—ziprasidone can increase pressure inside the eye
- Parkinson's disease—Some Parkinson's symptoms may be worsened
- Breast cancer—may increase risk of cancer progression
- Overweight/obesity—ziprasidone can cause weight gain
- Diabetes—ziprasidone can make this condition worse
- Elevated lipid (cholesterol and triglycerides) levels—ziprasidone can make this condition worse

- High blood pressure—ziprasidone can make this condition worse

ZOLPIDEM (ZOLE-pi-dem)

Drug Category: Insomnia medicine
Requires prescription, controlled substance, moderate potential for abuse

COMMONLY USED BRAND-NAME PRODUCTS

Tablets
Ambien 5mg, 10mg
Tablets, extended release
Ambien CR 6.25mg, 12.5mg

GENERAL INFORMATION

Used to treat insomnia. *Even when taken as prescribed, zolpidem may cause psychological and/or physical dependence. Not intended for long-term use.*

BEFORE TAKING THIS MEDICATION

Talk to your doctor about the benefits and risks associated with zolpidem. Make sure you understand how to take it safely and effectively. You and your family members should be very familiar with the side effects and signs of having too much in your system. Make sure your doctor has the following information in detail:

- Any allergic or bad reactions you have had to zolpidem or any other medication
- All prescription and over-the-counter medicines you are taking
- Your complete medical history, including mental health conditions

- If you are pregnant, could be pregnant, or are planning a pregnancy in the near future, zolpidem should not be taken
- If you are breast feeding, zolpidem can pass into breast milk and affect the baby

USUAL ADULT DOSAGE RANGE

5–10 mg at bedtime (regular tablets) or 6.25–12.5mg at bedtime (extended release tablets).

Older adults are more susceptible to side effects and will generally require lower dosages.

DIRECTIONS FOR PROPER USE

- *Take exactly as prescribed. Do not take more or less than prescribed. Zolpidem levels that are too high can cause serious toxicity.*
- If you take zolpidem regularly for an extended period of time, do not stop taking it unless told to do so by your doctor. It may be necessary to gradually reduce the dose before stopping completely.
- Take on an empty stomach.
- Take immediately before bedtime and only if you are sure you will get a full night's sleep of at least 7 to 8 hours.
- If you are taking the extended release form, swallow the tablet whole; do not crush, break, or chew.

PRECAUTIONS

- Zolpidem can cause drowsiness and slowed reaction times. Be cautious when driving, operating machinery, or doing jobs requiring alertness.
- Alcohol can cause extreme drowsiness when taken with zolpidem. *Alcohol should be avoided while taking zolpidem.*
- Zolpidem may cause a severe allergic reaction and/or

severe facial swelling, which can occur as early as the first dose.

- Zolpidem can cause complex sleep-related behaviors, which may include sleep-driving, making phone calls, and preparing and eating food (while asleep).

SIDE EFFECTS

Not all side effects will occur. Many side effects will diminish with time. *However, some side effects may be warning signs of toxicity and will require attention from your doctor.* Check with your doctor immediately if you experience any of the following:

- Confusion, severe drowsiness, slurred speech, severe weakness, unusual thoughts, shortness of breath, excitement, hyperactivity, memory problems

Some side effects appear when you first start taking zolpidem and go away for most people. If the following side effects continue, contact your doctor.

- Dizziness, lightheadedness, daytime drowsiness, blurred vision

DRUG INTERACTIONS

Zolpidem can adversely interact with the following frequently prescribed medications:

- Oral antifungal agents—can cause high zolpidem levels
- HIV protease inhibitors—can cause high zolpidem levels
- Serotonin-type antidepressants—can increase effects of zolzpidem
- Drugs that depress certain functions of the nervous system, when combined with zolpidem, cause extreme drowsiness and slowed reaction times. Examples of these medicines are antihistamines, narcotics, muscle relaxants, and barbiturates.

MEDICAL CONSIDERATIONS

If you have any of the following medical conditions, make sure your doctor is aware of it.

- Liver disease or alcoholism—zolpidem levels may be higher than expected
- Kidney disease—zolpidem levels may be higher than expected
- Drug or alcohol dependence—dependence on zolpidem may occur
- Chronic lung disease—zolpidem may make breathing more difficult

APPENDIX 1
Directory of Brand Names

If you want information about a particular medication and you have only the brand name, look at the directory below. Brand names are all listed in the left-hand column. To the right of the brand name, you will see the generic name or a general drug category. First, find the generic name under which the drug will be found. Then, turn to the alphabetized entry.

BRAND	GENERIC
Abilify	aripiprazole
Adapin	doxepin
Adderall	amphetamine
Ambien	zolpidem
Anafranil	clomipramine
Artane	trihexyphenidyl
Asendin	amoxapine
Atarax	hydroxyzine
Ativan	lorazepam
Aventyl	nortriptyline
Benadryl	diphenhydramine
BuSpar	buspirone
Catapres	clonidine
Celexa	citalopram
Clozaril	clozapine

BRAND	GENERIC
Cogentin	benztropine
Corgard	nadolol
Concerta	methylphenidate
Cymbalta	duloxetine
Dalmane	flurazepam
Daytrana	methylphenidate
Depakene	valproate
Depakote	valproate
Desoxyn	methamphetamine
Desyrel	trazodone
Dexedrine	dextroamphetamine
Doral	quazepam
Effexor	venlafaxine
Elavil	amitriptyline
Equetro	carbamazepine
Eskalith	lithium
Focalin	dexmethylphenidate
Geodon	ziprasidone
Halcion	triazolam
Haldol	haloperidol
Inderal	propranolol
Invega	paliperidone
Klonopin	clonazepam
Lamictal	lamotrigine
Lexapro	escitalopram
Librium	chlordiazepoxide
Lithobid	lithium
Lopressor	metoprolol
Loxitane	loxapine
Ludiomil	maprotiline
Lunesta	eszopiclone
Luvox	fluvoxamine

BRAND	GENERIC
Mellaril	thioridazine
Metadate	methylphenidate
Methylin	methylphenidate
Moban	molindone
Nardil	phenelzine
Navane	thiothixene
Norpramin	desipramine
Orap	pimozide
Pamelor	nortriptyline
Parnate	tranylcypromine
Paxil	paroxetine
Pristiq	desvenlafaxine
Prolixin	fluphenazine
ProSom	estazolam
Prozac	fluoxetine
Remeron	mirtazapine
Restoril	temazepam
Risperdal	risperidone
Ritalin	methylphenidate
Rozerem	ramelteon
Serax	oxazepam
Seroquel	quetiapine
Serzone	nefazodone
Sinequan	doxepin
Sonata	zaleplon
Stelazine	trifluoperazine
Strattera	atomoxetine
Surmontil	trimipramine
Symbyax	olanzapine/fluoxetine
Symmetrel	amantadine
Tegretol	carbamazepine
Tenormin	atenolol

BRAND	GENERIC
Thorazine	chlorpromazine
Tofranil	imipramine
Topamax	topiramate
Tranxene	clorazepate
Trilafon	perphenazine
Trileptal	oxcarbazepine
Valium	diazepam
Valrelease	diazepam
Visken	pindolol
Vistaril	hydroxyzine
Vivactil	protriptyline
Vyvanse	lisdexamfetamine
Wellbutrin	bupropion
Xanax	alprazolam
Zoloft	sertraline
Zyprexa	olanzapine

APPENDIX 2
Caffeine Consumption Questionnaire

CAFFEINE CONSUMPTION QUESTIONNAIRE			
		AVERAGE NUMBER OF OUNCES/ DOSES/ TABLETS PER DAY	AVERAGE TOTAL PER DAY
Beverages/snacks			
Coffee (6 oz.)	125 mg	x _____	_____
Decaf Coffee (6 oz.)	5 mg	x _____	_____
Espresso (1 oz.)	50 mg	x _____	_____
Tea (6 oz.)	50 mg	x _____	_____
Green tea (6 oz)	20 mg	x _____	_____
Hot cocoa (6 oz.)	15 mg	x _____	_____
Energy drinks (12 oz.) equivalent	200 mg +	x _____	_____
Caffeinated soft drinks (12 oz.)	40–60 mg	x _____	_____
Chocolate candy bar (2 oz.)	20 mg	x _____	_____

(continued)

CAFFEINE CONSUMPTION QUESTIONNAIRE (continued)

			AVERAGE NUMBER OF OUNCES/ DOSES/ TABLETS PER DAY	AVERAGE TOTAL PER DAY
Over-the-counter medications				
Anacin	32 mg	x	_____	_____
Appetite control pills	100–200 mg	x	_____	_____
Dristan	16 mg	x	_____	_____
Excedrine	65 mg	x	_____	_____
Extra-strength Excedrine	100 mg	x	_____	_____
Midol	132mg	x	_____	_____
NoDoz	100mg	x	_____	_____
Triaminicin	30 mg	x	_____	_____
Vanquish	33 mg	x	_____	_____
Vivarin	200 mg	x	_____	_____
Prescription medications				
Cafergot	100 mg	x	_____	_____
Fiorinal	40 mg	x	_____	_____
Darvon compound	32 mg	x	_____	_____
Total milligrams of caffeine per day			_____	_____

More than 250 mg per day may interfere with deep sleep.

APPENDIX 3
General References

Akiskal, H. S. et al. "Re-evaluating the prevalence of and diagnostic composition within the broad clinical spectrum of bipolar disorders." *J. Affective Disorders, 59* (2000), Suppl: 55–530.

American Psychiatric Association. *Diagnostic and Statistical Manual of Mental Disorders: Fourth Edition: Text Revision.* Washington, D.C.: American Psychiatric Association, 2000.

American Society of Health-System Pharmacists. *American Hospital Formulary Service Drug Information.* Bethesda, Md.: American Society of Health-System Pharmacists, 2004.

Baxter, L. R. "PET studies of cerebral function in major depression and obsessive-compulsive disorder: The emerging profrontal cortex consensus." *Annals of Clinical Psychiatry* 3 (1991): 103–109.

Benet, L. Z. et al. "General principles." In *Goodman & Gilman's: The Pharmacological Basis of Therapeutics.* A. G. Gilman, T. W. Rail, A. S. Nies, and P. Taylor, eds. New York: Pergamon Press, 2007.

Bloomfield, H. et al. *Hypericum and Depression.* Los Angeles: Prelude Press, 1996.

Brotman, A. *Practical reviews in psychiatry* (audiotape). Birmingham, Ala.: Educational Reviews, 1992.

Burton, T. M. "Anti-depression drug of Eli Lilly loses sales after attack by sect." *Wall Street Journal* (April 19, 1991), A1–A2.

Castellanos, F. X. et al. "Quantitative morphology of the caudate nucleus in Attention Deficit Hyperactivity Disorder." *American Journal of Psychiatry* 151 (1994): 1791–1796.

Facts and Comparisons. St. Louis, Mo.: Wolters Kluwer Health, 2008.

Goodwin, F. K., and K. R. Jamison, *Manic Depressive Illness: Bipolar Disorders and Recurrent Depression.* Oxford University Press: New York, 2007.

Gordon, B. *I'm Dancing as Fast as I Can.* New York: Bantam, 1990.

Journal of Clinical Psychiatry. "Consensus development conference on antipsychotic drugs and obesity and diabetes." *Journal of Clinical Psychiatry* 65 (2004): 267–272.

Katzung, B. G. "Basic Principles." In *Basic and Clinical Pharmacology.* B. G. Katzung, ed. New York: McGraw-Hill, 2006.

Kessler, R. C. et al. "Lifetime and 12-month prevalence of DSM-III-R psychiatric disorders in the United States." *Archives of General Psychiatry* 51 (1994): 8–19.

Ketter, T. A. *Advances in the Treatment of Bipolar Disorder.* Washington, D.C.: American Psychiatric Publishing, Inc., 2005.

Kramer, P. D. *Listening to Prozac.* New York: Viking, 1993.

Kreisinan, J. J., and H. Strauss. *I Hate You, Don't Leave Me: Understanding the Borderline Personality.* New York Avon Books, 1989.

Lieberman J. A. et al. "Effectiveness of antipsychotic drugs in patients with chronic schizophrenia." *New England Journal of Medicine* 353 (2005): 1209–1223.

Norden, M. J. *Beyond Prozac*. New York HarperCollins, 1995.

———. "Fluoxetine in borderline personality disorder." *Progress in Neuropsychopharmacological Biological Psychiatry*, 13 (1989): 885–893.

Preston, J. D. et al. *Handbook of Clinical Psychopharmacology for Therapists*. Fifth Edition. Oakland, Calif.: New Harbinger Publications, 2008.

Rosenthal, N. E. *Winter Blues*. Guilford Press: New York, 2006.

Safer, D. J., and J. M. Krager. "Effect of a media blitz and a threatened lawsuit on stimulant treatment." *JAMA* 268 (1992): 1004–1007.

Schwartz, J. M. *Brainlock*. New York: Reganbooks, 1997.

Susann, J. *Once Is Not Enough*. New York: Grove Atlantic, 1997.

Zisook, S. "Bereavement: grief, depression, anxiety." *Audio Digest Psychiatry* (audiotape). Glendale, CA: Audio Digest Foundation, 1996.

PRACTICE GUIDELINES AND MAJOR RESEARCH STUDIES

American Psychiatric Association: 2008.
PTSD, Bipolar Disorder, OCD, Alzheimers disease,
Eating disorders, Major Depression, Panic Disorder,
Schizophrenia.
http://www.psychiatryonline.com/pracGuide/pracGuide
Home.aspx

National Institute of Mental Health, 2008.
Sequenced Treatment Alternatives to Relieve Depression:
STAR-D.
www.nimh.nih.gov/health/trials/practical/stard/index
.shtml

National Institute of Mental Health, 2008.
Systematic Treatment Enhancement Program for Bipolar Disorder.
www.nimh.nih.gov/health/trials/practical/step-bd/index.shtml

Texas Department of Mental Health: Texas Medication Algorithm Projects, 2008.
Bipolar Disorder, Schizophrenia, Major Depression.
www.dshs.state.tx.us/mhprograms/TMAPover.shtm

APPENDIX 4
Resources

Alzheimer's Disease and Related Disorders Association
(This is a national organization for caregivers.)
919 North Michigan Avenue
Suite 1000
Chicago, IL 60611
312-335-8700

CHADD: Children and Adults with Attention Deficit/
Hyperactivity Disorder
www.chadd.org

National Alliance for the Mentally Ill (NAMI)
200 N. Glebe Rd., Suite 1015
Arlington, VA 22203-3754
703-524-7600, Fax 703-524-9094
Help Line 1-800-950-6264
www.nami.org

The National Depressive and Manic-Depressive Association
1-800-826-3632

National Mental Health Association, Campaign on Clinical
Depression
1-800-969-NMHA

Obsessive-Compulsive Foundation
P.O. Box 70
Milford, CT 06460-0070
203-878-5669

APPENDIX 5
Recommended Reading

ADHD

Barkley, Russell. *Taking Charge of ADHD;* Revised Edition. New York: Guilford Press, 2000.

AGGRESSION

McKay, Matthew. *The Anger Control Workbook.* Oakland, Calif.: New Harbinger, 2000.

ANXIETY

Greist, J. H., and J. Jefferson, *Panic Disorder and Agoraphobia: A Guide.* Madison, Wis.: Madison Institute of Medicine, 2001.

BIPOLAR DISORDER

Jamison K. R. *Unquiet Mind.* New York: Random House, 1997.

Miklowitz. D. *The Bipolar Disorder Survival Guide.* New York: Guilford Press, 2002.

Fast, J., and J. Preston, *Taking Charge of Bipolar Disorder.* New York: Warner Wellness Books, 2006.

BORDERLINE PERSONALITY DISORDER

Mason, P., and R. Kreger, *Stop Walking On Eggshells*. Oakland, Calif.: New Harbinger, 1998.

DEPRESSION

Preston, J. *You Can Beat Depression*. Atascadero, Calif.: Impact Publishers, 2004.

EATING DISORDERS

Sandbek, T. *The Deadly Diet: Recovering from Anorexia and Bulimia,* Second Edition. Oakland, Calif.: New Harbinger, 1993.

OBSESSIVE-COMPULSIVE

Steketee, Gail et al. *Obsessive Compulsive Disorder: The Latest Assessment and Treatment Strategies.* Kansas City, Mo.: Compact Clinicals, 2002.

PANIC DISORDER

Beckijeld, D. *Master Your Panic,* Third Edition. San Luis Obispo, Calif.: Impact Publishers, 2004.

POST-TRAUMATIC STRESS DISORDER

Greist, J. H. et al. *Post-Traumatic Stress Disorder: A Guide.* Madison, Wis.: Madison Institute of Medicine, 2000.

Schiraldi, Glenn. *Post Traumatic Stress Disorder Source Book.* New York: McGraw Hill, 2000.

SCHIZOPHRENIA

Torrey, E.F. *Surviving Schizophrenia: A Family Manual.* New York: Harper and Row Publishers, 2001.

Index

Page numbers in **boldface** refer to information in the Guide to Psychiatric Drugs

Abilify, 61, **258–62**
Adapin, 58, **329–34**
Adderall, 64, 99, 199, 217, **250–55**
addiction to drugs, potential for, *see* drug addiction, potential for
adolescents, *see* teenagers
aggression, 208–10, 228
  medications for, 209–10
  primary disorders associated with, 209
agranulocytosis, 177–78
akathisia, 176
alcohol, 18, 81, 151
  antidepressants and, 95
  bipolar medications and, 136
  depression and, 76, 77
  insomnia and, 182, 183, 184–85
  social anxiety and, 156
alcoholic dementia, 210
allergic reaction to drugs, 226
alpha-2 adrenergic agonists, 193, 195–96
  chart of, 197, 200

alprazolam, 62, **237–41**
Alzheimer's disease and dementia, 210–11
amantadine, **255–56**
Ambien, 63, 188, **514–17**
American Psychiatric Association, 112, 117, 119
amitriptyline, 58, **241–46**
amnesia, 188
amoxapine, 58, **246–50**
amphetamines, 18, 194, 199, **250–55**
amygdala, 34
Anafranil, 58, 63, 217, **293–98**
anger, 34, 35–36
anhedonia, 41–42, 69, 71
anorexia, 200–03
antianxiety drugs
  addiction potential, 136, 151–52, 153, 154, 158
  caution about abruptly stopping, 150
  chart of, 62
  children and teenagers and, 217
  for daytime versus nighttime anxiety, 149

antianxiety drugs (*cont.*)
dependence on, potential for, 18, 99–100, 150, 153, 161
depression treated with, 102–03
dosages, 150, 151
efficacy of, 150
frequency of use, 150
for generalized anxiety disorder, 161–62
listing of, 149
for obsessive-compulsive disorder, 163
for panic disorder, 158, 159
for phobias, 154–55
pregnant and breast-feeding women, 221
for PTSD, 207
side effects of, 151
for situational anxiety, 148–52
for social anxiety, 156
see also individual drugs
anticholinergics, **255–56**
anticholinergic side effects of psychotic medications, 177
anticonvulsants, 205, 209, 210
for bipolar disorders, 120, 133–34
pregnant and breast-feeding women, 221
antidepressants
addiction potential, 99–100, 154
for ADHD, 193, 196, 197, 198, 200
adjustments to initial prescription, 101–02
augmentation approach, 101–02
bipolar disorders and, 117, 124–25, 135, 137
for borderline personality disorder, 205
chart of, 58, 197
children and teenagers and, 20, 95–98, 216–17
choosing, 88–90
doses, 90, 101
dual-action, 87
effectiveness of, 82–83
first prescribed, failure of, 101–02
for generalized anxiety disorder, 161, 162
generic and trade names of, 86–87
long-term safety of, 100–01
MAO inhibitors, *see* MAO inhibitors
nerve cell response to, 80–81, 87–88
for obsessive-compulsive disorder, 163, 164
for panic disorder, 158–59
phases of treatment, 91–93
precautions and contraindications, 94–95
pregnant and breast-feeding women, 220
side effects of, 82–83, 87, 89, 94
for social anxiety, 156
SSRIs, *see* SSRIs (Selective Serotonin Reuptake Inhibitors)
standard, 85–88
suicidality and, 20, 198
time needed to work, 81
tricyclic, 19, 83, 85
see also individual drugs
antidyskinetics, **255–56**
antihistamines, 152, **257–58**

antihypertensives, 76, 208
antimanic medications, 124–38
  addiction potential, 136
  augmentation approach,
    125–26, 133, 134, 137
  children and teenagers, 217
  first prescribed, failure of,
    137
  listing of, 57, 124, 125
  research on effectiveness of,
    126–27
  side effects of, 128–30, 131,
    132–33, 134
  time needed to work, 125,
    137
  see also individual drugs
anti-obsessional drugs, chart
    of, 63
anti-Parkinsonian drugs, 174,
    176
  depression and, 76
antipsychotics, 29–30, 171–79,
    209, 210
  addiction potential, 154
  atypical, 171, 173–74, 205,
    210, 211
  for bipolar disorders, 124,
    125
  chart of, 60–61, 172
  children and teenagers and,
    217
  choice of medication,
    173–74
  for dementia, 211
  drug addiction, potential for,
    179
  high-potency, typical, 171,
    174
  increasing dosages of, 174
  overview, 170–71
  phases of treatment, 175
  pregnant and breast-feeding
    women, 220

side effects of, 173, 175–79
  types of, 171
  see also individual drugs
anxiety disorders, 144–64
  drugs that may cause anxiety,
    147
  generalized anxiety disorder,
    145, 160–62
  medical causes of, 146–47
  obsessive-compulsive
    disorder, 145–46, 162–64
  overview, 144–47
  panic disorder, *see* panic
    disorder
  phobias, 145, 154–55
  physical exam to evaluate,
    147
  situational anxiety, *see*
    situational anxiety
  social anxiety, 145, 155–56
  statistics, 146
aripiprazole, 61, **258–62**
Artane, **255–56**
Asendin, 58, **246–50**
asylums, confinement in, *see*
    state psychiatric hospitals
Atarax, 62, 152, **257–58**
atenolol, 62, **266–68**
Ativan, 62, 99, 189, 217,
    388–91
atomoxetine, 59, 196, 200,
    262–66
attention, 35, 36
attention deficit hyperactivity
    disorder (ADHD), 18–19,
    36, 140, 190–200, 213
  the brain and, 193
  diagnosis of, 181–83
  inattentive subtype, 181–82
  medical treatments for,
    18–19, 192, 193–200
  treatment considerations,
    197–98

atypical psychosis, 165, 167
augmentation approach
    for antidepressants, 101–02
    for antimanic medications,
        125–26, 133, 134, 137
Aventyl, 58, **412–17**

barbiturates, 18
Baxter, L. R., 42
BDNF (brain protein), 81
Benadryl, 63, 189, 218,
    257–58
benztropine, **255–56**
bereavement, 69–70
beta blockers, 210, **266–68**
    for aggression, 209, 210
    for anxiety disorders, 152,
        155, 159, 162
    for PTSD, 207
bioavailability, 48–49
biological clock, 185
biotransformation, 50
Bipolar Child, The (Papolos
    and Papolos), 143
bipolar disorders
    addiction to medications for,
        136
    antidepressants and, 117,
        124–25, 135, 137
    antimanic medications, *see*
        antimanic medications
    antipsychotics for, 124, 125
    associated behaviors, 113
    atypical symptoms, 116
    bipolar I, 116–17
    bipolar II, 117
    brain function and, 119–20
    calcium channel blockers for,
        138
    children and teenagers and,
        139–43, 213
    clinical features of, 73–74
    cyclothymia, 118

diagnosis of, 113–19
drugs that can induce mania,
    118–19
education and lifestyle
    management, 121,
    122–23
electroconvulsive therapy
    (ECT) for, 138
genetic component to, 121
hypomania, 114
interval between cycles,
    111–12
kindling, 120
mania, diagnosing, 113
medical conditions that can
    induce mania, 118
medications to treat, 57,
    124–38
omega-3 fatty acids for, 139
physical exam to diagnose,
    119
precautions and
    contraindications for
    bipolar medications,
    135–36
psychiatric exam to diagnose,
    119
psychotherapy for, 121–22
psychotic symptoms, 113
rapid cycling, 117
research limitations, 120–21
response to treatments,
    112–13
SAM-e and, 104
St. John's wort and, 104
statistics, 111, 112, 117
subtypes of, 116–18
suicide and, 112, 126
symptoms of, 114–16
treatments for, 120, 121–43
birth control pills, 76
"black box" warnings, 97
blood-brain barrier, 48

Bly, Robert, 18
borderline personality disorder,
    203–05
    causes of, 204
    diagnosis of, 203–04
    medical treatment for,
        204–05
    psychotherapy for, 205
    statistics on, 203
brain
    abnormal chemistry, brain
        cells and, 36–37
    ADHD and, 193
    basic, 32–36
    central core of, 33–35
    cortex, 35–36
    emotions and, 28–43
    frontal lobes, 35–36
    generalized anxiety disorder
        and, 161
    hypothalamus, see
        hypothalamus
    imaging technologies, 31, 78
    limbic system, see limbic
        system
    obsessive-compulsive
        disorder and, 163
    panic disorder and, 158
    pleasure centers of, 41–42
    prefrontal cortex, 35–36
    reptilian, 33
    schizophrenia and, 170
brand names of drugs
    directory for locating generic
        drug names from, 519–22
    see also specific drugs
breast-feeding women, see
        pregnant and breast-
        feeding women
bromides, 18
bronchodilators, 182
Brotman, Andrew, 18–19
bulimia, 200–03

buproprion, 59, 200, 202–03,
    268–72
Bush, George H. W., 31
BuSpar, 62, 159, 217, 272–75
buspirone, 62, 159, 161–62,
    163, 209, 210, 272–75

caffeine, 182–83
    bipolar disorders and, 123
    consumption questionnaire,
        523–24
calcium channel blockers, 139
carbamazepine, 57, 124, 125,
    126, 130–31, 275–81
Catapres, 62, 195, 200,
    302–07
CATIE study, 174
Celexa, 59, 63, 216, 289–93
Centrax, 62
"chemical straightjacket,"
    13–14
children, 212–18
    with ADHD, see attention
        deficit hyperactivity
        disorder (ADHD)
    antidepressants and, 96–97,
        216–17
    bipolar disorders in, 139–43,
        213
    compliance in taking
        medications, 214
    depression in, 96–97
    dosages for, 215–18
    legal issues, 215
    psychotropic medication
        guidelines, chart of,
        216–18
    Ritalin and, see Ritalin
    safety issues for, 213–14
    social environment issues,
        214
    suicidality and antidepres-
        sants, 20, 95–96

chlordiazepoxide, 62, 177, **281–84**

chlorpromazine, 60, **285–89**

Churchill, Winston, 10

citalopram, 59, 63, **289–93**

clinical depression, *see* depression

clinical social workers, 23

clomipramine, 58, 63, **293–98**

clonazepam, 62, **298–302**

clonidine, 195, 198, 200, 209, 210, 218, **302–07**

clorazepate, 62

clozapine, 60, 177–78, **307–12**

Clozaril, 60, 217, **307–12**

Cogentin, **255–56**

Cognex, 211

cognitive-behavioral therapy, 12
  for bipolar disorders, 122
  for depression, 66, 80
  for obsessive-compulsive disorder, 164
  for panic disorder, 159–60
  for PTSD, 208

co-morbidity (co-occurrence), 10

compulsive behavior, *see* obsessive-compulsive disorder (OCD)

concentration, 35, 36
  schizophrenia and, 166

Concerta, 64, 199, **400–04**

Corgard, **266–68**

corticosteroids and depression, 76

corticotropin-releasing factor (CRF), 38

cosmetic psychopharmacology, 25–27

cost of medications, 226

counselors, licensed, 23

CT (computerized tomography), 31

Cylert, 64

Cymbalta, 59, **334–38**

Dalmane, 63

Daytrana, 64, 199, **400–04**

decongestants, 182

delusions, 109, 171
  bipolar disorders and, 113
  schizophrenia and, 166, 168

Dement, Dr. William, 180

dementia and Alzheimer's disease, 210–11

Depakene, 124, **498–502**

Depakote, 57, 124, 125, 217, **498–502**

depression, 65–110, 230
  alcohol and, 76, 77
  antidepressants, *see* antidepressants
  bipolar disorder, screening for, 73–74
  brain function and, 78–79
  characteristics of, 66
  cognitive therapy for, 12
  diagnosis of, 70–79
  drugs that can cause, 38, 75–77
  dysthymia, 107–08
  electroconvulsive therapy (ECT) for, 110
  exercise for, 105
  generalized anxiety disorder as precursor to, 161
  grief distinguished from, 69–70
  high-intensity light therapy for, 105–07
  ineffective treatments for, 102–03
  medical disorders related to, 74–75

misunderstandings about,
    67–68
"natural" treatments for, 103
nerve cells implicated in, 79
nonmedical treatments for,
    105–07
over-the-counter products
    for, 103–04
physical exam to diagnose,
    77–78
pleasure centers of the brain
    and, 41–42
premenstrual dysphoria,
    108–09
psychotherapy for, 43, 66,
    79–80
psychotic, 109–10
PTSD and, 207
as recurring illness, 67
seeking treatment, 66
signs and symptoms of,
    69–70, 71–73
statistics, 65
temporary sadness
    distinguished from clinical,
    65, 66, 68
treatment of, 79–107
see also bipolar disorders
desipramine, 58, **312–17**
Desoxyn, 199, **250–55**
desvenlafaxine, 59, **317–21**
Desyrel, 58, 189, **485–89**
Dexedrine, 64, 99, 199, 217,
    250–55
dexmethylphenidate, 64, 199,
    321–25
dextroamphetamine, 64, 199,
    250–55
diagnosis, *see individual
    disorders*
dialectical behavior therapy,
    205
diazepam, 62, **325–29**

diet
    as depression treatment, 104
    food and drug interactions,
        MAO inhibitors and,
        84–85
    "health foods" and herbs,
        103, 230–34
diphenhydramine, 63, 189,
    257–58
disorganized thinking, 166,
    167, 171
divalproex, 57
Doral, 63, **452–56**
dopamine nerve cells, 38, 80,
    87–88
dosages of drugs, *see individual
    drugs*
doxepin, 58, **329–34**
drug addiction, potential for
    antianxiety drugs, 136,
        151–52, 153, 154, 158,
        161
    antidepressants, 99, 154
    antipsychotics, 179
    bipolar medications, 136,
        154
    chart of medication type and
        abuse potential, 154
    historical perspective, 18
    stimulants, 99–100
    tranquilizers, 18, 99–100
    *see also specific psychiatric
        disorders and drugs*
drug interactions
    MAO inhibitors and, 84, 85,
        95
    pharmacist information on,
        24
    St. John's wort, 104
    see also individual drugs
duloxetine, 59, **334–38**
dysthymia, 107–08
dystonia, 176

eating disorders, 200–03
education and lifestyle
    management
  bipolar disorders, 121,
    122–23
Effexor, 59, 217, **502–06**
Elavil, 58, **241–46**
elderly, special issues for,
    223–25
electroconvulsive therapy
    (ECT)
  for bipolar disorders, 138
  for depression, 110
emotions and the brain,
    28–43
Emsam, 59
endorphins, 201
Equetro, 57, 124, 125,
    275–81
escitalopram, 59, 63, **338–42**
Eskalith, 57, **383–88**
estazolam, 63, **342–46**
eszopiclone, 63, 188, **346–49**
exercise
  alteration of brain function,
    43
  for depression, 105
  panic attacks and, 160
  sleep and, 185
exposure and systematic
    desensitization, 155, 164

family doctors, *see* primary care
    doctors
family-focused psychoeducation
  for bipolar disorders, 122
fight-or-flight response, 34,
    144, 147–48
fluoxetine, 57, 58, 63, **349–54**
fluphenazine, 61, **354–62**
flurazepam, 63
fluvoxamine, 59, 63, **362–66**
Focalin, 64, 199, **321–25**

Food and Drug
    Administration, 20, 97,
    198, 234
food and drug interactions,
    MAO inhibitors, 84–85
  see also diet
Freud, Sigmund, 11, 29

GABA neurotransmitter
    system, 39, 132, 133
gabapentin, 57, 62, 133–34
Gabitril, 57
gene mapping, 31
generalized anxiety disorder,
    145, 160–62
generic names of drugs
  directory for locating, from
    brand names, 519–22
  see also specific drugs
genetic predisposition, *see*
    heredity
Geodon, 61, **509–14**
glutamate, 39, 134
grief, 74
  distinguished from
    depression, 69–70
guanfacine, 62, 195, 200
Guide to Psychiatric Drugs,
    236–517
  brand names directory,
    519–22
  note on use of, 236

habit-forming drugs, 18
  antianxiety drugs, 18, 150,
    153, 161
  antidepressants, 153, 158
  antipsychotics, 179
  sleeping pills, 188–89
  stimulants, 194
  see also individual drugs
Halcion, 63, 188, **489–93**
Haldol, 61, **366–70**

half-life of medications, 51
hallucinations, 30, 109, 171
   bipolar disorders and, 113
   schizophrenia and, 166, 168
haloperidol, 61, 177, **366–70**
herbs and health foods, 103,
   230–34
heredity
   bipolar disorder and, 121
   predisposition to psychiatric
      disorders and, 212–13
high-intensity light therapy,
   105–07
historical perspective on
   psychiatric medication,
   9–20
hydroxyzine, 62, 152, 162,
   257–58
hypertension, 38
hyperthyroidism, 146
hypnotics, *see* sleeping pills
   (hypnotics)
hypomania, 114
hypothalamus
   depression and, 78
   functions of, 33

I Hate You—Don't Leave Me
   (Kreisman), 205
imipramine, 58, **370–75**
IMS America, 188
Inderal, 62, 218, **266–68**
insomnia
   causes of, 181–83
   depression and, 72
   secondary, 181
   situational anxiety and, 151
*Integrative Treatment for
   Borderline Personality
   Disorders* (Preston), 205
interpersonal therapy
   for bipolar disorders, 121
   for depression, 66, 80

Invega, 61, **425–29**
isocarboxazid, **375–80**

kindling, 120
Klonopin, 62, 99, 217,
   298–302
Korsakoff's syndrome, 230
Krager, J. M., 18–19
Kramer, Dr. Peter, 25–27

Lamictal, 57, 124, 134, 217,
   380–82
lamotrigine, 57, 124, 134,
   380–82
Lewy body dementia, 210
Lexapro, 59, 63, 216, **338–42**
Librium, 62, **281–84**
lifestyle management and
   education
   bipolar disorders, 121,
      122–23
light-headedness, as side effect
   of antipsychotics, 177
limbic system, 148
   functions of, 34–35
Lincoln, Abraham, 10
lisdexamfetamine, 64, 199,
   250–55
lithium, 57, 124, 125, 126,
   127–30, 205, 209, 210,
   217, **383–88**
   dosages, 127–28
   precautions and
      contraindications, 135
   pregnant and breast-feeding
      women, 221
   side effects, 128–30
Lithobid, **383–88**
Lithonate, 57
locus coeruleus (LC), 158
Lopressor, **266–68**
lorazepam, 62, **388–91**
loxapine, 60, **392–95**

Loxitane, 60, **392–95**
Ludiomil, 58, **396–99**
Lunesta, 63, 188, **346–49**
Luvox, 59, 63, 217, **362–66**

manager case, 25–26
managing your medications,
    52–56
mania, *see* bipolar disorders
manic depression, *see* bipolar
    disorders
manic psychosis, 165, 167
MAO inhibitors, 58, 83–85,
    204
    generic and trade names, 87
    for social anxiety, 156
maprotiline, 58, **396–99**
marijuana, 18
Marplan, **375–80**
media reporting on psychiatric
    medications, 18–20, 95
melatonin, 231–32
Mellaril, 60, **477–80**
mental health specialists
    choosing, 23–24, 122
    prescriptions, ability to write,
        21–22
    seeking help, 24–25
    types of, 23
mesoridazine, 60
Metadate, 64, 199, **400–04**
methamphetamine, 199,
    250–55
methlyphenidate, 194, 199
Methylin, 64, 199, **400–04**
methylphenidate, 64, **400–04**
metoprolol, **266–68**
Minipress, 62, 208
Mirapex, 187
mirtazapine, 59, 189, **404–08**
Moban, 60, **408–12**
modafinil, 64
molindone, 60, **408–12**

"mother's little helpers,"
    14–15
MRI (magnetic resonance
    imaging), 31
multi-infarct dementia, 210

nadolol, **266–68**
Nardil, 59, **439–43**
National Institute of Mental
    Health, 9, 66, 82, 174
National Sleep Foundation,
    188
natural rememdies, 103,
    226–34
Navane, 61
nefazodone, 58
negative stigma of psychiatric
    problems, 10
nerve cells (neurons)
    abnormal chemistry and,
        36–37
    antidepressants's effects on,
        80–81
    interference with functioning
        of, factors causing, 39–40
    method of functioning,
        37–39
    naming of types of, 38–39,
        80
neuroleptic malignant
    syndrome (NMS), 177
neurons, *see* nerve cells
    (neurons)
Neurontin, 57, 62, 133–34,
    217
neuroprotective proteins, 81
neurotransmitters
    bipolar disorder and,
        119–20
    functioning of neurons,
        37–38
New York Times, 187
Niramam, **237–41**

norepinephrine nerve cells, 38, 80, 87
  panic disorder and, 158
Norpramin, 58, **312–17**
nortriptyline, 58, **412–17**
NSF (National Sleep Foundation), 234

obsessive-compulsive disorder (OCD), 145–56, 162–64
  psychotherapy for, 42–43, 164
olanzapine, 57, 61, 124, **417–21**
omega-3 fatty acids, 64, 233
  for bipolar disorders, 139
  for depression, 104
Orap, 61, **444–47**
organic psychosis, 165, 169–70
Ornstein, Robert, 32
over-the-counter drugs, 231–34
  cautionary notes, 234
  chart of, 64
  for depression, 103–04
  see also individual drugs
oxazepam, 62, **421–25**
oxcarbazepine, 57, 124, 125

paliperidone, 61, **425–29**
Pamelor, 58, **412–17**
panic attacks, 155–56, 157, 207, 228
  the brain and, 158
  case study, 15–17
  exercise and, 160
  medical treatment for, 159
panic disorder, 145, 157–60
  diagnosis of, 157–58
  medical treatment for, 158–59
  psychotherapy for, 159–60

Papolos, Dr. Demitri, 143
Papolos, Janice, 143
Parkinsonian side effects, 174, 176
Parkinson's disease, 210
Parnate, 59, **481–85**
paroxetine, 59, 63, **430–34**
pastoral counselors, 23
Paxil, 59, 63, 216, **430–34**
pemoline, 64
periodic limb movements in sleep (PLMS), 187
perphenazine, 60, **434–39**
PET (positron emission tomography), 31
pharmacists, information on drug interactions from, 24
phenelzine, 59, **439–43**
phobias, 145, 154–55
physical examination, 39
  anxiety disorders and, 147
  bipolar disorders and, 119
  depression and, 77–78
Pick's disease, 210
pimozide, 61, **444–47**
pindolol, **266–68**
pleasure centers of the brain, 41–42
post-tramautic stress disorder (PTSD), 145, 206–08
pramipexote, 187
prazepam, 62
prazosin, 62
precautions and contraindications
  antidepressants, 94–95
  bipolar medications, 135–36
  see also individual drugs

pregnant and breast-feeding
women, 218–23
antidepressants and, 94
breast-feeding and drugs,
222–23
chart of classes of drugs and
their safety, 220–21
complications of pregnancy
and drugs, 222
determination of safety of
drugs during, 218–19
premenstrual dysphoria,
108–09
prescription drugs
authority to write, 21–22
"black box" warnings, 97
depression and, 38
nerve cell function and,
39–40
psychiatric, see psychiatric
medications
primary care doctors
ability to diagnose psychiatric
disorders, 22
prescriptions from, 21–22
referrals from, 22, 122
safety issues for younger
people taking psychiatric
drugs and, 213–14
Pristiq, 59, **317–21**
Prolixin, 61, **354–62**
propranolol, 62, **266–68**
ProSom, 63, **342–46**
protriptyline, 58, **448–52**
Provigil, 64
Prozac, 58, 63, 216, **349–54**
psychiatric medications
absorption of, 48–49
basic pharmacology: how
drugs work, 46–51
brand names, directory for
locating generic names
from, 519–22

cost of, 226
distribution of, 49–50
excretion of, 51
goal of, 40–41
guide to, alphabetic,
236–517
half-life of, 51
historical perspective, 9–20
managing your, 52–56
metabolism of, 50–51
note on use of guide to, 236
quick reference, 57–64
*see also individual drugs,
categories of drugs, and
psychiatric disorders*
psychiatrists, 23
psychologists, 23
psychotherapists, ability to
diagnose and prescribe
medications, 22
psychotherapy
alteration of brain function,
42–43
for borderline personality
disorder, 205
general effectiveness of,
11–12
for generalized anxiety
disorder, 161, 162
group, 156
historical perspective, 11–12,
29
limitations for severe mental
illnesses, 29
medication combined with,
22–23
for obsessive-compulsive
disorder, 42–43, 164
for panic disorder, 159–60
for phobias, 155
for PTSD, 208
for situational anxiety,
152–53

see also types of therapy, e.g.
  cognitive therapy; *specific
  psychiatric disorders*
psychotic depression, 109–10,
  165, 167
psychotic disorders, 165–79
  antipsychotics, *see*
    antipsychotics
  atypical psychosis, 165,
    167
  manic psychosis, 165, 167
  medical conditions causing,
    165, 169–70
  organic psychosis, 165,
    169–70
  overview, 165–66
  psychotic depression,
    109–10, 165, 167
  schizophrenia, *see*
    schizophrenia

quazepam, 63, **452–56**
quetiapine, 60, 124, 189,
  456–61

ramelteon, 63, 188, 189,
  461–64
Remeron, 59, 189, **404–08**
reptilian brain, 33
Requip, 187
reserpine, 38
response prevention, 164
restless legs syndrome (RLS),
  187
Restoril, 63, **473–77**
Risperdal, 61, 217, **464–68**
risperidone, 61, **464–68**
Ritalin, 18–19, 64, 99, 192,
  194, 199, 217, **400–04**
ritualistic behavior, *see*
  obsessive-compulsive
  disorder (OCD)
ropinirole, 187

Rosenthal, Dr. Norman, 107
Rozerem, 63, 188, 189,
  461–64

Safer, D. J., 18–19
safety of medications, *see* drug
  addiction, potential for;
  habit-forming drugs; side
  effects of psychiatric
  medications; *specific
  medications and classes of
  medications*
St. John's wort, 64, 104,
  232–33
SAM-e, 64, 104, 233
Sarafem, 58
schizophrenia, 30, 230
  antipsychotics for, *see*
    antipsychotics
  the brain and, 170
  diagnosis of, 166–69
  distinguishing from psychosis
    caused by medical illness
    or drugs, 169–70
  overview, 165–66
  phases of, 166, 167
  resistance to treatment,
    patient's, 169
  signs and symptoms of, 168
  statistics, 166
seasonal affective disorder
  (SAD), 105–07
selegiline, 59
self-harming behaviors, 205
Serax, 62, **421–25**
Serentil, 60
Seroquel, 60, 124, 189, 217,
  456–61
serotonin nerve cells, 38, 80,
  87, 161
  influencing serotonin levels
    in the brain, 228–30
sertraline, 59, 63, **469–73**

Serzone, 58
shock therapy, 110
side effects of psychiatric
    medications, 46–47
  antianxiety drugs, 162
  antidepressants, 82–83, 87,
    89, 94
  antimanics, 128–30, 131,
    132–33, 134
  antipsychotics, 173, 175–79
  children and, see children
  cosmetic
    psychopharmacology,
    25–27
  in the elderly, 224–25
  historical perspective, 12
  media reports on, 20
  stimulants, 195
  teenagers, see teenagers
  see also individual drugs;
    specific drugs
Sinequan, 58, 329–34
situational anxiety, 145,
    147–54
  antianxiety drugs for,
    148–52
  antihistamines for, 152
  beta blockers for, 152
  diagnosis of, 147–48
  medical treatment for,
    148–52
  psychotherapy for, 152–53
sleep disorders, 180–89,
    227–28
  amount of sleep needed,
    180
  effects of sleep deprivation,
    180–81
  functions of sleep, 180,
    227–28
  insomnia, see insomnia
  medical conditions that may
    cause, 183

medications and drugs
    affecting sleep, 182–83
  psychotherapy and, 43
  restless legs syndrome (RLS),
    187
  sleep apnea, 186–87
  sleep hygiene, 184–86
  stages of sleep, 183
sleeping pills (hypnotics), 63,
    182, 183, 187–89
  side effects of, 188–89
social anxiety disorder, 145,
    155–56
social rhythm therapy, 121–22
Sonata, 63, 188, 506–09
Sparlon, 64
SPECT (single photon
    emission computerized
    tomography), 31
SSRIs (Selective Serotonin
    Reuptake Inhibitors), 87,
    108–09, 163, 203, 204,
    207–08, 209, 210, 216,
    217, 228
  see also individual drugs
state psychiatric hospitals, 28,
    30
  confinement in, 11
  release of patients from, 14,
    30
statistics
  anxiety disorders, 146
  on bipolar disorders, 111,
    112, 117
  on borderline personality
    disorder, 203
  on dementia and memory
    impairment, 210–11
  on depression, 65
  on psychiatric disorders in
    the U.S., 3, 9
  on schizophrenia, 166
Stelazine, 60

steroids, 182
stimulants
    as addictive or habit-
        forming, 99–100
    for ADHD, 193–95, 199
    chart of, 64, 195, 199
    children and teenagers and,
        217
    depression treated with, 103
    safety of long-term use,
        200
    side effects of, 195
    see also individual drugs
Strattera, 59, 196, 200, 217,
    262–66
stress
    brain function and, 43
    insomnia and situational,
        181
    see also anxiety disorders
substance abuse, *see* drug
        addiction, potential for;
        habit-forming drugs
suicidality
    antidepressants and, 20,
        95–96, 97–99, 198
    antidepressant use in
        children and teenagers,
        20, 95–96, 97–98
    bipolar disorders and, 112,
        126
    psychotic depression and,
        110
    reserpine and, 38
Surmontil, 58, **493–97**
Symbyax, 57, 124
Symmetrel, **255–56**
Szasz, Dr. Thomas, 14

Tacrine, 211
talk therapy, *see* psychotherapy
tardive dyskinesia, 173,
    178–79

teenagers, 212–18, 215
    antidepressants for, 96–97,
        216–17
    bipolar disorders in, 73,
        139–43, 213
    compliance in taking
        medications, 214
    depression in, 96–97
    dosages for, 215–18
    psychotropic medication
        guidelines, chart of,
        216–18
    safety issues for, 213–14
    social environment issues,
        214
    suicidality and
        antidepressants, 20,
        95–96, 97
Tegretol, 57, 124, 125, 217,
    275–81
temazepam, 63, **473–77**
Tenex, 62, 195, 200
Tenormin, 62, **266–68**
therapists, *see* mental health
        specialists
thioridazine, 60, **477–80**
thiothixene, 61
Thorazine, 30, 60, **285–89**
tiagabine, 57
Tofranil, 58
Topamax, 57, 217
topiramate, 57, 134
tranquilizers, 81
    addiction potential, 18,
        99–100
    historical perspective, 13–15
    minor, or antianxiety drugs,
        see antianxiety drugs
    sleep and, 182, 183
    see also individual drugs
Tranxene, 62
tranylcypromine, 59, **481–85**
trazodone, 58, 189, **485–89**

Treatments for Adolescents with Depression Study (TADS), 96
triazolam, 63, 188, **489–93**
tricyclic antidepressants, 19, 83, 85
trifluoperazine, 60
trihexyphenidyl, **255–56**
Trilafon, 60, **434–39**
Trileptal, 57, 124, 125
trimipramine, 58, **493–97**
Trofanil, **370–75**
tryptophan, 230
tyrosine, 230

USP (United States Pharmacopeia), 234

Valium, 62, 99, **325–29**
valproate, 57, 124, 125, 126, 132–33, **498–502**
venlafaxine, 59, **502–06**

violent behavior, *see* aggression
Visken, **266–68**
Vistaril, 62, 152, **257–58**
vitamins
    deficiencies, 230
    supplements, 230–31
Vivactil, 58, **448–52**
Vyvanse, 64, 199, **250–55**

Wellbutrin, 59, 196, 200, 216, **268–72**
    panic symptoms and, 158–59

Xanax, 62, 99, 189, 217, **237–41**

zaleplon, 63, 188, **506–09**
ziprasidone, 61, **509–14**
Zoloft, 59, 63, 216, **469–73**
zolpidem, 63, 188, **514–17**
Zyprexa, 61, 217, **417–21**